LIBRARY IN A BOOK

PRESCRIPTION DRUGS

Fred C. Pampel

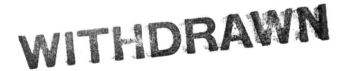

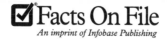
Facts On File
An imprint of Infobase Publishing

Prescription Drugs   MAR 1 0 2011

Copyright © 2010 by Fred C. Pampel

Facts On File, Inc.
An imprint of Infobase Publishing
132 West 31st Street
New York NY 10001

Library of Congress Cataloging-in-Publication Data
Pampel, Fred C.
   Prescription drugs / Fred C. Pampel.
      p. cm. — (Library in a book)
   Includes bibliographical references.
   ISBN 978-0-8160-8014-4 (alk. paper)
   1. Drugs—Popular works. 2. Drug development—Popular works. I. Title.
   RM301.15.P36 2010
   615'.19—dc22   2009036173

Facts On File, Inc. books are available at special discounts when purchased in bulk quantities for businesses, associations, institutions, or sales promotions. Please call our Special Sales Department in New York at (212) 967-8800 or (800) 322-8755.

You can find Facts On File on the World Wide Web at http://www.factsonfile.com.

Text design by Ron Monteleone
Composition by Hermitage Publishing Services
Cover printed by Art Print, Taylor, Pa.
Book printed and bound by Maple Press, York, Pa.
Date printed: July 2010
Printed in the United States of America

10 9 8 7 6 5 4 3 2 1

This book is printed on acid-free paper.

CONTENTS

PART I
OVERVIEW OF THE TOPIC

PART II
GUIDE TO FURTHER RESEARCH

PART III
APPENDICES

PART I

OVERVIEW OF THE TOPIC

CHAPTER 1

INTRODUCTION TO PRESCRIPTION DRUGS

If popularity is any indication, prescription drugs have become one of the great medical success stories of the last few decades. According to figures from the National Center for Health Statistics, 45.3 percent of adults used a prescription drug in 1999–2002, up from 39.1 percent in 1988–1994.[1] One of science's finest achievements, prescription drugs have become a routine and widespread form of treatment. Popular drugs help deal with severe depression and daily troubles of living, ease heart problems that come from high blood pressure and cholesterol, and make it possible to live with chronic diseases of asthma, arthritis, and diabetes. Sometimes lifesaving, sometimes comforting, these prescription drugs have helped millions of Americans and others across the world live a healthier, more enjoyable life.

Or have they? Consider two common, yet in some ways conflicting, criticisms.

First, critics say that prescription drugs often do not get to the people who need them most. Drug companies price new prescription drugs, those not available in generic form, at levels beyond the reach of many patients. With large parts of the population lacking access to them, prescription drugs do not have the benefits they should. Some Americans who don't have insurance coverage for the prescription drugs they need cross the border to buy them at lower prices in Canada or Mexico. Others trying to buy cheaper products end up with counterfeit drugs.

On the other side, critics suggest that many drugs are overhyped, over-prescribed, and misused. Rather than too little access, the public has too much access to prescription drugs. Overuse of prescription drugs wastes resources, according to the critics. Worse, all prescription drugs have side effects, sometimes quite dangerous, that can outweigh any benefit. The more prescription drugs a person takes, the more likely the drugs will inter-act in ways that harm health. Despite risks of overuse, pharmaceutical

3

companies aim through advertising to create new worries about diseases and conditions that in turn call for prescription drugs.

Some popular prescription drugs are intentionally abused. People use pain medications, stimulants, and tranquilizers for recreational rather than medical use. Adults and teens alike can become addicted to drugs such as OxyContin, Vicodin, and Demerol. Sometimes misuse has even more serious consequences. The actor Heath Ledger died on January 22, 2008, from an accidental overdose of legitimately prescribed drugs, including oxycodone, hydrocodone, diazepam, temazepam, alprazolam, and doxylamine. More recently, Michael Jackson appears to have died from taking a powerful anesthetic drug, one restricted to use in hospitals under continuous monitoring, to help him sleep.

Are these problems overstated? Are prices too high? Has prescription drug use gotten out of control? Policies need to balance two goals: (1) to make prescription drugs available to those who need them by keeping prices reasonable; and (2) to limit the overuse, misuse, and abuse of prescription drugs. As the Harvard physician Jerry Avorn says, "Taking drugs can hurt you; not taking drugs can hurt you."[2] The question remains as to whether drug manufacturers, physicians, the government, and patients have managed to find the proper balance in use of prescription drugs.

This chapter examines these questions and the debates they generate. By offering an overview of the basic facts and the competing interpretations of the facts, it provides the background for understanding debates over the proper use of prescription drugs. However, the chapter avoids technical issues relating to the chemical and biological workings of prescription drugs and medical details on recommended usage and doses. Recommendations to take or not take prescription drugs should come from physicians and qualified health care providers. Other reference books on prescription drugs cover these topics. Instead, this book presents a balanced view of social, economic, and political controversies over prescription drug use.

THE GROWTH OF PRESCRIPTION DRUGS

A prescription is an order or plan, usually involving the taking of medicines, that a physician or medical practitioner gives to a patient. The physician or medical practitioner has the responsibility to ensure the effectiveness and safety of the prescription, while the patient has the responsibility to follow directions in taking the prescription. Based on a written or e-mailed prescription, pharmacists provide the medications to the patients. Prescription comes from the terms *pre* ("before") and *script* ("written"), indicating that the prescribed medication is written before so the drug can be prepared by a pharmacist. Prescription drugs differ from over-the-counter (OTC) drugs, which consumers can buy without approval by a medical professional. The symbol *Rx* also means prescription.

Prescription drugs typically have two names, a generic name indicating the active ingredient and a brand name used by the maker to promote and sell the drug. Being generally more familiar, brand names are used in the discussion when possible.

EARLY HISTORY

Throughout history, people have prepared and used folk medicines and herbal remedies. In Europe during the Middle Ages, local apothecaries set up shops to measure, mix, and sell these remedies, often providing medical advice with their products. By at least the 1800s, however, new ways of selling medicines emerged that brought both benefits and problems. In terms of benefits, the rise of newspapers in many countries led to mass advertisements that acquainted people with possible treatments for their problems. In terms of problems, the mass advertisements also led to misleading claims and fraud.

As one response to the problems, national boards began to assume some responsibility for the safety of drugs and accuracy of claims. Experts collated information on medicines into books called pharmacopoeias. These books mostly listed available drugs but eventually started to include information on proper ingredients and quality. In the United States, 11 physicians met in Washington, D.C., in 1820 to create a U.S. Pharmacopeia. This new reference source helped reduce misuse of drugs but did not eliminate it. In 1846, Lewis Caleb Beck called attention to the many problems concerning drug quality in *Adulteration of Various Substances Used in Medicine and the Arts*. His book provided the scientific evidence in support of concerns about drug impurities. In 1848, Congress responded to these concerns by passing an act to require the U.S. Customs Service to inspect and bar entry of any adulterated drugs imported from overseas.

Despite these efforts, the use of nonstandard, impure drugs persisted, even worsened. During the late 1800s, so-called patent medicines became increasingly popular. These medicines actually did not have patents; the term referred instead to products with a trademark or brand name. For a variety of reasons, patent medicines came to be associated with dishonesty. The products often claimed to have secret ingredients and made excessive claims about their benefits. As described by an exhibit of collections at the Hagley Museum and Library in Wilmington, Delaware,

> *Their advertising and labels were very enticing: "Eckman's Alterative for all throat and lung diseases"; "Cerralgine Food for the Brain, a safe cure for*

headache, neuralgia, nervousness, insomnia, etc."; and "Drs. Mixer, sole manufacturers and proprietors of Mixer's Cancer and Scrofula syrup; the world renowned blood purifier."[3]

Despite little evidence that the patent medicines worked, the advertising increased sales.

Patent medicines often included a large amount of alcohol and sometimes opium, cocaine, or morphine. One group of patent medicines contained snake oil, a supposed treatment for a variety of ailments. (Today, the term *snake-oil salesman* means a swindler or fraud.) With companies and salespeople advertising them for all kinds of ailments ranging from colic among children to tuberculosis, indigestion, and female complaints, patent medicines became popular. Even if harmless themselves, the patent medicines discouraged people from seeking the help of legitimate physicians and using proven drugs. In some cases, the ingredients made users sicker and even caused death.

In response to these wild claims and harmful side effects, medical societies called for regulation of patent medicines. The dean of the Harvard Medical School, Oliver Wendell Holmes, Sr., said in 1860 before the Massachusetts Medical Society that if all available drugs "could be sunk to the bottom of the sea, it would be better for mankind, and all the worse for the fishes."[4] An exposé of the patent drug industry called "The Great American Fraud" by Samuel Hopkins Adams appeared in *Collier's Weekly* in 1905. Hopkins accused the industry of relying on fake testimonials and fraud to poison the public.

In contrast to patent medicines, a new chemical/pharmaceutical industry began in the late 1800s to produce "ethical drugs." These drugs followed accepted knowledge about treatments established by scientists and legitimate physicians but were produced on a large scale rather than by local apothecaries. One company founded in 1880 by two Americans, Silas Mainville Burroughs and Henry Solomon Wellcome, began to produce medicine in compressed form called a "Tabloid" and eventually a tablet. The tabloid put medicine in compact form that consumers found easy to take and set a new standard for precision in ingredients. Following on its success producing medicine, the company established a research lab in 1896 to develop new drugs. One of its early successful scientifically based products, a serum antitoxin, immunized people against various infections. Still, few truly beneficial drugs existed at this time. The most common drugs, morphine for pain, digitalis for ailing hearts, and aspirin for fever and inflammation, came from plants such as poppies, foxglove, and willow bark.

As more legitimate drug companies began to develop and market products and objections to the fraudulent claims of patent medicines escalated, the federal government took a more active role in regulation. In 1901, nine children in Camden, New Jersey, died from tetanus after receiving a commercially produced vaccine for smallpox, and in 1902, 13 children in St. Louis died from a contaminated diphtheria antitoxin. In response, Dr. Lyman F. Kebler assumed duties in 1903 as director of the drug laboratory in the Bureau of Chemistry, a government agency established by the Department of Agriculture that aimed to ensure the safety and purity of drug products. The American Medical Association (AMA) also became involved. In 1905, it set up a voluntary program for drug approval that required companies advertising drug products in the association's magazine to undergo a review by experts.

With the support of President Theodore Roosevelt, Congress passed the Biologics Control Act in 1902 to ensure the purity and safety of vaccines and serums. The Pure Food and Drug Act followed in 1906, which among many other things prohibited interstate commerce in adulterated drugs. By today's standards, the Food and Drug Act did little. It did not require manufacturers to prove the safety of their products. Rather, it required the government to prove a product was unsafe before removing it from the market. Even at that, government enforcement led to disputes over the meaning of the law. In 1911, the Supreme Court ruled in the *U.S. v. Johnson* that the law did not prohibit false claims about the benefits of a drug, only false claims about the ingredients. Congress then passed the Sherley amendment in 1912 to prohibit labeling of medicines with false claims about therapeutic value that intended to defraud the consumer. Once again, the burden of proof remained on the government. To prosecute unethical drugmakers, government authorities had to prove that manufacturers deliberately lied about benefits.

Another major step in the control of drugs came in 1914 with passage of the Harrison Narcotics Act. Until that time, few regulations controlled use of opiates and cocaine, and addiction had become a serious problem. In 1911, Dr. Hamilton Wright, the first U.S. opium commissioner, wrote, "Of all the nations of the world, the United States consumes most habit-forming drugs per capita. Opium, the most pernicious drug known to humanity, is surrounded, in this country, with far fewer safeguards than any other nation."[5] Along with taxing opium and cocaine products, the law used the medical profession to limit access to the narcotics. It allowed doctors to distribute the drugs only in the course of professional practice. The courts interpreted this to mean that, because opium dependence is not a disease, doctors could not give opium for treatment of addiction. The new law reduced abuse of these narcotics substantially, and a similar law applying to heroin passed in 1924.

MODERN DRUG POLICIES

By the 1930s, the 1906 Pure Food and Drug Act had become obsolete. Much wrangling among legislators followed in the efforts to revise it, but an event in 1937 made clear the urgency of passing a new law to protect drug users. In that year, 107 persons died, mostly children, from a contaminated medicine used to treat streptococcal infections. A company mistakenly used a poisonous chemical to put the drug in liquid form. At the time, the law neither required tests for the safety of new drugs nor made the selling of toxic drugs illegal. The commissioner of the Food and Drug Administration (FDA), Walter Campbell, pointed out how the inadequate law failed to prevent this disaster.

Congress responded with the 1938 Food, Drug, and Cosmetics Act. The law added something new in drug regulation: It required that companies demonstrate the safety of their drugs and receive approval from the FDA before marketing them. Further, the law required that labels give directions for use and warn of any habit-forming properties. In the years to follow, the FDA steadily took a greater role to ensure the safety of drugs. In 1941, the agency received responsibility for certifying the purity and effectiveness of insulin for treating diabetes, and in 1945 it received the power to test for the safety and effectiveness of penicillin products.

A problem with the 1938 law remained, however. Drugs available with and without a prescription from a physician were not well defined. Consumers did not know which drugs required approval of a physician and which did not. In 1951, the Durham-Humphrey amendment, known as the prescription drug amendment, defined two classes of drugs. First, prescription drugs required that a licensed health practitioner, usually a physician, supervise their use. Drugs in this class could be habit forming or potentially harmful unless dispensed under the supervision of a health practitioner. Second, the other class of less risky and harmful drugs, OTC drugs, did not need a physician's supervision. Under the law, manufacturers no longer decided which category their product fit.

The change in laws and regulations during the period from 1935 to 1955 coincided with scientific discoveries and the invention of a host of effective drugs—penicillin and other antibiotics, the polio vaccine, many other vaccines, antihistamines, tranquilizers, cortisone for arthritis, and drugs to help children suffering from leukemia. Almost miraculously, these medicines saved peoples' lives. Public attitudes toward many drugs changed, and sales more than doubled from the early 1940s to 1957. The untrustworthy reputation of patent medicines disappeared, and a new era of prescription medicines had begun.

The next major step toward more effective regulation of prescription drugs followed a well-publicized tragedy in Europe. A sedative drug called thalidomide that eased nausea became popular among pregnant women in Europe from 1957 to 1961. However, an FDA officer, Dr. Frances Kelsey, slowed approval in the United States, believing that its safety had not yet been adequately demonstrated. When thalidomide was found later to cause grotesque birth abnormalities such as malformed arms and legs, perhaps among as many as 10,000 babies, Dr. Kelsey became something of a hero for preventing the same tragedy in the United States. It also led Congress to pass the Kefauver-Harris Drug Control Act of 1962, which required that drugs approved by the FDA be proven both safe and effective. The law represented a major change. The FDA reviewed drugs beginning in 1966 that it had approved as safe from 1938 to 1962 to see if the drugs also had demonstrated effectiveness. Although manufacturers delayed in providing evidence, the amendment did much to eliminate the continued use of worthless products.

In one case, the FDA notified the Upjohn Company, manufacturer of an antibiotic drug called Panalba first used in 1957, that the drug was being removed from the approval list. A panel of experts concluded in 1968 that the drug and other similar antibiotics performed no better than other antibiotics and might be harmful. In defending the removal, the FDA said that there was no evidence in clinical trials of the drug's effectiveness. Upjohn claimed that the popularity of the drug and its high sales, rather than clinical studies, demonstrated its effectiveness. Why would doctors and patients use the drug so much if it failed to work? However, the Supreme Court upheld the FDA rules in *Upjohn v. Finch* (1970) and later in *Weinberger v. Hynson* (1973). In affirming the power of the FDA, this decision forced changes on drugmakers, who now needed to offer strong evidence that their drugs worked as advertised.

Still other regulations aimed to foster the proper use of prescription drugs. In 1968, the FDA first required drug manufacturers to include a patient package insert (PPI) with isoproterenol, a medicine that treated heart problems and asthma with an inhaler device. The insert explained to patients how to use the medication and inhaler properly and warned them to contact their physician immediately if breathing problems persisted. A similar PPI was required for birth control pills in 1970 and many other drugs in the 1970s. Aiming to further help consumers understand the drugs they were taking rather than relying just on guidance from prescribing physicians, the FDA set up regulations for clear drug labeling.

CLINICAL DRUG TRIALS AND EVIDENCE OF DRUG EFFECTIVENESS

As it had argued successfully in *Upjohn v. Finch*, the FDA needed something more scientific than personal accounts from patients and physicians to validate a drug's effectiveness. Informal evaluation by patients and doctors is subject to placebo effects (*placebo* is Latin for "I will please"). Originally, a placebo referred to a harmless substance given to please a patient complaining about symptoms that otherwise could not be treated. The belief of the patient in the effectiveness of the drug often led to an improvement in the symptoms. That the benefits come from the mind-set of the patient rather than the substance itself created problems for evaluating the effectiveness of new drugs. Improvements due to the placebo effect might easily though wrongly be attributed to a drug.

As the FDA began to evaluate the effectiveness of medications beginning in 1966, it increasingly relied on randomized clinical trials. Although these trials do not guarantee that tested drugs work well and are safe, they greatly improve on past methods of evaluation, and they became crucial to demonstrating the benefits of prescription drugs. As one physician says, the randomized clinical trial in the last 50 years "has transformed the way we understand medications . . . [and] is nothing less than the single most important development in the revolution of modern therapeutics."[6]

The randomized clinical trial has several characteristics. First, the clinical trial assigns volunteer subjects to two groups, one receiving the medication and one receiving a placebo, or a substance known to have no direct physiological effects. If the experimental medication is effective, the subjects receiving it should do better than those receiving the placebo. Improvement among those taking the medication is not enough by itself—the improvement should be greater than for those taking the placebo. If, for example, the group receiving an experimental drug for pain relief reports 50 percent less pain and the group receiving the placebo reports 20 percent less pain, this outcome would likely show the effectiveness of the new drug.

Second, the trial assigns patients randomly to the two conditions. Randomization or random assignment means that, at the start of the trial, the two groups differ only by chance, and preexisting differences likely cannot account for any differences in outcomes. The group receiving the pain relief drug therefore would not report less pain simply because these patients had milder symptoms at the start. Random assignment does not guarantee that the two groups are identical in the characteristics that affect the response to experimental drugs. Although chance can still produce some differences, random assignment helps eliminate alternative sources of group differences in outcomes.

Third, neither the subjects nor the researcher should know who received the real drug or the placebo. If they know, it could bias the outcomes. Patients might expect to get better because they receive the real drug, and researchers might expect those patients to get better. The design is called double-blind because both patients and researchers do not know the membership in the experimental and control groups until after the outcomes have been measured.

Fourth, tests for the effectiveness depend on probability and statistical significance. A drug may do better than the placebo by chance alone. Perhaps the experimental and control group differ by chance in characteristics that affect the outcomes or in how well subjects in the two groups follow rules for taking the drug. A small improvement, say 25 percent reporting less pain in the experimental group and 20 percent in the control group, may not be enough to establish the drug's effectiveness. Clinical trials require that improvements from an experimental drug do better than what might result from chance alone.

Even when meeting these conditions, clinical trials still face problems in determining whether a drug works safely. Sometimes the benefits or the harmful side effects of an experimental treatment take a long time to show; it is not always clear how long a clinical trial should last. Sometimes the drugs work for certain kinds of patients but not for others. To find out which patients benefit, trials might need to complete additional detailed studies of patient subgroups. And sometimes the drugs have benefits or side effects that are real but too small to measure accurately. Clinical trials need to follow procedures carefully to make sure they get reliable measurements and findings. Despite these limitations, however, the randomized clinical trial does much to avoid false conclusions about drug benefits and safety.

With the FDA and randomized clinical trials setting a tough standard to demonstrate effectiveness, the 1970s proved a difficult time for the drug industry. Makers of drugs fought the FDA requirements for proof of effectiveness but ultimately lost in the Supreme Court. Some companies delayed in providing information on effectiveness but risked having the FDA withdraw its approval of a drug. Some drug companies, unable to demonstrate effectiveness of profitable drugs, lost the right to sell them. For new drugs, the approval process became stricter. The companies had to generate new evidence of both safety and effectiveness of a new drug before the FDA would approve it.

With new FDA standards, many complained bitterly about the slow pace of approval of new drugs—nearly two years on average and often much longer. After years of development, including tests on animals, a new drug must then go through time-consuming clinical trials on humans to meet FDA standards. The long process affected the profitability of new drugs. Companies patented a new drug early in the process of discovery so that they could establish clear ownership and profit from the drug if it proved successful. However, a patent and right to make and sell the drug exclusively lasted 17 years from the issue date or 20 years from the filing date of the earliest application. If the company spent a good chunk of that time getting approval, it meant less time to sell the drug exclusively and make profits. Slipping profits led some industry leaders to worry about the survival of the drug industry over the next decades.

Worsening difficulties for drug companies, much of the population remained suspicious of prescription drugs through the 1970s. Physicians prescribed drugs sparingly, believing that excess use could be dangerous for patients. Patients also tended to avoid prescription drugs unless absolutely necessary. Some bad publicity perhaps worsened suspicions. For example, Valium, a tranquilizer used to treat anxiety and insomnia that was introduced in 1963, became popular. However, its addictive properties led to serious problems for patients and new concerns about drug abuse. The maker of the drug, Hoffman-La Roche, faced accusations that it failed to warn the millions of users of the risks they faced. Worries of addiction and side effects reinforced concerns about use of prescription drugs.

DRUG INDUSTRY AND REGULATION

Ronald Reagan entered the presidency in 1981 with a mandate for lowering taxes and removing government regulations and restrictions on business. The favorable climate for business and loosening of government restrictions that he cultivated in the 1980s helped the drug industry. The next decades were a period of growing acceptance of prescription drugs by the public and growing profits for the drug companies. Initially, however, one of the first steps in deregulation (or a lessening of government regulations) of the drug industry made things worse for the drug companies. Senator Orrin Hatch of Utah and Representative Henry Waxman of California aimed to lower consumer costs by making generic drugs easier to sell and buy. A generic drug is one whose patent has expired and can be sold under a name other than the trademarked brand-name version. A generic drug has the same active ingredients as the original and works much the same but costs less, has a different appearance, and can be made and sold by any company. The Drug Price Competition and Patent Term Restoration Act of 1984 sponsored by Hatch and Waxman made it easier for generic drugs to get approval from the FDA. Rather than requiring new clinical studies, the FDA could rely on previous studies for the brand-name product to prove the safety and effectiveness of the nearly identical generic product.

The increased competition from generic drugs worried the drug companies. To allay some of these concerns, the Hatch-Waxman bill dealt with a complaint of the drug companies. The slow FDA approval process reduced the patent period the companies had for exclusive marketing of their new drugs. The law therefore extended the patent period by up to five years, depending on how long the drug had taken to develop. The longer a new drug spent in the approval pipeline, the longer the granted patent extension and the longer the monopoly period a company had under the patent to sell a new drug without competition from generics.

To make sure that a generic drug did not infringe on an unexpired patent, another provision of the law aimed to protect drug companies. It allowed a company to obtain a 30-month stay—and sometimes multiple 30-month stays—from the FDA while it sued for patent infringement and disputed another company's right to sell a generic drug. A stay prevents sale of the generic drug until a court reaches a decision on the claim of patent infringement, or some other form of agreement is reached. According to some, companies abused this provision by finding technicalities to justify a suit and 30 months of continued sales without generic competition.

Under the new law, drug companies still had incentives to obtain speedy approval of their drugs—the sooner the drug went to market, the longer the companies had to sell it without competition. In this goal, the drug companies had new allies—patient groups. Beginning with AIDS activists wanting new drugs to treat this initially untreatable disease, patient groups suffering from deadly or debilitating diseases wanted new and potentially helpful drugs approved quickly. For example, protests by AIDS activists outside FDA headquarters carried signs that said "Red Tape Kills." Organizations representing people with diabetes, cancer, arthritis, asthma, and other conditions joined the call. Activists said that the slow research and approval process for potentially lifesaving drugs led to unnecessary suffering and death. When patients rather than drug company leaders testified before Congress demanding faster approval, the goal of fast-track drug approval gained much support.

The FDA took some steps on its own. In 1987, it made it easier for patients with serious diseases to participate in studies on experimental drugs. In 1991, the FDA published new regulations to accelerate reviews of drugs for life-threatening diseases. However, the FDA needed more funding and a larger staff to speed approvals. Such a change came with the Prescription Drug User Fee Act of 1992. Under the law, the pharmaceutical industry would pay user fees to the FDA in return for changes to reduce approval time. With the new funds, the FDA planned to hire 600 new workers for the Center for Drug Evaluation and Research and the Center for Biologics Evaluation Research. It adopted the goal of reducing the typical 22-month review to 12 months for standard reviews and six months for priority reviews.

Critics of the new law pointed out that the user fees provided no money to follow up on safety concerns. With many new drugs entering the market quickly, surveillance after the approval process became especially important. After all, the quick approval process might not catch all the dangerous side effects that a slower and longer review might. Yet most Americans viewed the new system favorably. Congress reauthorized the user fee system in 1997, added more funds for safety surveillance after approval in 2002, and added more funds for review of advertising in 2007.

The 1997 FDA Modernization Act reauthorized the Prescription Drug User Fee Act and the system of having drug companies subsidize reviews of new drugs. In addition, the act made several other changes to speed the approval of drugs and allow for their wider use. It simplified the paperwork for drugs being reviewed and allowed critically ill patients to use promising drugs still undergoing review and not yet approved. Of special importance, it allowed drug companies to make information available on unapproved, or "off-label," uses of drugs approved for other purposes. The potential to sell approved drugs for off-label uses widened the market for many drugs. The law required that companies commit to doing research on the off-label use and later apply for approval of the new use. Even so, the law gave companies wider latitude in the claims they could make on behalf of their drugs.

Through the decades of growth, Congress maintained its aim to keep prescription drugs safe. One problem it addressed was haphazard distribution of drugs. Over the years, free samples given to physicians and hospitals were being sold to patients, sometimes after a period of improper storage. Also, drugs exported to foreign countries were being reimported back to the United States for sale, again sometimes after periods of improper handling and storage. There were instances when the reimported drugs were counterfeit, misbranded, or expired. To safeguard the quality of drugs used by consumers, Congress passed the Prescription Drug Marketing Act of 1987. Along with some amendments in 1992, the law banned the sale of drug coupons, restricted the reimportation of prescription drugs, and set requirements for drug wholesalers. It also made it illegal for American citizens to go to other countries, Canada and Mexico in particular, to buy drugs for use in the United States. This last provision would become controversial in later decades—it prevented Americans from buying drugs at cheaper prices in other countries.

Since about 2004, when evidence became convincing that an approved and widely used drug for pain relief, Vioxx, caused serious heart problems, the government has given renewed emphasis to safety. Criticisms by Congress of the FDA for approving Vioxx and related drugs led to new congressional legislation and policy changes at the FDA. For example, the FDA now may approve drugs with restrictions that require doctors to have special training or experience before prescribing the drugs. It considers the potential for misuse of products rather than assuming patients will use products as directed. The FDA also increased its surveillance efforts to identify safety problems after drug approval.

DIRECT-TO-CONSUMER ADVERTISING

Along with quicker approval of new drugs and a longer time span for companies to profit from successful new discoveries, another change beginning in the 1980s and accelerating in decades to follow fueled the rise of prescription drugs. Direct-to-consumer (DTC) advertising slowly but steadily grew. No single change in laws made such advertising legal, but numerous smaller decisions led to the ever-present drug ads on television today.

Introduction to Prescription Drugs

Before the 1980s, ads for prescription drugs appeared only in magazines and journals for physicians. Since 1962, the FDA has had responsibility for regulating the advertising of prescription drugs (while the Federal Trade Commission [FTC] has regulated advertising for OTC drugs). Advertising of drugs in the mass media was legal, but most companies thought that medical professionals and the public would reject products advertised to consumers. Medicines differed from heavily advertised products like cars, beer, and laundry soap. Besides, it seemed to make little sense to advertise to consumers when physicians made decisions about the drugs to prescribe. Most sales efforts accordingly targeted physicians and medical students.

Attitudes started to change in the 1980s. In 1981, Boots Pharmaceuticals, a British company with a subsidiary in the United States, advertised its prescription pain reliever Rufen (an ibuprofen product) in American magazines. Merck Sharp & Dohme soon followed with a second print ad for consumers on its pneumonia vaccine Pneumovax. A larger-scale effort that began in 1982 took a different approach and had greater influence. Hoping to garner publicity for its new arthritis drug Oraflex, Eli Lilly and Company sent out press kits to outlets such as television and radio stations, newspapers, and magazines. Although not advertised directly to consumers, the kits made claims that the drug could delay the progress of the disease. Despite FDA concerns about the claims, the publicity kits worked. Some 500,000 prescriptions were written for the drug. The overstated, inaccurate claims angered many physicians, who rightly noted that the press kits left out information on potential side effects. The next year, Lilly withdrew Oraflex from the market for causing liver- and kidney-related deaths.

In 1983, the FDA called for a moratorium on DTC drug ads while it studied the issue. Given the FDA's power to regulate the content of the ads, drug companies followed the voluntary moratorium. Yet backers of the ads worked to overcome resistance. They argued that making information available to consumers was for the best. Because advertisers might reach patients in ways that doctors could not, the public would benefit. The ads might get people with some conditions to learn of treatments and go to their doctors rather than think nothing could be done. Legal precedent existed for informing consumers. In a case decided by the Supreme Court in 1976, the Virginia Citizens Consumer Council sued the Virginia Board of Pharmacy for prohibiting pharmacists from advertising drug prices. The Supreme Court ruled in favor of the council that the public had the right to know truthful information about prescription drugs.

In 1985, the FDA ruled to allow DTC ads but stipulated that they must provide the same information as ads directed at physicians. Ads must present a fair balance of information on the drug, including a brief summary of possible side effects and risks. That made it difficult to advertise drugs on television and radio, where commercials were too short to include the summary information. Most in the FDA believed that these conditions would greatly restrict DTC advertising.

Advertisers managed to find ways around the restrictions, however. For example, Merrill-Dow, the maker of a new antihistamine called Seldane, claimed that its product made users less drowsy. Ads for the drug did not mention it by name and therefore did not need to summarize risks and side effects. Rather, the ads merely said that a new drug for allergies was out, it did not make users drowsy, and doctors could provide more information. The 1988 ad campaign was hugely successful, and sales of Seldane soared.

Other ads aptly named reminder ads mentioned the brand name of the prescription drug but not the condition it treated. Again, that limited the need to describe all the risks and side effects. One 1996 ad for Claritin, an allergy medication, showed balloons rising in the sky and the face of a young woman. In the background, words to a famous song went "Blue skies, shining on me/ Nothing but blue skies do I see." The ad simply told viewers to ask their doctor about Claritin. If nothing else, it piqued the interest of viewers, who did indeed try to find out more and ask their doctors. Claritin became remarkably successful. Sales rose 20 percent following the $185 million ad campaign.

Changing views within the AMA helped legitimate the new ads. Historically, this organization of physicians had worried that DTC ads would harm the closeness of the doctor-patient relationship. During the 1980s, however, some AMA leaders began to see the value of patients taking more control of their own health, of actively striving to improve rather than passively waiting to do what the doctor told them. Toward that end, having more information would help rather than hurt. In 1992, the AMA voted to rescind its opposition to DTC ads. The 1992 change opened the door for more DTC advertising.

Drug advertisements mushroomed. In 1989, companies spent $12 million on ads, a large number compared to the past. The figure reached $313 million in 1995—26 times greater than only six years earlier. It would go to $2.38 billion by 2001. Overwhelmed by all the ads, the FDA held hearings on what steps were needed to regulate all this activity. On one side, industry representatives called for the FDA to relax its regulations further. Patients, they said, craved more information and, with information, could become better advocates for themselves in dealing with the health bureaucracy and health maintenance organizations. On the other side, opponents of DTC ads said that, although having more information is good, the information must be accurate. Too many ads presented incomplete, misleading information and used emotion rather than facts to attract users to their products. According to a leading critic, Dr. Sidney Wolfe, the FDA made more than 150 requests for drug companies to pull ads for false or misleading information from 1995 to 1996. With such information, ads did little to help consumers learn more about drugs and act in ways to benefit their health.

Introduction to Prescription Drugs

The FDA commissioner from 1990 to 1997, Dr. David Kessler, agreed with the critics. Reflecting his opposition, the FDA issued draft guidelines in 1997 that were finalized in 1999. The regulations allowed for broadcast advertisements, but the television ads now had to include a major statement of risks and benefits and make provision for distributing FDA-approved information on risks and benefits to consumers. For example, ads could list a toll-free number that consumers could call for more information. Of course, the ads were obligated to present only scientifically valid information and to fairly balance benefits and risks. Some kinds of ads could avoid these restrictions. Help-seeking ads that merely encouraged patients to see their doctors about a drug and reminder ads that made no claims about the effectiveness of the drug were exempted from the brief summary and fair balance requirements.

During this time, Washington Legal Foundation, a nonprofit organization with conservative leanings, had taken action to eliminate restrictions on DTC advertising. Lawyers with the foundation argued that First Amendment rights to free speech included commercial speech such as advertising for prescription drugs. In a suit against the FDA *(Washington Legal Foundation v. Friedman)*, a district court ruled in 1999 that the FDA could not restrict truthful, non-misleading speech. That decision and another 2002 decision, *Washington Legal Foundation v. Henney*, broadened the freedom of manufacturers to disseminate information about their products. Although the FDA can regulate advertising of prescription drugs, free speech rights make it hard for the government to block such advertising altogether.

Along with the continued growth of DTC advertising, another practice grew. Off-label use of drugs involves prescription of a product for a condition other than that approved by the FDA. For example, the antidepressant Paxil might be used for shyness, or the epilepsy drug Neurontin might be used for chronic pain or attention deficit disorder. For patients with a fatal illness, experimentation with different drugs might help and do little harm. In addition, drug companies encouraged physicians to try their products for promising, even if unproven, treatments on a wider range of conditions. The FDA Modernization Act of 1997 allowed manufacturers to distribute information about unapproved uses of drugs and medical devices. However, they needed to then agree to conduct research and file a supplemental application for approval of these off-label uses so that new information could be added to the official product labeling.

DTC ADVERTISING TODAY

Simply watching television reveals the massive amount of advertising for prescription drugs that has developed over the decades. By 2005, spending on DTC ads for prescription drugs had reached $4.2 billion. The ubiquitous ads continue to create controversy. Even if they say nothing wrong, the ads may give viewers misleading impressions about the benefits of the drugs and aim to replace the judgment of doctors in determining the right drug. Some critics even say that drug companies, in effect, are practicing medicine without a license. Drug companies continue to say that the ads inform consumers and improve health.

The United States remains unusual in allowing such advertising. The only other high-income nation not to ban DTC ads for prescription drugs is New Zealand. The European Union has rejected proposals to allow ads for drugs that treat diseases such as AIDS, asthma, and diabetes, and new proposals to ease the ban, which emerge regularly, have had little success. Canada bans DTC ads but allows ads that either name the drug but not the condition it treats or name the condition but not the drug.

In 2006, the AMA reversed the position it took in 1992 in support of DTC ads. It called for a moratorium on DTC ads for newly approved drugs and suggested new, stricter guidelines on what ads can say when they are allowed. The AMA wanted the ads to be more understandable and informative to consumers and to give physicians more time to understand the pros and cons of new drugs.

In response to the concerns, the FDA announced in October 2007 that it would study consumer reactions to drug ads. Congress has not passed any restrictions but some congressional representatives have asked drug companies to accept a voluntary moratorium on advertisement of new drugs. While not agreeing to the request, drug companies have made some changes. On June 19, 2008, four companies, Johnson & Johnson, Pfizer, Merck, and Schering-Plough, agreed to a six-month moratorium on advertising of new drugs and to modify payment of celebrities and experts who endorse their products. Yet nothing permanent followed.

BENEFITS OF PRESCRIPTION DRUGS

Despite criticism of drug companies and their advertising to consumers, most Americans agree that prescription drugs have brought enormous benefits to the population. According to one study, new medicines accounted for about 40 percent of the two-year gain in life expectancy that occurred across 52 countries between 1986 and 2000.[7]

To make this point, it is worth summarizing the views of several experts. Dr. Jerry Avorn of Harvard University lists these benefits of prescription drugs:

- Anticoagulants (drugs to prevent clotting of the blood or thin the blood) reduce the risk of stroke by 67 percent in patients with a certain kind of irregular heart rhythm.

- Medications to strengthen bones reduce the risk of breaking a hip by 50 percent among patients with osteoporosis (or loss of bone density).
- Antipsychotic medications greatly improve the lives of patients with severe mental illness.
- Beta-blocker drugs that reduce the force of the heart's pumping and lower blood pressure markedly reduce the chance of death among heart attack patients.
- ACE-inhibitor medications for diabetics slow the development of kidney failure, a common cause of death among patients with diabetes.
- ACE-inhibitor medications also lower the death rate among patients with congestive heart failure (the inability of the heart to pump blood effectively throughout the body).
- Antibiotics have made once-dangerous infectious diseases into a source of sickness rather than death.
- Drugs to lower cholesterol called statins reduce the risk of a heart attack by 20–30 percent and stroke by about 17 percent.
- A variety of medications to lower high blood pressure reduce the risk of stroke and heart attack by 25 to 40 percent.[8]

Dr. Marcia Angell, former editor of the *New England Journal of Medicine*, adds a few others to the list of highly beneficial prescription drugs. Vaccines against infectious diseases, insulin for diabetics, chemotherapy agents for treating cancer, drugs to suppress the secretion of stomach acids, and painkillers for injuries and chronic diseases help people get and stay healthy. Less commonly needed but still helpful drugs include:

- Epogen, a genetically synthesized drug for treatment of anemia in patients on kidney dialysis;
- Gleevec, a drug that inhibits production of a certain enzyme and treats some forms of cancer;
- cyclosporine, an ingredient in many drugs that suppresses the immune system of persons receiving organ transplants; and
- protease inhibitors and other antiviral agents for treatment of HIV/AIDS.[9]

Many of these drugs were developed during the last 10 to 20 years and have benefited from easing of restrictions on patents, approval, and advertising.

In the last decade, a class of drugs called biologics has seen special promise. Biologic medicines are produced by living organisms rather than chemical synthesis, and the newest forms come from genetic engineering. These medicines include Avastin and Gleevec for cancer, Enbrel and Orencia for rheumatoid arthritis, Epogen for anemia, and Tysabri for multiple sclerosis. However, biologics tend to have major side effects and are expensive to produce and to buy. Even so, their benefits have made them one of the fastest-growing classes of drugs and an area of new drug development by pharmaceutical companies.

The dramatic growth in sales of prescription drugs has coincided with another trend that everyone views positively—the decline in mortality and the increase in longevity. Based on mortality rates in 1980, the average years lived from birth equaled 73.7. By 2004, the number reached 77.8. Although it is difficult to be precise about the benefits of prescription drugs for longevity, healthier living and better medical care (other than drug use) obviously contribute to the steady progress, and many prescription drugs for chronic pain, erectile dysfunction, and depression do more to make life better rather than longer. Yet drugs for HIV/AIDS, diabetes, infections, high blood pressure, and heart disease extend the lives of many.

MOST PRESCRIBED AND BEST-SELLING DRUGS

IMS Health, a company that gathers market data on global health care, reports on the top 10 classes and top 10 individual prescription drugs in the United States for 2007 (the most recent year available).[10] Here are the top 10 classes of most prescribed drugs, the number of prescriptions (in millions) given during the year, and a brief description of the uses of each class:

1. antidepressants, 232.7 million (for depression and related problems)
2. lipid regulators, 220.9 million (for high blood cholesterol)
3. codeine and combinations, 181.6 million (for pain)
4. ACE inhibitors, 157.9 million (for high blood pressure)
5. beta blockers, 132.5 million (for high blood pressure)
6. proton pump inhibitors, 108.4 million (to reduce production of stomach acid)
7. seizure disorder treatments, 101.8 million
8. thyroid hormones, 101.4 million (to treat thyroid hormone deficiency)
9. calcium blockers, 87.4 million (for high blood pressure)
10. benzodiazepines, 82.9 million (sedatives)

The most prescribed drugs do not always have the highest sales income. Sales depend in addition on the prices paid for the drugs. Following are the top 10 classes for total U.S. sales in billions.

1. lipid regulators, $18.4 billion (to lower blood cholesterol)
2. proton pump inhibitors, $14.1 billion (to reduce production of stomach acid)

3. antipsychotics, $13.1 billion (for mental disorders)
4. antidepressants, $11.9 billion (for depression and related problems)
5. seizure disorders treatments, $10.2 billion
6. erythropoietins, $8.6 billion (for treatment of anemia)
7. antineo monoclonal antibodies, $6.8 billion (for cancer treatment)
8. angiotensin II antagonists, $6.6 billion (for high blood pressure)
9. antiarthritis drugs, $5.3 billion
10. bisphosphonates, $4.6 billion (for osteoporosis or loss of bone mass)

While they are often prescribed, the lower costs of codeine, ACE inhibitors, beta-blockers, thyroid hormones, calcium blockers, and benzodiazepines keep them off the list of top sales. Conversely, the higher cost of erythropoietins, antineo monoclonal antibodies, angiotensin II antagonists, antiarthritis drugs, and bisphosphonates put them on the list of top sales but not top prescriptions.

The list of top 10 products (rather than classes of products) gives further insight into the most popular and best-selling drugs. Here are the most prescribed prescription drugs, the number of prescriptions (in millions) given during the year, and a brief description of the use of the drug:

1. hydrocodone/acetaminophen (HYCD/APAP), 119.1 million (for pain relief)
2. lisinopril, 70.5 million (an ACE inhibitor for high blood pressure)
3. Lipitor, 65.1 million (for high cholesterol)
4. levothyroxine sodium, 55.3 million (thyroid hormone)
5. amoxicillin, 53.2 million (antibiotic)
6. hydrochlorothiazide, 47.8 million (a diuretic for high blood pressure)
7. simvastatin, 47.7 million (for high cholesterol)
8. azithromycin, 46.3 million (antibiotic)
9. atenolol, 44.2 million (for high blood pressure and cardiovascular diseases)
10. furosemide, 43.8 million (for fluid retention and swelling associated with heart disease)

Drugs that have the greatest sales and reflect high prices include:

1. Lipitor, $8.1 billion (for high cholesterol)
2. Nexium, $5.5 billion (for excess stomach acid)
3. Advair Diskus, $4.3 billion (for asthma)
4. Plavix, $3.9 billion (protects against heart attacks)
5. Seroquel, $3.5 billion (for bipolar disorder)
6. Singulair, $3.4 billion (for asthma and allergies)
7. Enbrel, $3.4 billion (for arthritis)

8. Prevacid, $3.4 billion (heartburn and acid reflux)
9. Aranesp, $3.2 billion (for anemia associated with kidney disease)
10. Epogen, $3.1 billion (for anemia associated with kidney disease)

Although not prescribed as often as many other drugs, prescriptions for stomach problems and arthritis have high sales.

THE HIGH COST OF PRESCRIPTION DRUGS

Spending on prescription drugs has grown faster than other medical costs for hospital care and clinical services. Americans spent $216.7 billion on prescription drugs in 2006, up from $40.3 billion in 1990. From 1994 to 2004, drug prices rose 8.3 percent per year, well above the inflation rate of 2.3 percent per year. Private health insurance programs cover much of the increase, but out-of-pocket expenditures remain high. In 2006 out-of-pocket costs for prescription drugs reached $47.7 billion, or 22 percent of the $216.7 billion spent on prescription drugs.

Most of the increase in spending comes from more people taking more drugs. Figures for 2007 show that Americans purchased 3.8 billion prescriptions, 12.6 per person. These numbers represent substantial increases from the 1990s. In addition, prices per drug have increased. The average price per prescription increased from $35.72 in 1997 to $69.91 in 2007. The journalist Melody Peterson helps puts the spending on prescription drugs in perspective:

> *Americans spent more on prescription drugs in 2004 than they did on gasoline or fast food. They paid twice as much for their prescription medicines that year as they spent on either higher education or new automobiles. . . . Americans spend more on medicines than do all the people of Japan, Germany, France, Italy, Spain, the United Kingdom, Australia, New Zealand, Canada, Mexico, and Argentina combined.[11]*

Even if health insurance pays for much of the cost, patients still pay indirectly with higher premiums and taxes.

An article in the *AARP Bulletin* gives several examples of high costs that further illustrate the problem.[12] Specialty drugs that are made in the lab from living cells rather than from chemicals and require sophisticated techniques of genetic engineering are particularly expensive. The article lists several examples of these specialty drugs. The cost for a three-month supply of the cancer drug Tykerb is $10,000. The drug Avonex for multiple sclerosis costs about $24,000 a year. The arthritis drugs Enbrel and Humira cost from $15,000 to $45,000 a year. It cost $300,000 a year in 2006 for two cancer drugs, Herceptin and Avastin. Insurance covers most of the costs of these drugs, but patients often have to pay substantial out-of-pocket expenses. Although not typical, high-cost specialty drugs are becoming a more important part of medical treatment today.

Americans rely on several types of insurance to pay for prescription drugs but do not always have complete coverage. Private insurance covers most costs but can require substantial co-pays for expensive or rarely used drugs and sometimes excludes needed drugs from their coverage. As prices rise, insurers can raise monthly premiums or require patients to pay a higher proportion of the cost. Medicare, a federal insurance program for qualifying persons age 65 and over, allows recipients to sign up for private prescription drug plans approved by the government. These plans require a monthly fee, however. Medicaid, an insurance program run by the states for those too poor to qualify for private medical insurance programs, covers prescription drugs, but only the poorest of the population qualify for these benefits. Otherwise, paying for prescription drugs without some form of insurance is an expensive proposition.

Rising drug prices can affect the health of patients. According to a poll from the Kaiser Family Foundation and the Harvard School of Public Health, about 41 percent of Americans say they struggle to pay for prescriptions, 29 percent have not filled a prescription because of costs, and 23 percent have cut pills in half (to take half the prescribed dose) or skipped doses. Doctors say that, particularly with the economic downturn that began in 2008, patients are skimping even more on their prescriptions. Yet not taking the prescribed dose of drugs endangers the health of patients.

Patients having trouble paying for prescriptions should search for lower prices rather than cut back on prescriptions. They should aim to purchase generics whenever possible, perhaps use OTC remedies, and discuss alternative and cheaper prescriptions with their physician and pharmacist. Sometimes buying in larger doses or different-sized pills is cheaper. Discount stores such as WalMart, Sam's Club, and Target offer low-price prescriptions for generic drugs. Comparison shopping can save significantly on drug prices.

Some Americans take more drastic action to purchase lower-cost prescription drugs. Buying drugs online or going to Canada or Mexico to buy drugs can reduce costs substantially, but there are risks. The quality of drugs online may be compromised, and reimportation of drugs is illegal (although that may change with the Obama administration). Still, millions of Americans obtain drugs in these ways. For those without insurance, drug prescription cards made available by charitable organizations provide discounts on purchases at participating pharmacies. Low-income persons may qualify for discounted drugs from several state and private programs. The Partnership for Prescription Assistance, NeedyMeds.org, and Access to Benefits Coalition help patients find programs to pay for all or part of their drugs. Most drug companies also provide drugs at reduced costs to needy patients.

The public not surprisingly has negative views of the high costs of prescription drugs. According to the Kaiser Public Opinion Spotlight, most Americans (73 percent) agree that prescription drugs developed in the past 20 years have improved the lives of people in the United States.[13] Despite this, 44 percent have an unfavorable impression of pharmaceutical companies. Nearly 80 percent believe that drug prices are unreasonable and that profits for the drug companies cause the high prices for prescription drugs. About two-thirds believe that the government can do more to regulate prices.

Why are drugs so expensive? The drug industry, consumer groups, politicians, and scholars tend to give different answers. The answers nonetheless tend to fall into two groups. One put forth by drug companies and many supporters of the free market says that the cost of discovering and inventing new drugs is enormous. High prices are needed to recoup these high costs and fund future discoveries. In this view, the pharmaceutical industry helps to save lives and improve health. Another view, put forth by consumer groups and supporters of more government control of private business, says that profits of drug companies are too high, and too much money goes into marketing rather than research. Polls show that patients largely accept this view, blaming pharmaceutical companies that set the prices and get the profits.

DRUG COMPANIES CITE EXPENSES
FOR DISCOVERY AND TESTING

In June 2005, a trade organization for the pharmaceutical industry named the Pharmaceutical Research and Manufacturers of America (PhRMA) published a booklet on what goes into the high cost of prescription drugs.[14] The booklet makes the case for what many consider high prices for brand-name products. The industry and the booklet argue that drug companies and patients have the same goal—to fight disease and the burden it places on people, businesses, the health care system, and society. According to the booklet, the costs of prescription drugs ultimately go toward helping patients. Here are some of the reasons for high costs for prescription drugs according to the pharmaceutical industry.

First, unlike for most products, the costs of prescription drugs depend on new discoveries and knowledge rather than on ingredients and manufacturing. These costs are huge. It takes on average from 12 to 15 years and $800 million to develop a new medicine. Making it even more costly, many efforts to develop new drugs fail. Only five of 10,000 compounds researched by drug companies make it far enough to undergo clinical trials with humans. Of those five, only one eventually receives approval for patient use. Prices for the successful drugs must cover the costs of the failed but necessary research: "Revenues from one successful medicine must cover the costs of the vast number of 'dry holes.'"[15] Of the drugs approved for patient use, only three of 10 recover their research costs and help support research on other drugs. Some drugs face stiff competition from similar drugs, serve a small population of patients, or do not become popular enough to make up their costs. The few very successful drugs need to have a high price to help develop new drugs. And profits to drug companies from sales of drugs attract investments, which in turn fuel more development and research.

Second, for most patients, the drugs are well worth the cost in terms of better health, less discomfort and pain, and prevention of future health problems. Drugs that prevent deaths from strokes, heart attacks, diabetes, and HIV/AIDS make an enormous contribution to the well-being of patients, their families, and society more generally. Drugs to treat depression, arthritis, erectile dysfunction, sleeping problems, excessive urination, and chronic pain save no lives. Yet they make living better, more enjoyable, and less pain ridden. As the U.S. population gets older, the need for prescription drugs grows, as do their benefits. It is hard to estimate the number of lives saved or the amount of mental and physical pain avoided, but the benefits of prescription drugs greatly exceed the costs.

Third, use of prescription drugs lowers costs for more expensive hospital treatments. Preventing death and pain brings other economic benefits. It saves money in lost work time, lower hospital admissions, less clinical treatment, and less use of government health and welfare programs. For example, treatment by antidepressant drugs saves on costs for expensive therapy and time spent in psychiatric hospitals. According to one study by a Columbia University economist, "Each additional dollar spent on using a newer prescription medicine (instead of an older one) saves roughly $7.20 in other health care costs."[16] Statistics show that for every dollar spent on health care costs, only about 11 cents goes to prescription drugs. In turn, the 11 cents reduce other costs.

Fourth, in trying to sell more prescription drugs though advertising and marketing, the drug companies increase awareness of disease. People with health problems might think that nothing can be done to help them, but they may learn of drug solutions through advertising and talking to friends and relatives who have seen the advertising. Their conditions may stay undiagnosed until consumer advertising of prescription drugs encourages people to visit their doctors. According to data reported by PhRMA, about 25 percent of patients who visit a doctor in response to an ad then receive a diagnosis of a new condition. As a result, much new spending on prescription drugs comes not from higher prices per pill but from greater use of available medication. Americans pay more for drugs largely because they use them more. This fact supports the view of drug companies that they are meeting the needs of the public.

Along with offering justifications for high drug prices, defenders of the drug industry note that companies cannot charge whatever price they want. To the contrary, they must deal with many pressures to keep prices low. Governments in many countries limit prices, and large health insurance companies negotiate for lower prices. Other companies may develop a drug much like another successful drug, changing only a few chemical details but also increasing competition. High prices may discourage doctors from prescribing a product or patients from taking it. Companies need to charge prices that cover research and development, but most drugs face counter-pressures to keep prices reasonable.

Competition among drug companies seems in some instances to keep prices lower. In an article in *New Yorker* magazine, the writer Malcolm Gladwell cites research showing prices for brand-name drugs are higher in the United States. At the same time, however, prices for generic drugs are lower in the United States. The many drug companies in the United States compete fiercely to sell generic forms of drugs once the patents for the brand-name drugs run out. In Gladwell's words:

> *It is not accurate to say, then, that the United States has higher prescription-drug prices than other countries. It is accurate to say only that the United States has a different pricing system from that of other countries. Americans pay more for drugs when they first come out and less as the drugs get older, while the rest of the world pays less in the beginning and more later.*[17]

Because many popular drugs have gone off their patent in recent years, Americans now pay less for these drugs than Europeans do.

The Bush administration, an advocate in general for free-market policies, largely agreed with the drug companies about not interfering with drug prices. The former commissioner of the FDA, Dr. Mark McClellan, argued that lower drug prices in other nations came from innovation spawned by high prices in the United States. He called for other countries to stop regulating drug prices rather than for the United States to increase price regulation. For the same reason, the Bush administration and many in Congress also opposed limits on the prices paid by Medicare for its prescription drug plan. They believe that limiting prices will slow innovative research and development.

DEBATE OVER RESEARCH AND DEVELOPMENT COSTS

Critics dispute the figures presented by drug companies on research and development costs. The drug companies keep their records private, so it is hard for an independent auditor to calculate the figures directly. In 1983, the industry won a nine-year battle with the U.S. General Accounting Office to prevent release of its research and development records. The reported figure of $800 million per drug comes from figures provided by drug companies to researchers, without independent verification of the figures.

Even without detailed data from the drug companies, critics say the figures appear inflated in at least two ways. One, nearly half the expenses claimed to go to research and development do not involve actual research expenditures. Instead, the expenses come from a calculation to consider the cost of capital. This cost involves the income lost by investing money in research rather than stocks. For example, if $100 million in research funds could have earned $10 million in the stock market, the calculations treat that $10 million as a research expense. Two, the figures do not adjust expenses downward to take account of federal tax benefits for research spending. According to Public Citizen, the costs of bringing a drug to market in the 1990s ranged from $57 million to $71 million per new drug.[18] While certainly expensive, the cost is lower than the claim of $800 million to develop a new drug.

Drug companies often take advantage of basic science discoveries that come from research funded by the federal government. The journalist Melody Peterson gives an example: "Bristol-Myers Squibb's bestselling cancer drug Taxol was discovered by scientists funded through government grants. The federal government then paid to manufacture the drug and test it in patients, before granting a license to Bristol-Myers to sell it."[19] The Bayh-Dole Act of 1980 (or the University and Small Business Patent Procedures Act) gave universities and small businesses ownership of patents that resulted from funding by the federal government. The major drug companies license many new drugs from universities and small businesses that had relied on funding by the federal government. The law encourages innovation among organizations that received government funding but also indirectly supports pharmaceutical company research with government funds.

Although counted as research, companies may do additional testing on FDA-approved drugs for the purposes of advertising and marketing. This research involves something less than development and discovery. In testimony before Congress, a former vice president of Abbott Laboratories noted another way to inflate research expenditures.[20] Companies sometimes count as research the expenses used to promote a drug before it receives FDA approval. The distinction between research and marketing may seem clear, but reports can blur the figures.

Even if the cost of discovering new drugs reaches the high levels claimed by drug companies, most drugs are not completely new discoveries. Much of the research goes toward developing drugs that imitate a popular drug already discovered and made by another company. It costs much less to find a small variation on an existing product than to discover something completely original. These kinds of "me-too" drugs are quite profitable but do not involve decades of failed efforts before discovering something new and successful.

Rather than devoting most of their resources to research, drug companies spend much on advertising and marketing. The drug companies present figures showing marketing to be a small part of the total, but new estimates published by the *Public Library of Science (PLoS)* offer something more.[21] The authors of this study present a more encompassing measure of marketing expenditures for 2004. It includes $15.9 billion for distributing free samples, $20.4 billion for visits by sales reps, and $14.4 billion for unmonitored promotional activity. The total expenditures reach $57.5 billion. The figure is twice the size of yearly research and development expenditures. The study concludes that the new figures give evidence of the need for the industry to do more research and less promotion.

CRITICS POINT TO HIGH PROFITS
FOR DRUG COMPANIES

Critics also note that, despite the costs of developing some new drugs, the pharmaceutical industry remains one of the most profitable—rather than the most risky—in the United States. Price competition, a process that normally moderates profits, sometimes works differently in the drug industry than in other industries. For example, in 1983 the British drug company Glaxo introduced an ulcer medicine call Zantac in the United States. The new product was actually quite similar to an existing product called Tagamet (both are now available for purchase without a prescription). Glaxo executives decided to price Zantac up to 50 percent higher than Tagamet, implying that it was different and better.[22] Along with intense promotion to encourage those with heartburn or more serious ulcers to take the product, Zantac sold well at the higher price. In 1986, Zantac passed Tagamet to become the world's biggest-selling prescription drug.

Given the success of Zantac and other best-selling drugs, pharmaceutical companies have adopted a strategy for producing and selling drugs. They aim for a few "blockbuster" drugs with enormous sales and profits rather than many drugs with smaller sales. A blockbuster drug is defined as one with more than $1 billion in sales. Revenues for blockbuster drugs come from both a large number of users and high prices. Heavy advertising and marketing of the drugs often contribute to their success.

The real problem, according to critics, is that drug companies have the power to exploit their customers with higher prices. For most purchases, consumers can search out the best prices or do without expensive products altogether. For pharmaceuticals, however, customers do not have the expertise or information to evaluate fairness in prices and effectiveness of alternatives. If they need a drug for health, they must pay the cost in one form or another. The desire for health is so great that customers feel they have no choice but to pay whatever prices companies charge. Under most circumstances, they do not want to risk their health by forgoing expensive drugs.

Although patients may not realize it, some heavily advertised and expensive new drugs work no better than the older, cheaper forms. One commonly cited example involves prescription drugs for high blood pressure. A study in *JAMA*, the journal of the AMA, compared several drugs—calcium channel blockers, alpha-adrenergic blockers, and angiotensin-converting enzyme (ACE)—made and sold by the top drug companies with a 50-year-old generic diuretic or water pill.[23] The older, cheaper water pill did just as well as the others to hold down blood pressure and perhaps did even better in preventing strokes and heart attacks. Even so, the more expensive, heavily advertised, and newer drugs are more commonly prescribed. This finding demonstrates how advertising and marketing rather than drug effectiveness can push up prices.

Given these kinds of studies, some experts recommend that the FDA require different types of studies to help identify the best-working drugs. Typically, companies demonstrate the effectiveness of their drugs by comparing them to placebos. If a drug does better than a placebo, it demonstrates effectiveness in comparison to doing nothing. Approving a new drug might instead use the standard of whether it does better than existing or cheaper drugs, rather than a placebo. Under this standard, some new and expensive drugs might not be approved, and drug costs might moderate.

Legislation introduced in 2008 proposes to use this new standard. The Comparative Effectiveness Research Act of 2008 would create an institute to review and publicize evidence on how to best treat diseases, disorders, and other health conditions. In evaluating the effectiveness of drugs and medical procedures, the institute would provide unbiased information to health care practitioners. Information on the most effective treatment rather than the most heavily advertised and expensive treatment would ideally reduce costs. The pharmaceutical industry also favors the legislation. A version of this legislation passed as part of the American Recovery and Reinvestment Act of 2009. The act provided funds to several agencies and created a Federal Coordinating Council for Comparative Effectiveness Research to advance comparative effectiveness research.

In addition, the United States might follow the lead of other high-income nations in regulating prices of prescription drugs. According to a study of 14 high-income nations, spending per person on drugs was 65 percent higher in the United States than in the other nations. For every $100 spent in, say England, Japan, or Germany, Americans spend about

$165.[24] Part of the high expense comes from higher prices in the United States, the only advanced industrial nation that does not regulate drug prices. However, many believe the high prices represent a strength rather than a weakness. They encourage innovation and discovery of new drugs. The research and development done in the United States and funded by the prices here lead to new products that other nations come to use.

PATENT LAWS AND DRUG COSTS

Much of the dispute over the costs of drugs relates to patent laws. In principle, patent rights give companies a period to own and profit from new discoveries before sharing the discoveries and sales with other companies. Exclusive marketing rights for a patented drug last 17 years from the issue of the patent or 20 years from the date of the first filing for the patent. During this period, companies will charge as much as possible to recoup the costs of research and development and make a profit. The FDA has similar rules that prevent it from approving a near-identical drug while the patent holds. After that, other companies can make and sell generic versions of the original drug. Since several companies can manufacture the generic drug and compete for customers, the prices are much lower than for brand-name drugs. Companies can still sell their brand-name drugs, but with the equivalent versions available at lower prices, sales and profits decline greatly. Ideally, the system encourages innovation by allowing for exclusive rights for a period but then allows for cheaper prices and widespread access to the drug.

According to critics, however, companies with patents abuse their rights by stretching the period of exclusivity. They sue for infringement when generic companies attempt to manufacture and sell a drug after a patent ends. These suits generally fail but can extend the patent for 30 months. In 2002 testimony before the Senate, Federal Trade Commissioner Timothy Muris summarized a report on the abuse of patent laws.[25] In 72 percent of cases, when a patent for a brand-name drug expired, the owner of the patent sued the first company to make a generic version. The suits seldom succeeded, but they slowed the sale of generic drugs. Legislation in 2003 curbed some of these kinds of suits, but the practice still contributes to higher drug prices.

In some extreme cases, drug companies have paid other companies not to produce generic forms of some drugs. In 2003, the FTC sued Bristol-Myers Squibb for blocking the sale of generic drugs, particularly the cancer drugs Platinol and Taxol and the antianxiety drug BuSpar. Among the accusations, the FTC suit contended that Bristol-Myers Squibb had offered another company $72 million to not market a generic version of one of its drugs. In a settlement of the suit, the company agreed not to engage in these types of unlawful behaviors.

Another strategy drugmakers use to get around patent laws is to make small changes in a popular drug that allow for a new patent but do little to improve the effectiveness of the drug. Dr. Marcia Angell cites several instances of this strategy to keep patent advantages.[26] This strategy is similar to the creation of me-too drugs, in which companies imitate the successful patented drugs of another company. In this case, a company develops a new patented drug that is like one of its own older drugs that has lost its patent. When the patent for its popular heartburn treatment Prilosec ended, AstraZeneca patented Nexium, with a formula very similar to that of Prilosec. When the patent ended for Claritin, the popular allergy medicine, Schering-Plough patented Clarinex, a drug that turns into Claritin once in the body. And when the patent ended for the popular antidepressant Prozac, Eli Lilly patented Sarafem, a form of Prozac used for premenstrual tension. Each of these new drugs received several years of exclusive marketing rights. With marketing to convince people that the revised versions performed better than the cheaper generics, companies could partly maintain sales.

Other laws and regulations help protect the patent rights and pricing strategies of companies. The Prescription Drug Marketing Act of 1987 made it against the law to reimport drugs from other countries (unless done by the original manufacturer or for emergency medical care). Reimportation refers to returning drugs to the United States after exporting them for sale in other nations. Because regulations in other nations keep prices lower than in the United States, consumers sometimes can save money by buying drugs outside the United States and bringing them back for use. People sometimes travel to Canada or Mexico to fill prescriptions or buy them from other countries via the Internet. The FDA has not consistently enforced the law, allowing individuals to get prescription drugs for personal use. However, custom agents on occasion have seized drugs bought in other countries for resale here.

Although the law keeps prices for prescription drugs in the United States higher than in other countries, it also helps ensure the safety of drugs. The FDA says that drugs reimported from other countries may have been improperly stored, passed their expiration date, or even be repackaged with counterfeit products. The agency says that it cannot guarantee the safety of reimported drugs. Critics respond that dealing with certified pharmacies and wholesalers in other countries could eliminate safety concerns, while at the same time give consumers a way to buy drugs at cheaper prices.

Congress has tried many times to end the restriction on reimported drugs but with no success. One law signed into law by President Clinton in 2000 allowed reimportation but required the Secretary of Health and Human Services to certify the safety of the drugs. Secretary Donna Shalala concluded, however, that reimportation would not be safe, effectively ending the program before it got started. During the Bush administration, proposals introduced in Congress to allow reimportation either failed to pass or required certification of safety that the government was unwilling to give.

If laws for drug patents and reimportation appear to favor the pharmaceutical industry, it may relate to the billions spent by the industry to lobby Congress. According to critics, the lobbying contributes doubly to high prices, through the actual cost of lobbying and through the higher prices protected by lobbying. For example, in three month from July 1, 2008, to September 30, 2008, the drug company Novartis spent $1.4 million in lobbying and Bristol-Myers Squibb spent $840,000. Drug companies also give millions to political campaigns. According to a report from the Center for Public Integrity, a critic of the drug industry, drug companies spent $675 million on lobbying between 1998 and 2005. That included paying 3,009 lobbyists, 1,014 former government officials who registered to lobby, and 75 former members of Congress who lobbied, and lobbying for 1,600 bills.[27] In 2006, PhRMA spent $18.1 million, Pfizer $11.8 million, and Amgen $10.2 million on lobbying.[28]

MEDICARE PRESCRIPTION ACT OF 2003

Until the last few years, the elderly objected most strongly to the high costs of prescription drugs. They tend to take more prescription drugs than younger persons, often expensive ones, and their health depends more on these drugs. Medicare, a government program to pay certain medical costs for qualifying elderly persons, covers persons age 65 and over. Until recently, however, the program typically covered only costs for hospital stays and medical services and supplies. As prescription drugs became an increasingly larger part of medical treatment over the past decades, out-of-pocket health care expenses that Medicare did not cover grew for elderly persons.

Federal legislation to deal with the problem, the largest reform in Medicare since its establishment in 1964, was enacted in 2003. The Medicare Prescription Drug Improvement and Modernization Act passed that year and set up a new prescription benefit to begin on January 1, 2006. The plan gave new assistance to program participants in buying prescription drugs through a mix of government funding, cost-sharing from beneficiaries, and service from private insurance companies.

Under the legislation, those eligible for Medicare can enroll voluntarily in a prescription drug plan called Medicare Part D. Private insurance companies rather than the government sponsor the plans that Medicare participants can select. The private plans compete for customers by offering discounts but receive reimbursement from the government. In this way, Medicare keeps costs low and gives program participants some choice in the companies they select.

Introduction to Prescription Drugs

Members of Medicare prescription drug plans pay a monthly premium that entitles them to savings of 10 to 25 percent on the drugs they buy. The premium varies depending on the plan and the company but on average costs about $28 a month in 2009. Costs for drugs also include deductibles and co-payments. The plans thus lower but do not pay all costs of prescription drugs. Low-income groups get additional subsidies to help with out-of-pocket expenses. Alternatively, those who belong to a Medicare-approved HMO, called Medicare Advantage, get prescription drug benefits as part of HMO membership rather than Medicare Part D. Others get drug coverage through employers or unions but must choose between private and public plans. Retirees who have prescription drug coverage from an employer or union lose these benefits if they join Medicare Part D. To encourage participation in the private sector, employer and union-sponsored plans receive government subsidies for the prescription-drug discounts they offer to members.

Given that it lowers the costs of prescription drugs, Medicare Part D appears popular among the elderly. According to figures from the Centers for Medicare and Medicaid Services, more than 90 percent of those eligible have enrolled in prescription plans. About 8.3 million have done so through Medicare Advantage plans. By some estimates, older persons save an average of $1,200 per year through the program (at the cost to the government of about $558 billion over a 10-year period).

The drug companies also benefited from the legislation. It likely increased purchases of drugs, as some elderly persons can afford drugs on insurance that they could not afford on their own. At the same time, it did not lead to price controls. To get broad support for the legislation in Congress, the law prevents the federal government from negotiating lower prices for drugs with pharmaceutical companies. This provision angered many who believe that the drug companies had too much control over the legislation. They say that the reliance on profit-seeking insurance companies and Medicare Advantage HMOs for the prescription drug benefits rather than on direct government payments hurts elderly consumers. However, others counter by noting that competition for Medicare enrollees among the profit-seeking companies has kept prices down.

The AARP (formerly the American Association of Retired Persons) notes big increases in prescription drug costs for Medicare enrollees in 2009.[29] The most popular stand-alone plans (those not part of Medicare Advantage HMO plans) raised monthly premiums by 8 to 63 percent. For example, the Humana Standard plan, the second largest in the country, rose from $9.51 per month in 2006, the first year, to $40.83 per month in 2009. The plan also raised required co-payments for brand-name drugs, while it lowered them for generic drugs. Also in 2009, there is an initial limit on payment for prescription drugs of $2,700. Those enrolled must pay all the costs for drugs beyond that amount until total expenses reach $4,350, after which catastrophic coverage pays for costs. This gap in coverage (informally called the donut hole) can cost elderly persons up to $1,650 in prescription drug costs. However, President Obama recently reached an agreement with the pharmaceutical industry to help reduce the donut hole costs paid by seniors.

Much debate has occurred in recent years over using Medicare Part D to control drug prices. After the 2006 elections, Democrats in Congress called for legislation that would allow the government to negotiate with drug companies over the prices of drugs for Medicare beneficiaries. The Bush administration opposed the change, arguing that price negotiation by the government would lead to price controls and reduce the incentives of companies to develop innovative drugs. Advocates deny wanting price controls but believe the government should get a discount for buying Medicare drugs in bulk. Although the legislation failed, the prospects for passing similar legislation look stronger with a Democratic Congress and president.

PHARMACEUTICAL INDUSTRY

The pharmaceutical industry is both big and profitable. The peak in profits occurred in the 1990s. The top 10 drug companies had profits of nearly 25 percent of sales in 1990 and 18.5 percent of sales in 2001. These profits substantially exceeded those for other industries. The second most profitable industry, commercial banking, had profits that were 13.5 percent of sales. Although still high, profits have not kept up at the same level during the 2000s. According to the Kaiser Family Foundation,

> *From 1995 to 2002, pharmaceutical manufacturers were the nation's most profitable industry (profits as a percent of revenues). They ranked third in profitability in 2003 and 2004, 5th in 2005, 2nd in 2006, and 3rd in 2007, with profits of 15.8% compared to 5.7% for all Fortune 500 firms in 2007.*[30]

Part of the slowdown in profits comes from the lack of new blockbuster drugs. Innovative drugs have come out more slowly than in the 1980s and 1990s. In 2007, for example, the Pharmaceutical Business Review reported that the FDA "approved just 19 new products, the lowest level for over 20 years."[31] At the same time, the patents of many of the most profitable drugs have ended. Since 2001, the antidepressant Prozac, the stomach acid medicine Prilosec, the diabetes drug Glucophage, and the allergy drug Claritin could be made in generic form and sold at lower prices. According to the Pharmaceutical Business Review, the top 50 pharmaceutical companies face the expiration of patents between 2007 and 2015 on drugs worth $115 billion in sales.[32]

The companies have yet to develop new, equally profitable drugs to replace these best sellers. According to a recent story from *Forbes* magazine, the sales of new drugs approved by the FDA since the mid-2000s have been slow. "In 2008, the Food and Drug Administration approved 24 brand new medicines, the most in three years. But medicines approved through June produced lower sales than had been seen in the preceding decade."[33] Many hoped that smaller biotechnology start-up companies using recombinant DNA techniques and molecular biology to develop new drugs would help the industry overcome sluggish sales of new products. Biotechnology companies have developed several successful prescription drugs and have become a crucial part of the pharmaceutical industry. Still, these kinds of innovations have not led to a new boom for the pharmaceutical industry.

Also putting pressure on profits of the pharmaceutical industry, buyers of prescription drugs have tried to cut their costs. Private health insurers bargain for discounts from sellers and encourage people to use the cheapest drugs. For example, they may fully cover generics, partially cover brand-name drugs, and exclude expensive drugs with limited evidence of value over cheaper drugs. In addition, insurers have a list of preferred drugs called formularies. Ideally, the evidence of safety and effectiveness for preferred drugs is strong and costs are reasonable. Patients covered by the formulary need to get prescriptions for these preferred drugs, and insurers can negotiate better prices with drug companies in return for including their drugs in the formulary. State governments that pay for drugs as part of Medicaid health care programs for the poor have also begun to negotiate better prices. A 2003 Supreme Court decision based on a case in Maine ruled that states had the right to control prices in certain ways.

On the other hand, the new Medicare prescription drug program has helped drug industry profits. A report from the office of Representative Henry Waxman, a Democrat from California who has been critical of the drug industry, analyzed profits during the first six months of the drug program. The analysis found that profits during the first half of 2006 increased by $8 billion or 27 percent over the same period in 2005.[34] The new coverage of drugs led many Medicare recipients to purchase what they could not afford before and led drug companies to increase some prices.

Moreover, drug companies are expected to weather the recent recession and debt crisis better than most. Despite the 2008 and 2009 drop in stock prices, the pharmaceutical industry has an advantage over many other industries—they have taken on little debt. They also have considerable cash on hand. Pharmaceutical stocks consequently have outperformed others during a period of huge stock losses.

Prescription Drugs

Here are thumbnail sketches of the companies with the largest global sales in 2006.[35]

1. Pfizer ($45 billion in sales). Founded by cousins Charles Pfizer and Charles Erhardt in Brooklyn, New York, in 1849, the company now has headquarters in New York City. During the 1800s, Pfizer produced several successful drugs and a variety of popular food additives. It later became know for mass-producing penicillin during World War II. In the 1980s and 1990s, it developed several popular drugs that account for its leadership in sales. The anticholesterol statin drug Lipitor is the world's best-selling drug. The antidepressant Zoloft and the erectile dysfunction drug Viagra are also best sellers. Several mergers in recent years with other large drug companies also contributed to the company's size. In 2000, Pfizer merged with Warner-Lambert, which had acquired Parke-Davis in 1970. The merger gave Pfizer full rights to Lipitor. In 2002, Pfizer merged with Pharmacia, which had earlier merged with Upjohn and G. D. Searle. Among the other drugs it produces are Celebrex for arthritis, Chantix for stopping smoking, Depo Provera for birth control, Aromasin for prevention of breast cancer, osteoporosis, and symptoms of menopause among women, Detrol for overactive bladder, Aricept for Alzheimer's disease, Norvasc for hypertension, Caduet, which combines Lipitor and Norvasc, and Lyrica for fibromyalgia.

2. GlaxoSmithKline ($37 billion in sales). Headquartered in London, England, but with major operations in North Carolina and Pennsylvania, this company represents the merger of several large companies over past decades. Glaxo was founded in New Zealand in 1904, Burroughs Wellcome in 1880 in London (but developed a strong presence in the United States), and SmithKline Beecham as the Beecham Group in England in 1843. GlaxoWellcome formed in 1995 with the merger of Glaxo with Glaxo Canada and Burroughs Wellcome, and GlaxoSmithKline was formed in 2000 with the merger of Glaxo-Wellcome and SmithKline Beecham (which formed earlier from SmithKline Beckman and Beecham). The company makes Paxil to treat depression, Advair for asthma and chronic obstructive pulmonary disease (COPD), Avandia for diabetes, Levitra for erectile dysfunction, Tagamet for stomach acid, Wellbutrin for depression and smoking cessation, AZT for treatment of HIV/AIDS, Requip for restless leg syndrome and Parkinson's, Avodart for enlarged prostate, and Valtrex for genital herpes.

3. Sanofi-Aventis ($36 billion in sales). Headquartered in Paris, this company resulted from the takeover of Aventis in 2004 by Sanofi-Synthélabo. The company has strong sales in developing countries.

It makes Allegra for allergies, Ambien for sleep problems, Plavix to prevent formation of blood clots that lead to heart attacks and strokes, Taxotere for treatment of breast cancer, Actonel for osteoporosis, Arava for rheumatoid arthritis symptoms such as joint swelling and tenderness, Lovenox for certain kinds of blood clots, Eligard for treatment of prostate cancer, and Lantus for diabetes.

4. Novartis ($29 billion in sales). Headquartered in Basel, Switzerland, this company was formed in 1996 from the merger of two Swiss companies, Ciba-Geigy (formed in 1970 from the merger of J. R. Giegy and Ciba) and Sandoz Laboratories. Sandoz is the generic pharmaceuticals division of the company, which makes Novartis one of the leaders in both patented and generic drugs. It makes Diovan for hypertension, Gleevec for chronic myeloid leukemia, Zometa for cancer complications, Sandostatin for excess production of growth hormone, Femara for breast cancer, and Enablex for an overactive bladder.

5. Roche ($27 billion in sales). Hoffman-La Roche, Roche for short, has its global headquarters in Basel, Switzerland, and U.S. headquarters in Nutley, New Jersey. It introduced a new class of tranquilizers in the 1960s, including Valium, and makes the antibiotic Rocephin, Invirase for HIV/AIDS, Xenical for treatment of obesity and absorption of fat, Tamiflu for influenza, and Boniva for treatment of osteoporosis.

6. AstraZeneca ($26 billion in sales). The result of a merger of Swedish AB and the British Zeneca Group in 1999, the company has headquarters in Södertälje, Sweden, and London. It has formed alliances with the smaller American companies Abbott Laboratories and Bristol-Meyers Squibb. Its products include Arimidex for treatment of certain types of breast cancer, Crestor for high cholesterol, Nexium for heartburn relief, Zomig or Seroquel for nervous system problems such as migraine, schizophrenia, and epilepsy, Atacand for hypertension, Zoladex for bowel and prostate cancers, Diprivan and Xylocaine for surgical anesthesia, and Pulmicort for asthma.

7. Johnson & Johnson ($23 billion in sales). With business in consumer products and medical devices as well as pharmaceuticals, this American company was founded in 1886 by Robert Wood Johnson and his brothers and now has its headquarters in New Brunswick, New Jersey. It is known more for selling OTC health products such as Band-Aids, Benadryl, Imodium, Listerine, Motrin, Nicoderm, Nicorette, Pepcid AC, Rogaine, Rolaids, Sudafed, Tylenol, and Visine. Among its prescription drugs are Haldol for treating schizophrenia, Topamax to treat epilepsy, Remicade for a variety of immune system diseases, Zyrtec for allergies, Orthoclone for preventing the rejection of

transplanted organs, Procrit for treatment of anemia associated with chronic renal failure, Risperdal for treatment of autism and bipolar disease, and Razadyne for treatment of confusion associated with moderate Alzheimer's disease.

8. Merck ($23 billion in sales). Headquartered in Whitehouse Station, New Jersey, this company was originally a division of the German company Merck KGaA but became an independent American company during World War I. It has received much negative publicity of late for its product Vioxx, a drug for treating arthritis that was withdrawn from the market after studies showed it caused heart problems. The company has been criticized for not withdrawing the drug earlier and faces some 50,000 suits over the drug. It makes Cozaar and Hyzaar for hypertension, Vytorin, Zetia, and Zocor to lower cholesterol, Propecia for male pattern baldness, Singulair for asthma, Fosamax for osteoporosis, and Gardasil, a vaccine for cervical cancer. It also makes many other childhood and adult vaccines.

9. Wyeth ($16 billion in sales). Formerly known as American Home Products, this company headquartered in Madison, New Jersey, makes many well-known OTC drugs such as Robitussin and Advil. The company first used machines to mass-produce tablet pills in 1872 and supplied the polio vaccine for early trials in the 1950s. It produced a diet drug called fenfluramine that when combined with other drugs into a form known as fen-phen caused health problems and was withdrawn from the market. It makes Premarin and Prempro for estrogen replacement, Effexor for depression and anxiety disorders, Ativan for anxiety and insomnia, and Enbrel for arthritis.

10. Eli Lilly ($15 billion in sales). Founded by Eli Lilly in 1876 in Indianapolis, where it still has its headquarters, the company is known for its breakthrough antidepressant drug, Prozac, and its many drugs for psychiatric and mental health conditions. It also became famous for one of the first ads explicitly discussing erectile dysfunction for its drug Cialis during the 2004 Super Bowl. It also makes Cymbalta for depression and anxiety, Gemzar for pancreatic cancer, methadone for treatment of drug addiction, Seconal for epilepsy and insomnia, and Zyprexa for schizophrenia and bipolar disorder.

Sales in the United States are dominated largely by the same companies. Ranked by most U.S. sales, the top 10 companies are Pfizer, GlaxoSmith-Kline, Merck, Johnson & Johnson, AstraZeneca, Amgen, Novartis, Hoffman-LaRoche, Sanofi Aventis, and Eli Lilly.[36] Amgen is a California-based biotechnology company that has developed successful drugs based on recombinant DNA such as Epogen for anemia. Hoffman-LaRoche is the U.S. prescription drug unit of Roche, headquartered in Basel, Switzerland.

However, mergers and buyouts have further changed the landscape of competition among drug companies. First, Pfizer agreed to buy Wyeth for $68 billion on January 26, 2009. With the addition of Wyeth, the world's largest pharmaceutical company will become even larger. However, the merger will result in substantial job cuts to improve the performance of the combined company. It will need to deal with declining sales of its top-selling anticholesterol drug, Lipitor, at the end of the drug's patent in 2011. Second, Merck and Schering-Plough announced a merger on March 9, 2009, making it one of the largest pharmaceutical companies in the world. Merck is paying $41.1 billion for the smaller company. Schering-Plough makes Clarinex, the biotech arthritis drug Remicade, a variety of other prescription medications, and popular consumer products such as Coppertone and Dr. Scholl's foot products. The two companies have $47 billion in combined revenues. A third buyout was the March 2009 purchase of the biotech company Genentech for $48 billion by Roche. Genentech, a company that developed cancer drugs through genetic engineering, has some promising drugs in the pipeline that may help Roche.

Experts predict that other mergers may follow, as drug companies attempt to deal with sluggish growth in sales, the lack of new blockbuster drugs, and a worldwide economic recession. Companies hope that consolidation will make them more efficient through sharing of research offices and sales force. They also hope that combining traditional pharmaceutical companies focused on chemical research with new biotechnology companies focused on genetic and molecular research will strengthen both.

Besides pharmaceutical companies, another key component of the drug industry has enjoyed success and growth. Drugstores such as Walgreens, CVS, and Rite-Aid, the three biggest chains in the United States, have grown over the past decades with increases in prescriptions. Grocery stores and discount stores such as Walmart and Costco also have pharmacies that have substantial sales and offer steep discounts for many generic drugs. A burgeoning market for Internet sales also exists. Figures for 2004 show that 36 percent of retail drug sales come from chain stores; 23 percent from hospitals, long-term care facilities, and clinics; 14 percent from independent stores; 14 percent from mail services; 9 percent from food stores; and 4 percent from other sources.

OVERUSE OF PRESCRIPTION DRUGS

Although concerns about the high cost of prescription drugs and the lack of access to needed drugs dominate much of the discussion, others point to the opposite problems. They say the benefits of prescription drugs are overstated or overhyped. The public has too much access to prescription drugs rather than too little access. America has become a pill-popping nation, looking for quick, easy, and unrealistic fixes to any and every problem. While most prescription drugs benefit certain patients, the huge increase in use extends well beyond the likely gain. Dr. Arnold Relman, the former editor of the *New England Journal of Medicine* and professor emeritus at Harvard University, makes the point strongly. The United States has become a "grossly overprescribed nation." He further says that "The average senior in America is probably taking twice or three times the medications they require."[37]

The National Center for Health Statistics does surveys that ask respondents about prescription drug use. The center has not yet released more recent figures, but their reports for two periods, 1988–1994 and 1999–2002, show a steep increase. During the first period, 39.1 percent of adults reported using at least one prescription drug in the last month; during the second period, usage rose to 45.3 of adults.[38] Among the elderly, 84.7 percent used at least one prescription drug in the last month during the 1999–2002 period. About 17.7 percent of all adults and 51.6 of the elderly used three or more prescription drugs. A more recent survey from the pharmacy benefit company Express Scripts relies on a different kind of data and reports even higher figures. The percentage of people in private health care plans using at least one prescription drug rose from 67 percent in 2000 to 74 percent in 2006.[39]

ADVERTISING AND PRESCRIPTION DRUG USE

The drug companies argue that the rising use of prescription drugs reflects the health needs of the population. New prescription drugs help treat health problems in ways that improve on past treatments. Both physicians who prescribe the drugs and patients who take them value these benefits. Demand for prescription drugs has risen with their effectiveness. By this account, drugs are appropriately used rather than overused.

Others take a different viewpoint. They identify multiple sources of the excessive growth of prescription drugs. Drug companies make exaggerated claims for their products. With sometimes unrealistic hopes, patients demand drugs they see on commercials. Managed health care organizations find that prescribing pills is cheaper and easier than other treatments. Physicians readily respond to demands for prescriptions. The government fails to adequately regulate drug companies and the claims they make. However, according to critics, the major driver of overuse is the drug companies. Rather than discovering new drugs to meet the needs of patients, they put the most effort into marketing and selling. Ads, sponsorships, and salespeople have had much success in selling products. The growth of DTC ads has become especially important. Although some see this claim as controversial, critics contend the excessive growth comes from selling drugs to people who have little need for them.

In May 2008, the Committee on Energy and Commerce held a hearing in the House of Representatives to examine what representatives and witnesses described as misleading ads sponsored by drug companies for their prescription drugs. Mollyann Brodie of the Kaiser Family Foundation testified that 91 percent of adults have seen or heard advertisements for prescription drugs.[40] Nearly a third of adults say they have talked to their doctor about a prescription drug after seeing or hearing an ad, and 80 percent of physicians say that patients have asked them for drugs they heard about from advertisements. While some argue that the ads lead people to get needed drugs that they otherwise would not know about, others say that it leads people to ask for—and often receive—drugs they do not need.

Sometimes drugmakers mislead consumers by making false statements. The FDA has warned several companies about misleading information in ads. For example, Bristol-Myers Squibb made false claims that its cholesterol-lowering drug Pravachol prevented strokes in all people rather than just those with heart disease. Pfizer falsely claimed in some ads that its cholesterol-lowering drug Lipitor was safer than other drugs used to lower cholesterol. Novartis Pharmaceuticals made false claims about the superiority of Lamisil, a treatment for fungus, and removed the ads after a warning from the FDA. A drug called Procrit made by Johnson & Johnson was approved for treating severe anemia for cancer patients undergoing chemotherapy, but commercials wrongly implied that the drug could reduce fatigue and weakness among a much larger group of people.

Rather than present false information, the ads more often exaggerate with images and music. The activities of attractive healthy people shown in the ads imply that the drugs can make users more active, healthier, and happier, when the scientific evidence is usually much more modest. Sometimes ads oversimplify the science in ways that make solutions to problems sound easier than they really are. Claims made in ads that an antidepressant can correct a chemical imbalance in movement of molecules in the brain have some validity but oversimplify a complex problem with multiple sources. Also, the optimistic, cheerful, and glowing parts of ads can overshadow the risks associated with the drugs—sometimes intentionally. The FDA told Procter & Gamble to stop some ads for its osteoporosis drug Actonel that listed the risks of its product but obscured these risks with rapidly changing images that distracted viewers.

Sometimes ads use evidence from scientific studies to publicize the benefits of the drugs. Again, however, the ads hide some important information—the drug companies often sponsor and control these studies.

Prescription Drugs

According to critics, drug-sponsored studies tend to ignore negative findings and highlight positive findings. According to a report in *JAMA*, a study sponsored by drug companies is three to four times more likely to report favorable findings about a drug than research sponsored by the independent National Institutes of Health. The authors of the report conclude that "Financial relationships among industry, scientific investigators, and academic institutions are widespread. Conflicts of interest arising from these ties can influence biomedical research in important ways."[41]

An editorial from the *New England Journal of Medicine* makes similar criticisms about prescription drug research:

> *The ties between clinical researchers and industry include not only grant support, but also a host of other financial arrangements. Researchers serve as consultants to companies whose products they are studying, join advisory boards and speakers' bureaus, enter into patent and royalty arrangements, agree to be the listed authors of articles ghostwritten by interested companies, promote drugs and devices at company-sponsored symposiums, and allow themselves to be plied with expensive gifts and trips to luxurious settings. Many also have equity interest in the companies.*[42]

These financial arrangements may skew research in ways that help in marketing products but not in identifying the best prescription drugs for patients.

Ads to consumers, which sometimes overstate the benefits of a prescription drug and the science behind the claims, do influence the public. According to Michael S. Wilkes, vice dean of the medical school at the University of California, Davis, "DTC advertising may cultivate the belief among the public that there is a pill for every ill."[43] As a result, patients may decide for themselves that they want the drug and not disclose all the information a physician might need to prescribe something else. This places physicians in a difficult position. They need to spend time to convince patients that the drug they saw advertised is not right for them. Changes in diet, exercise, and stress may better deal with problems, but patients convinced of the value of a heavily advertised drug may hope for an easier, though unrealistic solution.

All these complexities, ways around regulations, and tendencies to emphasize benefits over risks make regulation of prescription drug advertising challenging. Companies and advertisers can more quickly come up with new methods of publicizing their products and new ways to attract users than the FDA can control the ads.

Besides attempting to satisfy patients, physicians face other pressures to overprescribe drugs. The drug companies put enormous resources into persuading physicians of the value of their drugs. In fact, most of the marketing expenses of drug companies are targeted at physicians rather than the public. Large sales forces of drug reps visit doctors and promote the benefits of the prescription drugs their company makes. Besides providing free samples, companies often offer gifts, free meals, or consulting fees to doctors. For example, educational programs sponsored by drug companies describe their product and the benefits of prescribing it to patients—usually involving free meals at nice restaurants. Physicians say they evaluate the information objectively and remain unswayed by exaggerated sales pitches or gifts. Others wonder, however, if these efforts of drug companies contribute to overuse of pharmaceuticals.

CREATING DISEASE

Advertising to the public and marketing to physicians focus on certain types of health conditions. Drugs that make the most money treat conditions that meet three criteria. First, they are common in the population, ensuring a large market. Drugs designed for more specialized populations, such as persons with epilepsy, have less potential for high sales. Second, they last a long time. Drugs to treat chronic conditions such as arthritis, depression, high blood pressure, elevated cholesterol, stomach problems, allergies, and erectile dysfunction are most profitable. Drugs do not cure these conditions and involve continued use. Third, people needing the drug must have resources, through insurance, government aid, or personal income, to pay for it. Drugs for diseases common in poorer nations of the developing world such as malaria or sleeping sickness make little profit.

Companies tend to compete for the same set of conditions that produce the most sales. This encourages the development of me-too drugs that differ little from popular existing drugs. For example, the many similar drugs for high cholesterol—Mevacor, Crestor, Lipitor, Zocor, Pravachol, Lescol—have high sales but can offer little evidence that one is considerably better than the others. Competition for sales among these drugs then leads to more sales efforts to increase market share. The goal of taking market share away from existing and successful drugs diverts resources from the goal of making innovative discoveries for untreated conditions.

Another strategy for high sales involves transforming common problems of living into diseases that medications can treat. Critics call this strategy creating disease. The journalist Melody Peterson argues the point in her book on the drug industry:

> *Once I thought I knew what disease was. It had seemed black and white. A person was either healthy or sick. . . . Then I listened to the drug marketers and learned that the definition of disease was less certain. It was malleable, even slippery, in fact. A disease could be invented if one had the money, the power, and an adman's knack for salesmanship.*[44]

43

Scholars had long noted a tendency in modern societies to treat personal and social problems of daily living as medical diseases. Problems such as alcoholism, misbehavior of children, and sadness, once viewed as personal or social failings, came to be seen as diseases or disorders. More recently, however, drug companies have contributed to the process by identifying and publicizing new conditions that their drugs can treat. The strategy redefines normal aspects of living into something more serious and, according to critics, contributes to overuse of prescription drugs.

EXAMPLES OF POSSIBLE OVERUSE

Rather than speak of generalities, it helps to have examples of overuse. Although the following claims are themselves the subject of dispute, these examples show up often in discussions of prescription drugs. Each shows how drugs may help some people but also how exaggerated claims about the drugs may increase both sales and overuse.

Ritalin. According to the National Institutes of Health, attention deficit/hyperactivity disorder, or ADHD (formerly called attention deficit disorder), affects 3 to 5 percent of children.[45] It is a condition characterized by excessive restlessness or fidgeting, short attention span, inability to concentrate, impulsiveness, and disruptive behavior. The condition creates special problems at school, where learning requires sitting still, listening carefully, organizing tasks, and taking turns. The problems of children with ADHD are serious, ones that make life difficult for parents and teachers as well as the child. The symptoms can last through adulthood and make success in advanced schooling, jobs, and relationships difficult.

Ritalin is the brand name for a prescription stimulant made by Novartis used to treat ADHD. The drug comes in a variety of forms with other names, generic versions, and slow-release forms (e.g., Concerta). Other amphetamine drugs such as Dexedrine and Adderall also treat the condition. The stimulants affect underactive parts of the brain needed for concentration and goal-directed activities. Although many disagree, reports generally suggest that Ritalin and similar drugs moderate symptoms of ADHD. The drug has certainly grown in popularity. For example, from 1987 to 1999, the daily consumption of methylphenidate, the active ingredient in Ritalin, rose from about 50 million doses per day to more than 350 million. In 2004, about 2.5 million children were taking prescription drugs for ADHD, with levels reaching about 10 percent of all 10-year-old boys.

Critics of Ritalin and other stimulants say that overdiagnosis and overprescription results from the broad form of the symptoms. Many symptoms such as restlessness and impulsiveness characterize most children but moderate or disappear with age. Some children—boys in particular—show more extreme levels of these symptoms than others do, but it can be hard to say when the symptoms produce a condition that needs treatment by drugs. Even gifted children bored by normal activities exhibit symptoms of ADHD. The difficulties in diagnosis of the condition can result in widely varying rates of prescription. Reports from England show that prescription rates were 23 times higher in some areas than others. In one area, there were 14.4 prescriptions per 100 children under age 15—well above the average of 4.3 prescriptions per 100 children.[46] Such differences likely reflect the varied interpretations of the criteria for diagnosing ADHD rather than differences in behavior.

Given difficulties in diagnosis, some psychiatrists reject claims that ADHD is really a biological problem in the brain. They believe that behavior problems may result instead from poor diet and sleep, vision and hearing problems, or lack of discipline at home. Treating the behaviors with drugs replaces efforts to identify the social or physical sources of the problem. Counseling, behavior change, and parenting classes for the children and their parents may work better. Studies suggest that allowing children more play time in parks and recreation areas, activities that provide an outlet for their energy and desires for movement, reduces ADHD. Less time spent watching television may help as well. Other ways exist to improve the environment for children with ADHD without resorting to drugs.

Even when effective in controlling behavior, Ritalin and other stimulants have side effects common with use of amphetamines. These include nervousness, insomnia, and perhaps some more long-term problems such as dependency, slowed growth, or depression. Critics sometimes note the similarity between cocaine and the active chemical ingredient in Ritalin, methylphenidate. Both stimulate the dopamine system of the brain, but cocaine does so quickly and methylphenidate does so slowly. The similarities show in the abuse of Ritalin for its pleasure-inducing qualities.

Although experts recommend a full clinical evaluation to diagnose ADHD, that does not always occur. Indeed, the advertising of drugs for ADHD in magazines for parents suggests that it can make caring for children easier. According to a 2001 story from *Time* magazine,

> *In one ad, drug maker Celltech shows a smiling boy and his mom with the message: "One dose covers his ADHD for the whole school day," plus the drug's name, Metadate CD. The ad is running in a dozen magazines, including* Ladies' Home Journal, *which has two more ADHD drug ads in the same issue—from Shire Pharmaceuticals (maker of Adderall) and McNeil Consumer HealthCare (Concerta). These ads do not name any medications, but they do give toll-free numbers for more information. McNeil also has a similar ad on cable TV.[47]*

Prescription Drugs

The pharmaceutical industry defends the ads as valuable information for parents about risks of a serious medical problem among some children. Others say, however, that they encourage parents to ask for drug prescriptions when unnecessary. In support of the critics, the FDA sent five warning letters to drug companies on September 25, 2008, about false, misleading, or incomplete promotional materials.

Parents of children with ADHD vigorously defend use of the drugs and dispute claims of overuse. One organization, Children and Adults with Attention Deficit/Hyperactivity Disorder (CHADD), views the disorder as a serious disability (in some cases serious enough to warrant disability benefits from the government) that is treatable with prescription drugs. They advocate greater awareness of the problem and better treatment with all suitable methods, including Ritalin and similar drugs.

SSRIs. Selective serotonin reuptake inhibitors (SSRIs) are a class of prescription drugs used for treatment of depression, anxiety disorders, and other problems such as insomnia. Prozac was the first and is still perhaps the most famous SSRI, while other popular forms include Zoloft, Paxil, and Cymbalta. A related class of nonselective serotonin reuptake inhibitors also treats depression. Antidepressant SSRIs have become one of the most commonly prescribed drugs in the United States. From 1995 to 2002, prescriptions of the drugs rose by 48 percent. Of the 2.4 billion drugs prescribed in 2005, 118 million were antidepressants. The increase in usage has even occurred among kids, including some under age six. Some HMOs recommend therapy for patients with depression only after attempts to first deal with the problem through SSRIs have failed.

Are these prescription rates justified? One 1997 study of 1,080 patients found that 56 percent of those taking SSRIs did not have the conditions for which the FDA had approved the drugs.[48] While studies show that people with clinical depression and some forms of anxiety disorders benefit from SSRIs, many take the drugs for problems with sexual performance, timidity, eating disorders, low self-esteem, irritability, stress, and a host of problems people face in daily life. People want to believe that the pills can make them happier, but the evidence for the benefits of SSRIs are limited to a few specific conditions. Few studies examine the effects, beneficial or harmful, of SSRIs on generally healthy people. The brain chemistry of people with mild or usual problems may differ enough from those with clinical depression that SSRIs have little benefit. Even so, the tendency to prescribe the drugs to large parts of the population for a variety of difficulties can lead to overuse.

Drug companies encourage the widespread use of SSRIs. The money spent on ads is huge. For example, GlaxoSmithKline spent $91.8 million in advertising its SSRI Paxil in 2000. The ads typically mention conditions that affect large parts of the population, though only mildly, such as the blues, anxiety, and premenstrual disorders. Some ads say that the SSRIs correct a chemical imbalance in the brain that causes depression and other conditions. Scientists admit they have a limited understanding of the physiological sources of depression and that ads about the SSRIs oversimplify, perhaps in a misleading way, the causes of mental problems.

For serious and mild problems alike, the reliance on SSRIs may do harm as well as good. One harmful result is that people come to rely on a pill rather than using therapy to help deal with problems or changing their ways of living to make life more satisfying. Along with deterring people from doing more to help themselves, the drugs have side effects. There are claims, although disputed, that SSRIs induce suicidal thoughts and actions, especially among the young. In 2004, the New York attorney general Eliot Spitzer sued the maker of Paxil, GlaxoSmithKline, for fraud in concealing the dangers of the drug for children under age 17. The suit was settled when the company agreed to publish all its results. Another claim, also disputed, is that the drugs lead to violence and murder among some users. A list of less serious side effects includes problems with sleep, weight, and nausea. Many also say that going off some SSRIs causes uncomfortable withdrawal symptoms.

Of course, a key source of the popularity of SSRIs is that people like them. Many say the drugs make their life better. One famous 1993 book by the psychiatrist Peter Kramer, *Listening to Prozac*, says the drugs can make people feel better than well. If large parts of the population without clinical depression can cope better with life by taking the drugs, then the makers and prescribers are doing a real service for the mental health of Americans. Yet, others say the benefits are widely overstated, the side effects are minimized, and the huge number of prescriptions shows overuse.

Drugs for an Overactive Bladder. Overactive bladder is defined as a condition that leads to a sudden and intense urge to urinate. Although not life threatening, it can be embarrassing and limit activities. The need to drop everything to go to the bathroom is disrupting, as is having to wake up several times at night to urinate. The problem stems from the involuntary contraction of the muscles of the bladder. The causes of this involuntary contraction are varied and often unclear, but it occurs more often among older persons. Figures suggest that overactive bladder affects 15 to 20 million people in the United States, and about one in four women and one in 10 men aged 65 and over. Although the condition becomes more common in old age, older persons should not consider it a normal part of aging. Visits to a urologist who specializes in urinary diseases can lead to several tests to diagnose the problem and treatment.

The treatment can involve a variety of changes in behavior, including exercise, weight control, and diet, but increasingly medications are used to relieve the symptoms. Prescription drugs for the condition include Ditropan,

Prescription Drugs

Detrol, Sanctura, Vesicare, and Enablex. A test of these drugs by *Consumer Reports* found that they are only modestly effective and have unpleasant side effects such as dry mouth, constipation, and mental confusion.[49] Another heavily advertised drug called Flomax improves urination among men with benign prostatic hyperplasia (an enlargement of the prostate that commonly occurs among older men).

The widespread popularity of these drugs reflects recent changes in public and medical views. In the past, the need for more frequent urination as one grew older was regarded as part of the aging process. While perhaps annoying, the problem did not create serious medical or health concerns. Avoiding caffeine, drinking liquid in moderation, and using the bathroom regularly could help deal with one of the outcomes of growing old. Only the worst cases of incontinence or accidental urination among adults required treatment. The change toward acceptance of overactive bladder as a disease that warrants treatment, usually by prescription drugs, occurred only since the late 1990s.

What led to the change? According to the journalist Melody Peterson, a marketing campaign by the drug manufacturer Pharmacia for its drug Detrol played a major role.[50] Approved as a drug for treating incontinence, Detrol greatly helped persons subject to accidentally wetting their pants. The company saw that the market of incontinent adults was a small one, however. To become more profitable, the drug needed to be used by a larger segment of the population. Pharmacia (later purchased by Pfizer) developed a plan to market the drug for a condition they called overactive bladder. Peterson notes that Pharmacia hired physicians to help define the new disease and held conferences to acquaint other doctors with it. The company also needed to convince the public that going to the bathroom often involved something more than an annoyance and required medical treatment. Magazine and newspaper articles, brochures, and television ads warned consumers about the condition and encouraged them to talk to their doctors about getting help. The Olympic gold medalist in gymnastics Mary Lou Retton became a spokesperson for Detrol. Following these efforts, both prescriptions for Detrol and profits for the company grew. In essence, the company identified or created a new disease of overactive bladder. Other companies also came to offer similar products.

Increasing treatments in recent years for overactive bladder raise questions about overuse. On one hand, drug manufacturers say that the need for the drug always existed, but people did not know of treatments to help deal with their urination problems. Advertising served the purpose of informing people of the condition and ways to deal with it. On the other hand, advertising may create a need where none existed before. According to critics, the treatment does much to increase the profits of drug companies but less to help patients. The drugs may have modest benefits, but widespread use has drawbacks as well. They have unpleasant side effects and direct people away from making changes in their behavior and lifestyle to deal with the problem. Demand for drugs to treat overactive bladder may stem more from drug company advertising and marketing than real need.

Drugs for Fibromyalgia. Fibromyalgia is a disorder characterized by widespread chronic pain, extreme sensitivity to touch, and a variety of other symptoms. Patients diagnosed with the disease say it is extremely debilitating. However, it has come under scrutiny as a diagnosis. The diagnosis depends fully on reports of patients and has no objective test or imaging technique to confirm the diagnosis. The disease has no known cause, although some evidence suggests it stems from an abnormality in the central nervous system. The symptoms overlap with those of many other diseases and occur commonly among people with a history of mental illness, economic disadvantage, and high stress. The symptoms of fibromyalgia may relate to psychological and social problems rather than a physical disease, although many disagree with this assessment.

The controversy over the disease stems in good part from efforts of drug companies to promote the medications they make for the disease. The FDA has approved two drugs, Lyrica and Cymbalta, for treatment of fibromyalgia, and companies aim to help those with this neglected health problem by creating awareness of the disease through advertising and marketing. The drugmakers point out that the American Society of Rheumatology recognizes the disease and that patients with the painful symptoms suffer greatly. Their efforts help inform people of the disease, treat it with effective drugs, and reduce the pain many face.

The efforts of the companies have been both expensive and successful. First, extensive DTC advertising has publicized the disease and treatment by drugs. According to a report from the Associated Press, "Eli Lilly spent roughly $128.4 million in the first three quarters of 2008 on ads to promote Cymbalta, according to TNS Media Intelligence. Pfizer Inc. spent more than $125 million advertising Lyrica."[51] In addition, the Associated Press found that the two drugmakers contributed more than $6 million in the first three quarters of 2008 to nonprofit groups for medical conferences and education campaigns that publicize the disease and its treatment. The efforts seem to have paid off. Over the period from early 2007 to late 2008, sales rose for Cymbalta from $442 million to $721 million and for Lyrica from $395 million to $702 million.

Critics say that these two drugs are casebook examples of overuse. Advertising, more than demand from patients and physicians, led to the growing diagnosis of the disease and increasing use of drugs to treat it. The drug companies are creating awareness of a disease that may not even exist. In promoting drug treatment, they may direct people away from treatments for other diseases and changes in ways of living that could do more to help.

Others disagree with these conclusions but also recognize that promoting the disease and drug treatment raises profits and perhaps leads to overuse.

Antibiotics. The history of antibiotics is one of remarkable success in saving lives. Penicillin, although discovered earlier, began to be manufactured for sale as a drug in 1942. Tetracycline followed in 1955 and amoxicillin in 1981. These, other variants developed over the years, and some new recent classes of antibiotics treat bacterial infections by killing the bacteria or preventing them from multiplying. In the process, they save lives and speed recovery. Except for some products sold for external use, antibiotics require a prescription.

However, widespread use of antibiotics leads to bacterial resistance. After 50 years of use, many antibiotics do not appear to work as well as they once did. Although antibiotics kill most bacteria, those with mutations that protect them from antibiotics tend to spread. The Centers for Disease Control and Prevention (CDC) call antibiotic resistance one of the world's most pressing problems. Antibiotic resistance can be seen in the greater difficulty in recent years of treating bacterial diseases such as tuberculosis, malaria, gonorrhea, and childhood ear infections. It also shows in problems that hospitals have in controlling the spread of staph infections. According to statistics from the CDC, nearly 2 million patients in the United States get an infection each year while in the hospital, and about 90,000 of them die. About 70 percent of these infections are resistant to antibiotics. Patients with these infections must stay longer, must use more expensive and less effective drugs, and risk spreading their infection to others.[52]

Overuse of antibiotics comes from the desire to treat colds and other illnesses caused by viruses rather than bacteria. Unlike bacteria, viruses do not respond to antibiotics. Yet the symptoms of bacterial and viral infections are similar enough that patients often want antibiotics for both. For example, a study from Harvard University reports that more than a million children a year unnecessarily receive antibiotics for sore throats.[53] While 15 to 36 percent of children with sore throats have a bacterial streptococcal infection that antibiotics can treat, 54 percent of the children studied received an antibiotic. Other studies report similar overuse among adults for sinus infections. Although only a small portion of sinus infections result from bacteria, most patients visiting physicians for the problem get a prescription for an antibiotic.

In this instance, the motivation for drug use does not come, as in the other examples, from drug company ads or marketing. Rather, patients often demand antibiotics in the unlikely hope that it will have some benefit, and physicians often give the prescription. Parents worried about their children, in particular, may pressure their doctors to do something, and physicians may find it easier to reassure patients and parents with a prescription even if it likely will not help. Giving a prescription may make things easier in the short run, but in the long run, such overuse makes the antibiotics less effective.

THE CASE FOR HIGH USE OF PRESCRIPTION DRUGS

Makers of prescription drugs, the physicians who prescribe the drugs, and the patients who take them generally disagree with claims of overuse. They say that the drugs are helpful—what others call overuse actually means the drugs get to a wider part of the population that needs them. The problem of underuse, of people not knowing that drugs can help treat their health problems, creates consequences that are more serious.

Drugmakers argue that they have a right to present balanced information about their medicines to prescribers and patients. Given the FDA approval process and evaluations of effectiveness, the drugs the companies sell help people live longer, recover faster, and enjoy life more. Rather than misleading people, DTC ads for prescription drugs inform the public, increase knowledge of effective medical care, and allow patients to participate in their own treatment. Consumers of prescription drugs, like consumers of medical products, have the right to know about drugs that may help them. This is particularly so given a trend in doctor-patient relationships. Rather than viewing themselves as subject to doctor's orders, patients now desire an active role in their treatment and partnerships with doctors.

Patients who use the drugs must see some benefit from them. Drugs for childhood behavior problems, depression, and overactive bladders have costs as well as benefits, but patients along with their doctors can weigh both in making treatment decisions. The widespread popularity of prescription drugs for these conditions suggests patient satisfaction. Those who find that the drugs bring little benefit or have excessive side effects can—with their doctor's approval—stop taking them. Otherwise, defenders of widespread use can point to consumers for evidence of the value of popular prescription drugs.

In any case, physicians prescribing the drugs serve as a check on excessive consumer demands for prescription drugs. They best know the medical problems and history of the patients, the kinds of treatments they need, and the drugs that may work best. That the rising use of drugs has occurred through the treatment decisions of physicians gives some legitimacy to claims of the benefits of widespread prescription drug use.

DANGERS OF PRESCRIPTION DRUG USE

The possible overuse of many prescription drugs relates to other sets of concerns. Greater use increases dangers from side effects, errors in giving and taking the drugs, and risks of abuse for nonmedical purposes. These dangers stem from a variety of actions. Side effects are the undesired consequences of the proper usage of medications, whereas other kinds of harm result from improper use of medications. Sometimes doctors make mistakes in giving prescriptions, pharmacists make mistakes in filling them, and patients make mistakes in taking them. In these cases, the dangers are unintentional. In other cases, people intentionally take drugs improperly to get high or try to treat themselves.

SIDE EFFECTS

All prescription drugs have side effects, but in most cases the benefits outweigh unintended harm. While common, most side effects are not serious. Drugs to moderate the symptoms of allergies can make users sleepy; drugs to lower cholesterol can cause muscle pain and weakness; SSRI drugs to reduce depression can cause weight gain and decreased sex drive; and ACE inhibitors for high blood pressure can cause a dry cough. Consequently, prescription drugs come with detailed warning information about possible side effects, and physicians and pharmacists warn patients about possible problems. Even DTC ads briefly review common side effects. Patients experiencing more than mild side effects should discuss problems with the prescribing physician. Problems can lead to changes in dose, use of other prescription drugs, or other means of treatment.

Still, the use of prescription drugs has become so widespread that even rare side effects can affect thousands, even millions of people. The FDA operates the Adverse Event Reporting System to gather reports from patients and physicians of adverse reactions to prescription drugs. The numbers are high and getting worse. From 1998 to 2005, reports of adverse reactions increased from 34,996 per year to 89,842 per year.[54] Fatal adverse events rose during the same period from 5,519 to 15,107. The numbers of non-reported adverse reactions no doubt is even higher. According to the *Los Angeles Times*, "Studies have estimated that from as little as 3% of adverse events to a maximum of about 33% have been reported to the FDA."[55] Some of the increase comes from people taking more prescriptions, and some comes from people's greater willingness to report drug problems. More worrisome is the increase due to the greater side effects of some new drugs.

According to the FDA reports, painkillers are the most commonly reported cause of adverse reactions. The five drugs causing the most adverse reactions include oxycodone, fentanyl, morphine, acetaminophen, and methadone—all painkillers. The sixth most common cause of adverse reactions, clozapine is an antipsychosis drug. Other drugs reported to the FDA for adverse reactions include estrogens, insulin, paroxetine (the active ingredient in the antidepressant Paxil), interferon beta to treat multiple sclerosis and cancer, and the anticlotting agent warfarin.

For the first three months of 2008, the trend toward higher reporting has continued. According to an article from the Associated Press, "The Food and Drug Administration received nearly 21,000 reports of serious drug reactions, including more than 4,800 deaths."[56] Two drugs accounted for a large share of the recent reports. Heparin, a blood thinner that was contaminated during manufacturing in China, caused many adverse reactions. Chantix, a drug used to ease withdrawal symptoms of those who quit smoking, has led to reports of psychiatric problems.

How does the FDA use these reports of adverse events? The goal is to identify safety concerns for products it has already approved and alert the public. After all, clinical studies may not last long enough or have a large enough sample of cases to identify rare but major side effects. Safety procedures need to include vigilance after approval. Then, if products already approved later turn out to have more extensive and serious side effects than originally thought, the FDA can reevaluate the drug. In recent years, the agency has increased efforts to communicate safety information to the public through adding warnings to labeling information and issuing health alerts. In some cases, the FDA may restrict or ban use of a drug.

For example, the reporting system led the FDA in September 2008 to name 20 prescription drugs under investigation for safety problems. The agency publishes the list to inform health care providers and patients at an early stage about possible risks from the drugs. Officials advise doctors to keep giving and patients to keep taking the medicines but to be aware that the FDA is taking a closer look. According to the list,

- Cymbalta for depression may lead to urinary retention,
- Intelence for HIV may lead to bleeding into joints,
- Suprane for anesthesia may cause the heart to stop beating,
- Tykerb for advanced breast cancer may cause liver damage,
- Tyzeka for chronic hepatitis may lead to nerve damage,
- Heparin for thinning the blood may lead to serious allergic reactions,
- Tysabri for multiple sclerosis may lead to skin melanoma, and
- Tumor necrosis factor (TNF) blockers for juvenile arthritis may lead to cancers in children and young adults.[57]

The evidence of harm is not yet serious enough to ban the products, but it is serious enough to publicize the concerns.

Critics of the FDA say the problem is much worse than claimed. The journalist Stephen Fried, who investigated the extent of serious side effects in his book *Bitter Pills*, says that in the United States alone between 45,000 and 200,000 people die annually of reactions to legal drugs.[58] That number represents 2 to 9 percent of the 2.3 million Americans who die each year. By comparison, 5,000 to 10,000 die from illegal drug use. A study of hospital patients published in *JAMA* affirms the extent of the problem. It estimated that 106,000 died in 1994 from adverse drug reactions, making these reactions the fourth to sixth leading cause of death.[59] Greater use of drugs since 1994 likely has increased this number substantially.

Taking a more active role in investigating the possible side effects of medications can help reduce the problem. Stephen Fried offers advice based on personal experience. His wife suffered devastating side effects of seizures, delirium, insomnia, and later manic-depressive illness triggered by an antibiotic Floxin that she took for a urinary tract infection. He says prescription drug users must read packaged inserts more carefully. Although written for doctors and lawyers and sometimes hard to understand, these inserts contain important information. They identify precautions, warnings, and contraindications (or conditions the drug should not be used to treat). Black-box warnings, usually placed at the top of the inserts and surrounded by a black box to highlight their importance, can be especially important. The section on drug interactions lists other medications that cause problems when combined with the new medication. Although the detail of information is daunting, it is also essential for users.

Fried also recommends that patients engage in a more thorough discussion of drugs with physicians to minimize the potential harm from side effects. The doctor should know of all other medications being taken, and the patient should know the proper dose and possible adverse reactions of drugs being prescribed. Both should have the goal of taking the fewest medications at the lowest doses needed to deal with the problem. Pharmacists can help as well with advice about medications. Other writers such as Dr. Marcia Angell suggest asking doctors several direct questions: Is the drug better than older and cheaper alternatives? Can the drug be given effectively at a lower dose? Are the benefits worth the side effects? Although the questions sound confrontational, the answers can provide crucial information. Information obtained from physicians will be more reliable than information obtained from DTC ads.

DRUGS WITH DANGEROUS SIDE EFFECTS

Several drugs marketed since the late 1990s have had such serious side effects that companies and the FDA have removed them from the market or recommended restricting their use. A report from the PBS television show *Frontline* lists 12 drugs withdrawn between 1997 and 2001,[60] and several other high-profile withdrawals because of dangerous side effects have occurred since 2001—almost always because of lawsuits from persons claiming harm by them. Indeed, some highly publicized health damage led to new scrutiny of prescription drugs by Congress and the FDA since about 2004. Some of the high-profile examples include Vioxx, hormone replacement therapy drugs, fen-phen, Baycol, and Rezulin.

Vioxx. Merck received approval from the FDA on May 20, 1999, to market its anti-inflammation drug Vioxx for treatment of osteoarthritis and some other conditions causing acute pain. Vioxx, along with Celebrex, a drug made by Pfizer and approved by the FDA in December 1998, is part of a class of drugs called selective Cox-2 inhibitors. These drugs inhibit the body's production of enzymes that promote arthritis inflammation. The drug proved effective and highly successful. At one time, 80 million patients worldwide used the drug.

Controversy began with a study on Vioxx published in the *New England Journal of Medicine* in 2000.[61] The study found that patients taking Vioxx had four times as many heart attacks over 12 months as patients taking Aleve, an OTC pain reliever. It attributed the differences to the benefits of Aleve rather than the harm of Vioxx, but others viewed the results with more concern. In April 2002, the FDA changed the warning labels on Vioxx to highlight increased risk of heart problems. The next month, a woman sued Merck, claiming that Vioxx caused the fatal heart attack of her husband at age 59.

In 2004, Merck reported on another study showing that Vioxx doubled the risk of a heart attack or stroke over a period of 18 months. Combined with the earlier studies, these results led Merck to voluntarily remove the drug from the market. Pfizer also withdrew a similar drug, Bextra. The next year, an editorial in the *New England Journal of Medicine*, which published the earlier article on Vioxx, accused the study authors of not reporting all the instances of heart attacks among Vioxx patients. The additional evidence would have raised greater concerns about the drug early on, prevented its widespread use, and avoided some of its dangerous side effects. Another article in the British medical journal *The Lancet* said the company should have withdrawn the drug many years earlier. In the end, Vioxx likely caused 88,000 to 139,000 heart attacks during its five years on the market, with about 30 to 40 percent of the heart attacks causing death.

The suit against Vioxx brought in 2002 went to trial in 2005, and the jury awarded the plaintiff, the widow of a man who died of a heart attack while using Vioxx, $253.4 million in damages. Merck won an appeal, but by March 2006 it faced more than 10,000 individual suits and 190 class-action suits. Despite success in fending off many that went to trial, the enormity of the legal actions led Merck to reach a settlement. The company has set aside $4.58 billion for payments to those who have enrolled in the settlement program. The settlement amounts range from a minimum of $5,000 to several million for those most harmed by the drug.

Hormone Replacement Therapy. Several drugs prescribed to women going through menopause help moderate uncomfortable symptoms such as hot flashes by raising the levels of estrogen and progesterone in the body. For decades, many experts recommended the therapy, and several studies suggested (incorrectly it turns out) that the hormone replacement also reduced the risks of heart disease, osteoporosis, and other health problems commonly experienced by older women. According to advocates, the drugs not only made women feel better but could also lengthen their lives. By 2002, up to 6 million postmenopausal women were taking hormone replacement drugs such as Premarin and Prempro.

Beginning in 1992, new and better research began to reverse opinion on the safety of hormone replacement therapy. One randomized clinical trial called the Women's Health Initiative followed about 67,000 women age 50 to 79 over five years. The study concluded that those taking a combination of estrogen and progesterone experienced significantly more breast cancer, heart disease, stroke, blood clots, and Alzheimer's disease than those getting a placebo. After other studies replicated these results, the FDA in 2003 required Wyeth, the maker of Prempro, to add a new warning to its hormone replacement drug:

> *Estrogens with or without progestins should not be used for the prevention of cardiovascular disease. The Women's Health Initiative (WHI) study reported increased risks of myocardial infarction, stroke, invasive breast cancer, pulmonary emboli, and deep vein thrombosis in postmenopausal women (50 to 79 years of age) during 5 years of treatment with oral conjugated estrogens (0.625 mg) combined with medroxyprogesterone acetate (2.5 mg) relative to placebo.[62]*

These and warnings for other drugs such as Premarin greatly reduced their use.

Since 2002, users and their families have filed thousands of lawsuits against Wyeth for harm done by Prempro and Premarin. In one Nevada case, three women claimed that taking Prempro led to breast cancer. A jury awarded the victims $134 million, believing that the company knew its product could cause breast cancer but manipulated studies to minimize the apparent risk. In February 2008, the judge reduced the damages to $58 million—$23 million to compensate the women and $35 million for punitive damages. This makes it the largest award to date against the drug.

Referred to now as hormone treatment rather than hormone replacement therapy, use of estrogens is still prescribed for symptoms of menopause—though much less routinely than in the past. Recommendations from the Mayo Clinic, for example, suggest use of estrogen-based drugs for short-term relief of unpleasant symptoms of menopause.[63] For longer-term use, they note that the risks of heart disease, cancer, strokes, and blood clots increase by a small amount. The clinic thus recommends discussion of risks and benefits with physicians and suggests ways for some women to take the medicine with minimal risks.

Fen-phen and Redux. Fen-phen is the name for a combination of two drugs, fenfluramine and phentermine, that became popular for weight control in the early 1990s. Fenfluramine (under the brand name Pondimin) stimulates the body to release chemicals that give users a sense of being full, while phentermine (under several brand names) is a stimulant that helps counteract feelings of drowsiness that come from fenfluramine. Each drug is sold separately but can be combined for weight loss and control. Redux is the brand name of a drug made by American Home Products that is a newer version of fenfluramine. After some contentious debate, the FDA approved Redux in 1996. It had separately approved fenfluramine and phentermine for weight control but not in combination.

The use of fen-phen and Redux grew quickly.[64] *Time* magazine had a cover story on Redux, calling it a miracle drug that really works. According to the story, three months after introduction of Redux, physicians were writing 85,000 prescriptions a week. By 1996, the number of prescriptions reached an estimated 18 million for fen-phen and Redux. A $52 million marketing campaign for Redux contributed to its popularity, and sales for American Home Products reached $300 million with projections of $1 billion in sales.

Some experts warned early on about the side effects of these drugs, but in 1997 the evidence become stronger. As summarized by *Frontline*, an article in the *New England Journal of Medicine* reported that 24 patients taking fen-phen had an unusual form of heart disease that caused abnormalities in the heart valves.[65] After 75 more reports to the FDA of heart-valve disease among fen-phen patients, American Home Products voluntarily removed Pondimin and Redux from the market. The FDA recommended that patients taking the drugs see their doctors about possible evaluation for heart problems. Suits for the damage caused by the drugs followed, with reports that American Home Products (which changed its name to Wyeth in 2002) had paid out $13 billion in claims by 2003.

Baycol. Although many cholesterol-lowering statin drugs remain on the market, one caused severe enough side effects to be withdrawn. Baycol, a statin made by Bayer, received approval from the FDA in 1997. The drug cost less than competitors but, particularly when taken at high doses, had a serious albeit rare side effect. Reports accumulated that patients taking the drug developed rhabdomyolysis, a disease that destroys muscle tissue and can lead to renal failure and death. On August 8, 2001, Bayer withdrew its product from the market after analysis of new data showed that 31 patients taking the drug had died from rhabdomyolysis. According to reports from the company, more than 10,000 Baycol suits had been filed, and it had paid out nearly $1.2 billion in damages by April 2005. Other statin drugs still on the market do not cause the problems to the same extent, but patients must stay aware of possible side effects and undergo regular checkups.

Rezulin. A drug to control diabetes, Rezulin received approval from the FDA only after some controversy. One FDA scientist opposed approval because of the harm it did to the liver and heart in animal studies. However, the FDA approved the drug for sale in January 1997 without any requirements for tests of the drug's effect on the liver. By the end of the year, however, the FDA changed the drug's label because use of Rezulin led to liver failure. The FDA now recommended that patients taking the drug undergo regular liver enzyme tests to identify any problems. Those with elevated liver enzymes should stop taking the drug.

Beginning in 1998, reports of death and serious damage to the liver from Rezulin began to accumulate. A study of diabetes patients sponsored by the National Institutes of Health dropped the drug after one subject died from liver failure. After receiving reports of more deaths from liver failure of patients using Rezulin, the FDA more thoroughly investigated the problem. A report concluded that hundreds of Rezulin patients died from liver failure, and the FDA withdrew the drug from the market in March 2000. The maker of Rezulin, Warner-Lambert, had $2.1 billion in sales before the FDA prohibited the drug.

Pfizer, the current owner of Warner-Lambert, has faced numerous lawsuits over Rezulin. By 2003, the number of suits reached 8,700, and another 32,000 possible victims had given notice that they may sue. A 2008 Supreme Court decision, *Warner-Lambert v. Kimberly Kent,* allowed a Michigan class action suit against Pfizer over Rezulin to go forward.

ERRORS PRESCRIBING AND TAKING MEDICATIONS

By some counts, 1.5 million Americans are harmed each year by medication errors. These errors involve use of drugs of proven safety that are given or taken improperly. For example, the newborn twins of the actor Dennis Quaid nearly died in 2007 when they received adult rather than infant doses of a blood-thinning drug from hospital staff. According to reports in 2005, two patients died when they mistakenly received the Alzheimer's drug Reminyl instead of the similar-sounding diabetes drug Amaryl. Contamination of drugs during manufacturing, such as occurred in 2008 during the production in China of ingredients for the drug Heparin, can also cause severe reactions and sometimes even death.

Introduction to Prescription Drugs

Errors by patients in taking prescription drugs also contribute to the problem. Some reports suggest that half of all prescriptions are taken incorrectly. The complexities of treatment regimens often lead to mistakes such as taking the wrong dose. Or, when patients do not fully inform doctors about other drugs they take or conditions they have, they may end up getting drugs that can harm them.

According to a study in the *Archives of Internal Medicine,* deaths from errors in taking prescription drugs soared by 360.5 percent between 1983 and 2004.[66] Part of the problem came from mixing prescription drugs. For example, the actor Heath Ledger died from taking a lethal combination of prescription drugs, including painkillers, sleeping medications, and anti-anxiety drugs. These kinds of deaths rose by 555 percent during the period. Even worse, deaths from medications mixed with street drugs or alcohol rose by 3,196 percent. As a result, 12,426 deaths occurred in 2004 from all types of prescription errors.

Another example of the dangerous consequences of taking prescription drugs inappropriately has received much attention. Michael Jackson, who had in the past developed an addiction to painkillers, died on June 25, 2009, from taking a drug called propofol plus other sedatives to help him sleep. This dangerous drug should only be taken by a patient undergoing anesthesia in a hospital, under continuous monitoring. The coroner ruled the death a homicide, and Jackson's personal physician, Conrad Murray, has been charged with manslaughter for providing and giving the drug.

The Institute of Medicine recently provided new evidence of the extent of prescription errors. Responding to a new requirement passed as part of the Medicare Modernization Act of 2003, the institute brought together a panel of experts to investigate prescription drug errors in hospitals. Their report said that medication errors harm 1.5 million people each year and increase medical care costs by $3.5 billion.[67] The 1.5 million translates into one patient per hospital per day. The errors include writing prescriptions for drugs that interact in harmful ways with other drugs the patient takes, using the wrong dose, forgetting to take or give medications, and taking or giving the wrong medication. Sometimes patients make the mistakes, sometimes the nurses and doctors. In one example included in the report, a 39-year-old woman died when mistakenly given a high dose of a chemotherapy agent.

The report makes several suggestions for reducing prescription drug errors. Health care providers need to do more to inform patients about the proper way to take the drugs and avoid mistakes. Patients in turn should inform providers of other drugs they take, ask questions about possible problems with the drugs, and make sure they follow directions properly. The stronger the partnership between doctor and patient, the greater the likelihood of proper prescription drug use. Also, the FDA and drugmakers can do more to make the labeling and instruction information clearer and easier to follow. Hospitals can improve by requiring that prescriptions be submitted electronically so that nurses and health care workers can check with a standardized bar-code system to make sure they administer the drugs properly. Electronic prescriptions also help pharmacists filling the prescriptions. By some counts, about 15 percent of prescription errors result from bad handwriting.

Another problem results from the simple fact that many drugs have similar-sounding names. For example, Aciphex for stomach reflux sounds like Aricept for memory problems. The painkiller Celebrex sounds like the antidepressant Celexa, and the blood-clotting drug Amicar sounds like the cholesterol pill Omacor (now renamed Lovaza to reduce confusion). The FDA rejects more than one-third of proposed names for new drugs because they sound too much like existing ones, but manufacturers can do more to protect against confusion when they name their products.

Another source of error comes in manufacturing rather than dispensing and taking prescription drugs. A flu vaccine manufactured by Chiron in a German plant was found to be contaminated by bacteria in 2005. Hormone replacement drugs manufactured by Wyeth in a plant in Puerto Rico lacked quality controls and checks according to the FDA in 2006. And the blood thinner Heparin manufactured by Baxter in a plant in China contained chemicals that killed 81 people in the United States. The Heparin case in particular led to criticisms of the FDA for lack of controls over foreign manufacturing of prescription drugs. Congress has called for increases in the budget that would allow the government to inspect manufacturing plants more carefully.

ABUSE OF PRESCRIPTION DRUGS

Harm caused by prescription drugs from side effects and errors are unintentional. Another set of dangers involves the intentional misuse or abuse of prescription drugs. Prescription drug abuse refers to the illegitimate use of medications in ways not intended by the prescribing doctor. It ranges from taking mediations prescribed for someone else to using pills to get high. The motives range from the desire for self-treatment to an addictive or unhealthy dependence on the medications.

According to the Office of National Drug Control Policy, the abuse of prescription drugs—largely painkillers—ranks second to marijuana use among the nation's most prevalent drug problem. It ranks as more serious than the use of cocaine, heroine, and methamphetamine. The National Institute on Drug Abuse further highlights the problem:

Most people take prescription medications responsibly; however, an estimated 48 million people (ages 12 and older) have used prescription drugs for non-

medical reasons in their lifetimes. This represents approximately 20 percent of the U.S. population.[68]

The most commonly abused prescription drugs are opioids and opiates such as oxycodone and morphine, central nervous system depressants such as barbiturates and benzodiazepines, and stimulants such as dextroamphetamine and methylphenidate. Brand-name painkillers such as Vicodin and OxyContin, depressants such as Valium and Xanax, and stimulants such as Ritalin and Dexedrine are commonly abused (as are some OTC cough remedies). Although helpful and safe when used appropriately, these drugs can cause serious harm when taken in unapproved ways.

Opioids refer to a family of effective painkillers that come from opium products or are derived synthetically. The synthetic products can be taken orally or crushed into a powder for quicker release as a way to get high. Along with blocking pain, these drugs temporarily induce a sense of pleasure and well-being. When taken regularly, the drugs also result in painful withdrawal symptoms. Central nervous system depressants are taken orally and depress brain activity to give a drowsy or calming effect. If taken for prolonged periods, they also result in dependence and painful withdrawal symptoms. Stimulants increase alertness, attention, and energy and can induce a sense of euphoria. Once used commonly for a variety of disorders, stimulants are now prescribed mostly for ADHD, narcolepsy, and some forms of depression. Overuse results in dependence and can also lead to a dangerous irregular heartbeat, seizures, and paranoia.

The problem of prescription drug abuse has become serious among teens. In a survey of 12th graders in 2008, 9.7 percent reported using Vicodin and 4.7 percent reported using OxyContin over the past year.[69] A survey of youths ages 12 to 17 in 2005 and 2006 also indicates the extent of the problem.[70] Three percent of teens reported abusing prescription drugs (compared to 7 percent for marijuana and 0.4 percent for cocaine). With increasing use of prescription drugs by adults and the sale of prescription drugs through online pharmacies, teens find it easier to access drugs than in the past. Many obtain the drugs from parents' medicine cabinets or trade their own prescription pills for those of friends and acquaintances.

Adult abuse of prescription drugs occurs as well. Of the estimated 4.7 million who used painkillers, tranquilizers, sedatives, and stimulants for nonmedical purposes in 2002, 56 percent were ages 18 and over.[71] Many young adults use the drugs for recreation, but others aim to treat themselves medically with prescription drugs. According to the *New York Times*,

> *For a sizable group of people in their 20's and 30's, deciding on their own what drugs to take—in particular, stimulants, antidepressants and other psychiatric medications—is becoming the norm. Confident of their abilities*

61

and often skeptical of psychiatrists' expertise, they choose to rely on their own research and each other's experience in treating problems like depression, fatigue, anxiety or a lack of concentration.[72]

They obtain drugs both legitimately and illegitimately but then often trade unused prescription drugs with others. Because they take a larger percentage of prescription drugs, elderly persons are at risk for abuse as well. Although seldom interested in getting high, they can unintentionally become dependent on drugs they take.

Celebrities seem prone to misuse of prescription drugs—or at least to receiving publicity about the misuse. Among the famous abusers of prescription drugs are Michael Jackson (painkillers), Rush Limbaugh (Vicodin and OxyContin), Chevy Chase (painkillers), Elvis Presley (stimulants), Marilyn Monroe (sleeping pills), Matthew Perry (Vicodin), Betty Ford (painkillers), and Winona Ryder (painkillers). Alex Rodriguez, Floyd Landis, and Marion Jones are just a few of the athletes who have illegally used steroids to enhance performance.

Doctor shopping has emerged as a way for abusers to get access to excessive amounts of prescription drugs. It refers to obtaining care from multiple physicians, without informing each physician of the other treatments, in order to get multiple prescriptions, usually to feed an addiction. The Drug Enforcement Administration (DEA) says that doctor shopping is one of the primary ways for addicts to get prescription drugs for nonmedical uses. Often, nonaddicts will get multiple prescriptions to sell at higher prices to addicts.

Abuse of prescription drugs causes serious health problems. Figures on emergency room visits suggest that 25 percent are associated with abuse of prescription drugs. Opioid painkillers alone now cause more drug overdose deaths than cocaine and heroin combined. Yet, about 40 percent of teens and their parents think that abusing prescription drugs is safer than abusing street drugs. Many believe that there is nothing wrong with occasionally taking a prescription drug without a prescription.

The National Institute on Drug Abuse calls on physicians, pharmacists, and patients to do more to prevent prescription drug abuse. Doctors can screen for abuse when they meet patients and note unusual changes in the amount of drugs requested. Pharmacists can check carefully for fraudulent or altered prescriptions and the possibility of doctor shopping—moving from one provider to another to obtain multiple prescriptions. Patients need to follow instructions carefully when using prescription drugs so that they do not become dependent on them. They should also report problems of withdrawal and get help quickly. To help others avoid these problems, those with prescriptions should make sure that others do not use them.

The DEA has taken steps to monitor and control the illegitimate availability of prescription drugs. The Controlled Substances Act regulates the distribution and sales of prescription drugs. Manufacturers and distributors must provide information to a DEA database on sales of narcotics. Monitoring discrepancies between the amounts manufactured and amounts sold can identify diversion of prescription drugs for illegal purposes. The rise of Internet sales, a preferred means of many drug traffickers, makes this task harder, however. Difficulties in monitoring also occur because enforcers, in attempting to block illegal sales, must not prevent physicians from prescribing drugs for legitimate purposes.

DISPOSAL OF PRESCRIPTION DRUGS

Even nonusers of prescription drugs, both humans and animals, face some mild hazards from prescription drugs via environmental contamination. According to the Environmental Protection Agency (EPA), people dispose of about 19 million tons of active pharmaceutical ingredients each year by flushing them down the toilet, emptying them into sinks, or putting them in the garbage. According to a report from the *Washington Post*,

> *The EPA has identified small quantities of more than 100 pharmaceuticals and personal-care products in samples of the nation's drinking water. Among the drugs detected are antibiotics, steroids, hormones and antidepressants. Last year, the Associated Press reported that trace amounts of drugs had been found in the water supplies of 24 major metropolitan areas; water piped to more than a million people in the Washington area had tested positive for six pharmaceuticals.* [73]

Experts say that the water supply remains safe, but the buildup of hormones and opiates might cause long-term harm for animals and people. By affecting the environment and water supply, the increasing use of prescription drugs has consequences even for the people and animals not taking drugs.

The Office of National Drug Control Policy once recommended flushing drugs down the toilet. It now says the opposite: Flush only those drugs with explicit instructions on the label or package information to do so. Otherwise, the best alternative is to find community drug take-back programs that make collections. Many states have recently passed laws for disposing or recycling of unused prescription drugs, and local pharmacies sometimes collect the drugs. For those lacking access to a collection program, the Office of National Drug Control Policy suggests the following:

1. Take the prescription drugs out of their original containers.
2. Mix drugs with an undesirable substance, such as cat litter or used coffee grounds.

3. Put this mixture into a disposable container with a lid, such as an empty margarine tub, or into a sealable bag.
4. Conceal or remove any personal information, including Rx number, on the empty containers by covering it with black permanent marker or duct tape, or by scratching it off.
5. Place the sealed container with the mixture and the empty drug containers in the trash.[74]

Manufacturers may also need to do more to protect the environment. According to the Associated Press, "U.S. manufacturers, including major drugmakers, have legally released at least 271 million pounds of pharmaceuticals into waterways that often provide drinking water."[75] Manufacturers say they comply with all environmental laws and are not a significant source of water contamination, but few test regularly for the problem. Calls for the government to do more testing for the presence of pharmaceuticals in the water are increasing.

THE FUTURE OF PRESCRIPTION DRUGS

In the near future, government policies may be less supportive of the pharmaceutical industry than in the past. In the Bush administration, Secretary of Health and Human Services Michael Leavitt and FDA Commissioner Andrew von Eschenbach opposed federal efforts to negotiate lower prices for Medicare prescription drugs and to allow reimportation of prescription drugs at lower prices. In the Obama administration, Secretary of Health and Human Services Kathleen Sebelius, FDA Commissioner Margaret Hamburg, and FDA chief deputy Joshua Sharfstein will likely change these policies. New laws and policies may do more to favor consumers.

In the long term, however, the growing use of prescription drugs—or overuse according to some—will almost certainly continue. Although the growth will not likely continue at the fast pace of recent decades, several trends promoting use of prescription drugs will persist.

First, the aging of the population in the next decades will increase prescription drug use for the simple reason that older persons use drugs more than younger persons. According to figures from the National Center for Health Statistics, 84.7 percent of persons age 65 and over used a prescription drug in the last month, compared to 24.2 percent at ages under 18, 35.9 percent at ages 18 to 44, and 64.1 percent at ages 45 to 64.[76] Residents of nursing homes, in particular, receive a variety of drugs for health and mental problems. As the huge baby boom generation enters old age, prescription drug use will rise.

Introduction to Prescription Drugs

Many of the most popular drugs are well suited for use in old age. Age increases the need for statins to lower high cholesterol, beta blockers and ACE inhibitors to reduce high blood pressure, proton pump inhibitors to treat stomach acid reflux, bone density drugs to counter osteoporosis, drugs for bladder problems, pain relievers for osteoarthritis, and new drugs for Alzheimer's disease. Many see these drugs as doing more than preventing disease—they also make old age more enjoyable and people feel younger. The goal of slowing the aging process will drive the continued popularity of prescription drugs, despite some concerns about overuse and side effects. Many pharmaceutical companies accordingly concentrate their research and development on drugs suitable for a growing aging population with the greatest need for prescription drugs.

Second, attitudes among young and old alike have changed in ways that make reliance on prescription drugs more acceptable. Decades ago, patients used prescription drugs to treat acute conditions that lasted over a short time period. Today, many drugs aim not to cure a disease but to make chronic conditions safer and easier to tolerate. This goal requires users to take the drugs over long time periods, even a full lifetime. Once a patient discontinues SSRIs, statins, and ACE inhibitors, for example, the underlying conditions of depression, high cholesterol, and high blood pressure return. Drug companies focus their research and development on these kinds of drugs—those needed by large parts of the population over a long period and with the most potential for profit. The public as well has become increasingly accustomed to long-term use.

Advertising and marketing of pharmaceutical companies contribute to public acceptance of prescription drugs. The ads help make drug use common and normal. Ads and sales efforts sometimes aim to define new diseases and promote concern about problems that otherwise would receive little attention. They encourage people to go to the doctor about problems they had previously ignored. By promoting favorable public attitudes toward prescription drugs, commercials will foster high rates of future use.

Third, a new trend may encourage future use of prescription drugs still further. Drugs are increasingly taken for self-improvement rather than to deal with disease. Even those with no serious physical or mental problems may want to use prescription drugs to improve their feelings and performance. For example, SSRIs can deal with daily difficulties in life rather than clinical depression, statins can allow people to maintain low cholesterol while still eating rich and unhealthy foods, and tranquilizers such as Vicodin can moderate the stress and pressure of work. Similarly, recent trends show growing use of stimulants to improve performance. For example, some students take prescription drugs like Ritalin not to treat ADHD but to help them study. Provigil, a drug made by Cephalon and approved initially for treatment of narcolepsy, a disease that results in an uncontrollable urge to sleep, also improves concentration of those without the disease. Some people now use the drug to increase their job productivity. Even athletes find that stimulants improve their performance. For instance, there has been a huge increase in drug exemptions among major league baseball players for use of stimulants to treat ADHD. With nearly 8 percent of players having the exemption, some experts view the rise with suspicion—it may have more to do with aiding performance than dealing with a serious medical condition.

Some ethicists support the right of people to take pills to boost their brainpower. Martha Farah, a brain scientist at the University of Pennsylvania, says that improving brain function with pills is no more morally objectionable than eating right or getting a good night's sleep.[77] People need not have an illness to benefit from these kinds of prescription drugs. Of course, drugs used for improving performance should not have major side effects and risks of dependency, and people should have the right to freely choose to use them. Otherwise, however, the growing acceptance of prescription drugs for purposes other than treating disease will make them more common in the future.

All these forecasts are subject to a caution. If strong new evidence of serious harm from the side effects of popular prescription drugs emerges, attitudes may change. Because most popular drugs have been used by millions for more than a decade, problems should have appeared by now. The FDA tracks adverse drug results to remove harmful ones from the market. Yet some long-term harm could still result from taking multiple drugs over periods of decades. The liver, a critical organ that processes foreign substances in the blood, may show the most harm. Taking prescription drugs in large quantities can increase the burden on the liver and perhaps damage it.

Drug-induced liver disease is already a major problem. Rezulin for diabetes and Duract for pain caused liver failure and death before being removed from the market. Popular statins have the potential to cause liver problems severe enough that patients using the drugs need to undergo liver tests to make sure they can continue to use them. The evidence for widespread damage to people's livers from the growing long-term use of prescription drugs has not emerged yet. If it does, it will moderate the current high levels of enthusiasm and acceptance of prescription drug use.

---

[1] National Center for Health Statistics, *Chartbook on Trends in the Health of Americans.* Hyattsville, Md.: National Center for Health Statistics, 2007, Table 96. Also available online. URL: http://www.cdc.gov/nchs/data/hus/hus07.pdf#096. Posted November 2007. These are the most recent figures available. More recent figures no doubt would show higher usage.

[2] Jerry Avorn, *Powerful Medicines: The Benefits, Risks, and Costs of Prescription Drugs.* New York: Alfred A. Knopf, 2004, p. 17.

[3] Hagley Museum and Library, "Advertising and Branding," Patent Medicine. Available online. URL: http://www.hagley.org/library/exhibits/patentmed/history/advertisingbranding.html. Downloaded March 30, 2009.

[4] Quoted in Avorn, *Powerful Medicine*, p. 40.

[5] Quoted in Edward Marshall, "Uncle Sam Is the Worst Drug Fiend in the World," *New York Times*, March 12, 1911, p. SM12. Available online. URL: http://query.nytimes.com/gst/abstract.html?res=9906E4D71331E233A25751C1A9659C946096D6CF. Downloaded March 30, 2009.

[6] Avorn, *Powerful Medicine*, p. 53.

[7] F. R. Lichtenberg, "The Impact of New Drug Launches on Longevity: Evidence from Longitudinal, Disease-Level Data from 52 Countries, 1982–2001," National Bureau of Economic Research Working Paper No. 9754. Cambridge, Mass.: National Bureau of Economic Research, June 2003.

[8] Avorn, *Powerful Medicine*, p. 41.

[9] Marcia Angell, *The Truth about Drug Companies: How They Deceive Us and What to Do about It.* New York: Random House, 2004.

[10] IMS Health, "2007 U.S. Sales and Prescription Information," Top-Line Industry Data. Available online. URL: http://www.imshealth.com/portal/site/imshealth/menuitem.a46c6d4df3db4b3d88f611019418c22a/?vgnextoid=936d9df4609e9110VgnVCM10000071812ca2RCRD&vgnextfmt=default. Downloaded March 2, 2009.

[11] Melody Peterson, *Our Daily Meds: How the Pharmaceutical Companies Transformed Themselves into Slick Marketing Machines and Hooked the Nation on Prescription Drugs.* New York: Farrar, Straus, and Giroux, 2008, p. 5.

[12] Barbara Baler, "Million-Dollar Medicines," *AARP Bulletin*, October 2008, pp. 12–13.

[13] Kaiser Family Foundation, "Views on Prescription Drugs and the Pharmaceutical Industry," Kaiser Public Opinion Spotlight. Available online. URL: http://www.kff.org/spotlight/rxdrugs/upload/Rx_Drugs.pdf. Updated April 2008.

[14] PhRMA, *What Goes into the Cost of Prescription Drugs?* Washington, D.C.: Pharmaceutical Research and Manufacturers of America, 2005. Also available online. URL: http://www.phrma.org/files/Cost_of_Prescription_Drugs.pdf. Downloaded April 4, 2009.

[15] PhRMA. *What Goes into the Cost of Prescription Drugs?* p. 2.

[16] Quoted in PhRMA. *What Goes into the Cost of Prescription Drugs?* p. 6.

[17] Malcolm Gladwell, "High Prices: How to Think about Prescription Drugs," *New Yorker*, October 2005. Available online. URL: http://www.newyorker.com/archive/2004/10/25/041025crat_atlarge. Downloaded April 4, 2009.

[18] "Rx R&D Myths: The Case against the Drug Industry's R&D 'Scare Card,'" *Public Citizen*. Available online. URL: http://www.citizen.org/publications/release.cfm?ID=7065. Downloaded April 6, 2009.

[19] Peterson, *Our Daily Meds*, p. 130.

[20] Peterson, *Our Daily Meds*, p. 146.

[21] Marc-André Gagnon and Joel Lexchin, "The Cost of Pushing Pills: A New Estimate of Pharmaceutical Promotion Expenditures in the United States," *PLoS Medicine* 5, no. 1, 2008, p. e1. Available online. URL: http://medicine.

plosjournals.org/perlserv/?request=get-document&doi=10.1371/journal.pmed. 0050001&ct=1. Downloaded April 6, 2008.

[22] Peterson, *Our Daily Meds*, p. 137.

[23] ALLHAT Officers and Coordinators for the ALLHAT Collaborative Research Group, "The Antihypertensive and Lipid-Lowering Treatment to Prevent Heart Attack Trial," *JAMA* 288, no. 23, December 18, 2002, pp. 2,981–2,997.

[24] Organisation for Economic Cooperation and Development, *Health at a Glance.* Paris: OECD, 2001.

[25] Cited in Avorn, *Powerful Medicine*, pp. 225–226.

[26] Angell, *The Truth about Drug Companies*, p. 184.

[27] M. Asif Ismail, "Drug Lobby Second to None: How the Pharmaceutical Industry Gets Its Way in Washington," Center for Public Integrity. Available online. URL: http://projects.publicintegrity.org/rx/report.aspx?aid=723. Posted July 7, 2005.

[28] Robert Steinbrook, "Election 2008—Campaign Contributions, Lobbying, and the U.S. Health Sector," *New England Journal of Medicine* 357, no. 8, August 23, 2007, pp. 736–739. Also available online. URL: http://content.nejm.org/cgi/content/full/357/8/736. Downloaded April 7, 2009.

[29] Patricia Barry, "Medicare Part D: How to Avoid Bigger Bills," *AARP Bulletin*, December 2006, pp. 12–14. Also available online. URL: http://bulletin.aarp.org/yourhealth/medicare/articles/medicare_part_d_how_to_avoid_bigger_bills.html. Downloaded April 7, 2009.

[30] "Prescription Drug Trends," Kaiser Family Foundation, Available online. URL: http://www.kff.org/rxdrugs/upload/3057_07.pdf. Posted September 2008.

[31] "Opportunity Knocks for Big Pharmaceutical Companies in the Credit Crunch," *Pharmaceutical Business Review*. Available online. URL: http://www.pharmaceutical-business-review.com/article_feature.asp?guid=99C88B49-D9FA-412B-A7D9-8A665404A8A7. Posted October 9, 2008.

[32] "Opportunity Knocks," *Pharmaceutical Business Review*.

[33] Matthew Herper, "The Value of New Drugs Is Dropping," Forbes.com. Available online. URL: http://www.forbes.com/2009/01/07/pharmaceuticals-sales-biz-healthcare-cx_mh_0108drugssales.html?partner=alerts. Posted January 8, 2009.

[34] Henry A. Waxman. "Pharmaceutical Industry Profits Increase by Over $8 Billion after Medicare Drug Plan Goes into Effect," Committee on Government Reform. Available online. URL: http://oversight.house.gov/documents/20060919115623 70677.pdf. Posted September 2006.

[35] "Global Company Sales Summary 2006," PDR. Available online. URL: http://www.p-d-r.com/ranking/2006_Company_Sales.pdf. Downloaded April 10, 2009.

[36] "Top Ten Companies by U.S. Sales," IMS Health. Available online. URL: http://www.imshealth.com/deployedfiles/imshealth/Global/Content/Document/Top-Line%20 Industry%20Data/2007%20Top%20Companies%20by%20Sales. pdf. Downloaded April 10, 2009.

[37] Quoted in Peterson, *Our Daily Meds*, p. 7.

[38] National Center for Health Statistics, *Chartbook on Trends in the Health of Americans*, Table 96.

[39] "More Americans Are Using Prescription Drugs," Reuters. Available online: URL: http://www.reuters.com/article/pressRelease/idUS148673+13-Feb-2008+BW20080213. Posted February 13, 2008.

[40] Mollyann Brodie, "Testimony before the U.S. House of Representatives Committee on Energy and Commerce Subcommittee on Oversight and Investigations, May 8, 2008," Kaiser Family Foundation. Available online. URL: http://www.kff.org/kaiserpolls/upload/7774.pdf. Downloaded April 11, 2009.

[41] Justin E. Bekelman, Yan Li, and Cary P. Gross, "Scope and Impact of Financial Conflicts of Interest in Biomedical Research: A Systematic Review," *JAMA* 289, no. 4, January 22, 2003, pp. 454–465. Also available online. URL: http://jama.ama-assn.org/cgi/content/abstract/289/4/454. Downloaded April 11, 2009.

[42] Marcia Angell, "Is Academic Medicine for Sale?" *New England Journal of Medicine* 342, no. 20, May 18, 2000, pp. 1,516–1,518.

[43] Quoted in U.S. Food and Drug Administration, "Truth in Advertising: Rx Drug Ads Come of Age," *FDA Magazine*. Available online. URL: http://www.fda.gov/fdac/features/2004/404_ads.html. Posted July/August 2004.

[44] Peterson, *Our Daily Meds*, p. 15.

[45] National Institutes of Neurological Disorders and Stroke, "NINDS Attention Deficit-Hyperactivity Disorder Information Page," National Institutes of Health. Available online. URL: http://www.ninds.nih.gov/disorders/adhd/adhd.htm. Updated June 6, 2008.

[46] BBC, "'Wide Variations' in Ritalin Use," BBC News. Available online. URL: http://news.bbc.co.uk/1/hi/health/7509576.stm. Updated July 16, 2008.

[47] Viveca Novak, "New Ritalin Ad Blitz Makes Parents Jumpy," *Time* 158, no. 10, September 10, 2001, pp. 62–63. Available online. URL: http://www.time.com/time/magazine/article/0,9171,173468,00.html. Downloaded April 12, 2009.

[48] Cited in Jacky Law, *Big Pharma: Exposing the Global Healthcare Agenda*. New York: Basic Books, 2006, p. 105.

[49] Consumer Reports, "Overactive Bladder: Summary of Recommendations," Consumer Reports Health.org. Available online. URL: http://www.consumerreports.org/health/best-buy-drugs/bladder.htm. Downloaded April 12, 2009.

[50] Peterson, *Our Daily Meds*, pp. 15–17.

[51] Matthew Perrone, "$6 Billion Spent on 'Murky' Ailment," Associated Press. Available online. URL: http://seattletimes.nwsource.com/html/health/2008723050_fibro09.html. Posted February 9, 2009.

[52] Cited in Healthlink, "Antibiotic Overuse Fuels Drug Resistance," University of Wisconsin. Available online. URL: http://healthlink.mcw.edu/article/1031002561.html. Downloaded April 13, 2009.

[53] Jeffrey A. Linder, David W. Bates, Grace M. Lee, and Jonathan A. Finkelstein, "Antibiotic Treatment of Children with Sore Throats," *JAMA* 294, no. 18, November 9, 2005, pp. 2,315–2,322.

[54] Thomas J. Moore, Michael R. Cohen, and Curt D. Furberg, "Serious Adverse Drug Events Reported to the Food and Drug Administration, 1998–2005," *Archives of Internal Medicine* 167, no. 16, 2007, pp. 1,752–1,759. Also available online. URL: http://archinte.ama-assn.org/cgi/content/short/167/16/1752. Downloaded April 14, 2009.

[55] Thomas H. Maugh II, "Adverse Drug Reactions Rise Sharply, Study Finds—Reports Nearly Triple Since '98. Painkillers Are among the Key Culprits," *Los Angeles Times*, September 11, 2007, p. 13. Also available online. URL: http://articles.latimes.com/2007/sep/11/science/sci-drugs11. Downloaded April 14, 2009.

Prescription Drugs

[56] Ricardo Alonso-Zaldivar, "Reports of Serious Drug Reactions Hit Record," Associated Press. Available online. URL: http://lib.store.yahoo.net/lib/realityzone/UFNdrugdeathshigh.html. Posted October 22, 2008.

[57] U.S. Food and Drug Administration, "Potential Signals of Serious Risks/New Safety Information Identified from the Adverse Event Reporting System (AERS) between January–March 2008," FDA. Available online. URL: http://www.fda.gov/Cder/aers/potential_signals/potential_signals_2008Q1.htm. Updated February 4, 2009.

[58] Stephen Fried, *Bitter Pills: Inside the Hazardous World of Legal Drugs*. New York: Bantam Books, 1998.

[59] Jason Lazarou, Bruce H. Pomeranz, and Paul N. Corey, "Incidence of Adverse Drug Reactions in Hospitalized Patients: A Meta-Analysis of Prospective Studies." *JAMA* 279, no. 15, April 15, 1998, pp. 1,200–1,205. Also available online. URL: http://jama.ama-assn.org/cgi/content/abstract/279/15/1200. Downloaded April 15, 2009.

[60] Frontline, "A Dirty Dozen," Dangerous Prescription. Available online. URL: http://www.pbs.org/wgbh/pages/frontline/shows/prescription/etc/dozen.html. Posted November 13, 2003.

[61] Claire Bombardier, Loren Laine, et al., "Comparison of Upper Gastrointestinal Toxicity of Rofecoxib and Naproxen in Patients with Rheumatoid Arthritis. VIGOR Study Group," *New England Journal of Medicine* 343, no. 21, November 23, 2000, pp. 1,520–1,528. Also available online. URL: http://content.nejm.org/cgi/content/full/343/21/1520. Downloaded April 15, 2009.

[62] "Premarin I. V. (Conjugated Estrogens)—Summary," DrugLib.com. Available online. URL: http://www.druglib.com/druginfo/premarin-iv/. Downloaded April 16, 2009.

[63] "Hormone Therapy: Is It Right for You?" MayoClinic.com. Available online. URL: http://www.mayoclinic.com/health/hormone-therapy/WO00046. Updated February 19, 2008.

[64] Kate Cohen, "Fen Phen Nation." Frontline. URL: http://www.pbs.org/wgbh/pages/frontline/shows/prescription/hazard/fenphen.html. Posted November 13, 2003.

[65] Cohen, "Fen Phen Nation."

[66] David P. Phillips, Gwendolyn E. C. Barker, and Megan M. Eguchi, "A Steep Increase in Domestic Fatal Medication Errors with Use of Alcohol and/or Street Drugs," *Archives of Internal Medicine* 168, no. 14, July 28, 2008, pp. 1,561–1,566. Also available online. URL: http://archinte.ama-assn.org/cgi/content/short/168/14/1561. Downloaded April 17, 2009.

[67] National Academies of Science, "Medication Errors Injure 1.5 Million People and Cost Billions of Dollars Annually; Report Offers Comprehensive Strategies for Reducing Drug-Related Mistakes," News from the National Academies. Available online. URL: http://www8.nationalacademies.org/onpinews/newsitem.aspx?RecordID=11623. Posted July 20, 2006.

[68] Nora D. Volkow, "Prescription Drugs: Abuse and Addiction," National Institute on Drug Abuse Research Report Series. Available online. URL: http://www.nida.nih.gov/ResearchReports/Prescription/prescription.html. Downloaded April 20, 2009.

[69] National Institute of Drug Abuse, "Prescription and Over-the-Counter Medications." NIDA InfoFacts. Available online. URL: http://www.nida.nih.gov/infofacts/PainMed.html. Updated July 2009.

[70] Office of National Drug Control Policy, "Prescription for Danger," Executive Office of the President. Available online. URL: http://www.theantidrug.com/pdfs/prescription_report.pdf. Posted January 2008.

[71] National Institute of Drug Abuse, "Trends in Prescription Drug Abuse."

[72] Amy Harmon, "Young, Assured and Playing Pharmacist to Friends," *New York Times*, November 16, 2005, p. A1. Also available online. URL: http://www.nytimes.com/2005/11/16/health/16patient.html?_r=2&hp. Downloaded April 17, 2009.

[73] Susan Q. Stranahan, "For Old Drugs, New Tricks; Advice Veers away from Flushing Unused Pills," *Washington Post*, May 5, 2009, p. HE 1.

[74] "Proper Disposal of Prescription Drugs," Office of National Drug Control Policy. Available online. URL: http://www.whitehousedrugpolicy.gov/publications/pdf/prescrip_disposal.pdf. Posted 2009.

[75] Jeff Donn, Martha Mendoza, and Justin Pritchard. "Tons of Released Drugs Taint US Water." Associated Press. Available online. URL: http://abcnews.go.com/Technology/wireStory?id=7374412. Posted April 19, 2009.

[76] National Center for Health Statistics, *Chartbook on Trends in the Health of Americans*, Table 96.

[77] Quoted in Malcolm Ritter, "Scientists Back Brain Drugs for Healthy People," ABC News. Available online. URL: http://abcnews.go.com/Health/MindMoodNews/wireStory?id=6412215. Posted December 7, 2008.

CHAPTER 2

THE LAW AND PRESCRIPTION DRUGS

Laws covering prescription drugs have steadily strengthened the protection of the public from unsafe and ineffective products. During the 1800s, makers and sellers of patent medicines made exaggerated, even outrageous claims for their products with little more evidence of effectiveness than personal testimonials. Physicians had been compiling reliable information on legitimate drugs for many decades, but the loud and dishonest claims of ads and salespeople for illegitimate drugs tended to overwhelm that information. Federal and state laws slowly began to regulate medications and put patent medicines out of business. Refined by court decisions over the years and implemented by the Food and Drug Administration (FDA), federal and state laws now regulate drug production, approval, advertising, and sales. A brief overview of the laws and related court cases follows.

LAWS AND REGULATIONS

FEDERAL LEGISLATION

The first minimal laws to regulate drugs and medications emerged in the 1800s. In 1848, for example, Congress responded to concerns about impurities in drugs by passing an act to require the U.S. Customs Service to inspect and stop from entry any adulterated drugs imported from overseas. In 1902, Congress passed the Biologics Control Act to ensure the purity and safety of vaccines and serums. The modern age of regulation of medications began a few years later.

Pure Food and Drug Act of 1906

The Pure Food and Drug Act of 1906 prohibited the manufacture of and interstate commerce in adulterated or misbranded food and drugs. The law

72

defined drugs as "all medicines and preparations recognized in the United States Pharmacopeia or National Formulary for internal or external use, and any substance or mixture of substances intended to be used for the cure, mitigation, or prevention of disease of either man or other animals." It then defined as adulterated any difference in the standard of strength, quality, or purity, as determined by the United States Pharmacopeia or National Formulary, including products below standards of quality in strength or purity. However, if the bottle, box, or container clearly labels any difference from these standards, the drug is not deemed as adulterated. The law also made misbranding—false or misleading labeling—illegal. Labels needed to include information on the quantity of alcohol, morphine, opium, heroin, and other dangerous substances.

By today's standards, this act had major gaps. It did not require manufacturers to prove the safety of their products. Rather, it required the government to prove a product was unsafe or misbranded before removing it from the market. To get the proof, government agencies could collect products sold outside their state of manufacture, imported from foreign countries, or exported to foreign countries. The Bureau of Chemistry of the Department of Agriculture then could examine the product. Any findings of adulteration or misbranding would require the government to notify the maker of the drug. Without contrary evidence provided by the maker, the Department of Agriculture would turn over the information to the proper U.S. district attorney, who would prosecute the violation and enforce the penalties. Violators found guilty of a first offense faced a fine not to exceed $500 and imprisonment for one year.

Although modest in its regulations, the law signaled a major change in the goals of the government. In the past, laws allowed consumers to reach their own judgments about medications, and Congress avoided trying to control the choices individuals made in using the medications. The Pure Food and Drug Act took the step of outlawing dishonesty in ingredients and claims about medications. It set clear quality standards based on work done by a committee of physicians and pharmacists called the U.S. Pharmacopeia. It further gave new powers to the Bureau of Chemistry, a forerunner to the FDA.

Harrison Narcotic Act of 1914

With cocaine and opiates largely unregulated during the late 1800s, the use of the addictive products spread. Doctors sometimes recommended the drugs to patients for menstrual pain and a variety of other ailments, and others managed to obtain the drugs to feed an addiction. Congress responded with a law in 1914. It first required that "every person who produces, imports, manufactures, compounds, deals in, dispenses, distributes, or gives away opium or coca leaves or any compound, manufacture, salt, derivative, or preparation thereof, shall register with the collector of internal revenue of the district." Those registered had to pay an annual tax. Physicians could give written prescriptions to those who needed the narcotic for medical reasons but were required to keep track of what they dispensed or distributed. Those possessing the drug but not registered with the government or having a prescription from a physician, veterinarian, dentist, or nurse would be in violation of the law.

By requiring registration and taxes, the law curbed the use of cocaine and opium products. By putting limits on the kinds of drugs that the public could use without approval by health care personnel, the law took first steps toward requiring prescriptions. The narcotics remained available when needed for medical reasons, but the government interpreted the law to restrict the meaning of "medical reasons" and to regulate the purposes of these drugs. Responding to an addiction, for example, was not a valid medical reason for dispensing narcotics. To enforce the new regulations and warn others about violating the law, the government arrested and imprisoned several physicians for dispensing cocaine or opium products.

Federal Food, Drug, and Cosmetic Act of 1938

After more than 30 years, the 1906 Pure Food and Drug Act had become outdated. The Bureau of Chemistry, originally given powers to investigate drug adulteration and misbranding, became the Food, Drug, and Insecticide Administration in 1927 and the Food and Drug Administration in 1930. In 1933, the new agency called for an overhaul of the law that guided its actions. It identified several products that, despite concerns of the agency, remained on the market under current law:

> *Banbar, a worthless "cure" for diabetes that the old law protected; Lash-Lure, an eyelash dye that blinded some women . . . ; numerous examples of foods deceptively packaged or labeled; Radithor, a radium-containing tonic that sentenced users to a slow and painful death; and the Wilhide Exhaler, which falsely promised to cure tuberculosis and other pulmonary diseases.[1]*

Despite the legality of selling these dangerous products, congressional disputes prevented new legislation until a tragedy occurred. In 1937, the death of more than 100 persons, many of them children, from contaminated doses of a drug used to treat infections prodded Congress into action. The Federal Food, Drug, and Cosmetic Act of 1938 resulted.

The law gave the FDA new powers to regulate drugs. It required that new drugs be shown as safe before going on sale. This new form of regulation reversed past practices. Rather than removing unsafe drugs after they caused sickness and death, the FDA could prevent companies from selling unsafe drugs in the first place. The law also more clearly prohibited false health claims for drugs. In the past, the government had to prove that makers of misbranded drugs intended to defraud buyers to remove a drug. Rather than having to demonstrate that the makers had illegitimate motives, the government now had to meet a lower standard—show that the makers had misbranded or made false claims for the drugs.

The FDA needed to act quickly after Congress passed and President Franklin Delano Roosevelt signed the legislation. With the new powers came new responsibilities for the agency. Manufacturers had to prove the safety of their new drugs before they could sell them, but the FDA needed to review the evidence to give approval. The agency also moved closer to the current system of prescription drugs. It identified drugs such as sulfas for infections that patients could not use safely on their own. Like narcotics under the Harrison Act, these drugs under the authority of the FDA would now require a prescription.

Durham-Humphrey Amendment of 1951

A question emerged soon after enactment of the 1938 Federal Food, Drug, and Cosmetic Act—What drugs should require prescriptions from physicians and what drugs should consumers buy on their own? The FDA had concluded that use of some drugs such as sulfas needed the guidance of a physician, but many other drugs remained subject to dispute. Some observers thought that, with accurate and complete information on labels, consumers could decide what drugs to use. Others thought that consumers would misuse many drugs without physicians to guide them. Although drugmakers generally had the power to decide if their drug required a prescription, the lack of a clear rule led to disputes with physicians and pharmacists. The FDA had only one recourse in these disputes: It could sue for misbranding if, contrary to recommendations of the drugmaker, the drug warranted supervision by a physician or pharmacist.

The Durham-Humphrey amendment, known as the prescription drug amendment, aimed to settle the issue in 1951. Both the cosponsors, Representative Durham and Senator Humphrey, were pharmacists. The amendment distinguished prescription drugs from over-the-counter (OTC) drugs. Drugs required a prescription if they were unsafe because of toxicity, method of use, or habit-forming properties. In other words, evidence of the potential for serious harm through misuse of a drug meant it should be classified as a prescription drug. For example, a prescription would be required for drugs that caused serious harm when taken in the wrong dose or that misled patient into not seeking treatment from a doctor by hiding symptoms. Companies could no longer market both prescription and OTC versions of the same drug or market a drug as OTC when determined by the FDA to be prescription only. The distinction between prescription and OTC drugs remains central today but also depends on studies of safety and potential for misuse.

Kefauver-Harris Drug Control Act of 1962

After thousands of mothers in Europe taking a sedative drug called thalidomide gave birth to deformed infants, support for stronger regulation of drugs grew in the United States. The unwillingness of the FDA to approve the drug before reports of these problems had surfaced encouraged a more stringent strategy of evaluation, and new legislation in 1962 reinforced this strategy. The most important component of the Kefauver-Harris amendment to the Federal Food, Drug, and Cosmetic Act required that drugs approved by the FDA be proven safe but also effective. A safe drug that had little benefit to patients not only wasted time and money but might indirectly cause harm. It might prevent patients from receiving effective care from other drugs or treatments. Drugmakers now would have to provide evidence of effectiveness before the FDA could approve the drug. The law also required that advertisements about drugs in medical journals include information on side effects. It also outlawed the misleading practice of describing drugs without a patent as breakthrough drugs; makers had previously used this tactic to charge expensive prices for potentially less expensive drugs.

Requiring proof of effectiveness brought about major changes in consumer protection. First, it led to the widespread use of randomized clinical trials, a form of scientific study that proved crucial to obtaining accurate information on both safety and effectiveness. The method continues to guide evaluation of new prescription drugs today. Second, the FDA began to evaluate drugs already on the market to determine if evidence of either effectiveness or ineffectiveness existed. Thousands of existing drugs underwent review, and many failed to demonstrate the effectiveness needed to stay on the market. Efforts to remove ineffective, though still widely used drugs faced opposition from drugmakers, prescribing physicians, and users, but courts ultimately sided with the FDA in enforcing the law.

Comprehensive Drug Abuse Prevention and Control Act of 1970

The potential for abuse of several pleasure-inducing and habit-forming prescription drugs required that other agencies besides the FDA become involved in regulation. The FDA was largely a scientific agency, but abuse of some prescription drugs involved criminal activity. A patchwork of laws, including the Harrison Narcotics Act and the Pure Food, Drug, and Cosmetic Act, governed the use of dangerous prescription drugs. By the 1960s, multiple agencies carried out drug enforcement efforts. For example, the Bureau of Narcotics in the Department of the Treasury had responsibility for narcotics such as heroin, and the Bureau of Drug Abuse Control in the Department of Health, Education, and Welfare had responsibility for depressants, stimulants, and hallucinogens (such as LSD). A new agency in the Department of Justice, the Bureau of Narcotics and Dangerous Drugs, merged the separate organizations in 1968. Still, the variety of drugs that needed control, including those meant strictly for prescriptions, made for confusion and complexity. A single law that classified multiple drugs and set penalties for misuse followed.

The Comprehensive Drug Abuse and Control Act of 1970 classified drugs based on their potential for abuse and set criminal punishments for five different classes or schedules of drugs.

- Schedule I drugs such as heroin and LSD have no medical use.
- Schedule II drugs such as cocaine or morphine, although equally dangerous, have some carefully limited medical uses.
- Schedule III drugs such as barbiturates and codeine have limited medical uses and some danger for abuse and dependency but not as serious as cocaine and morphine.
- Schedule IV drugs such as diphenoxin, diazepam, and oxazepam have medical uses and limited potential for abuse and dependency.
- Schedule V drugs have medical uses and low potential for abuse and dependency.

Schedule I drugs were subject to the greatest level of control and most severe punishment for illegal possession and Schedule V drugs the least level of control and mildest punishment.

The law treated all drugs in the five schedules as controlled substances. Under the law, manufacturers and distributors of controlled substances needed to register with the U.S. attorney general and meet certain conditions. They needed to have controls in place to prevent diversion of the controlled substances for illegitimate use. The controls included sealed containers for prescription drugs with clearly labeled warnings and careful record keeping on who receives the controlled substances. Government agents checking on diversion of prescription drugs for nonprescription uses could then match the rate of production with the legitimate needs for the prescription drugs. Any inconsistencies would lead to an investigation.

The law focused new attention to the growing problem of abuse of prescription drugs. It gave responsibility for enforcement to the U.S. Attorney General, with help from the Department of Health, Education, and Welfare on determining the appropriate classification of drugs. A new agency created in 1973 under an executive order from President Richard Nixon, the Drug Enforcement Administration (DEA), came to have specific responsibility for enforcing the law.

Bayh-Dole Act of 1980

Also known as the University and Small Business Patent Procedures Act, this legislation gave universities, small businesses, and nonprofit organizations the intellectual ownership of property that resulted from government funding. Senators Birch Bayh and Robert Dole cosponsored the legislation. In the past, the government accumulated patents but licensed only a small number to commercial companies. The new law encouraged the commercialization of patents by the organizations that would profit from them and contributed to the growth of prescription drug discoveries in the decades to follow. However, the law also allowed companies to charge high prices for the newly discovered drugs. Critics of the law say that government discoveries should benefit the public rather than drug companies.

Orphan Drug Act of 1983

An orphan drug is defined as one that would serve fewer than 200,000 patients in the United States. It is uneconomical for a pharmaceutical company to devote expense to developing a drug that only a few will need or buy. The Orphan Drug Act of 1983 gives companies incentives to develop these drugs anyway. Companies gained some tax incentives for clinical trials and the exclusive right to sell orphan drugs for seven years, even without a patent. By some estimates, orphan drugs help 20 million Americans having any of 5,000 conditions, with some conditions affecting only a few hundred or few thousand people. By encouraging the development of drugs to treat patients with rare disorders, the law has helped in developing drugs for Gaucher's disease, rare cancers, hemophilia, multiple sclerosis, and Parkinson's disease.

From 1983 to 2004, the FDA approved 249 orphan drugs for sale. The National Association of Rare Disorders, a nonprofit group that pushed for the initial legislation, and companies that make the drugs praise the law for its success in bringing orphan drugs to market. With the special incentives provided by the law, many small biotechnology companies have focused on developing these drugs. However, some in Congress, including Representative Henry Waxman, believe that the law has made it too easy for companies to profit from the government incentives. Some drugs developed under the Orphan Drug Act have become hugely successful. For example, Gleevec, a drug for chronic myelogenous leukemia, has come to have many other uses and earns $2.5 billion in revenues for its maker, Novartis. According to a report in *Genetic Engineering and Biotechnology News*, "12 out of 19 leading orphan drugs had just one approval for an orphan indication but became blockbusters by expanding to nonorphan indications or by off-label usage."[2] This strategy brings high profits. Further, companies with exclusive marketing rights can charge high prices for their products. In the 1980s, Amgen developed a new orphan drug under the law called EPO to treat anemia in patients with kidney failure. Treatment at the time cost $4,000 to $8,000 per year, and first-year sales reached $200 million. EPO has gone on to become a highly used drug. Critics say that these expensive and profitable drugs should not benefit from government incentives. Overall, however, support for the law remains strong, and companies continue to develop orphan drugs.

Drug Price Competition and Patent Term Restoration Act of 1984

Known as the Hatch-Waxman Act, after the cosponsors Republican senator Orrin Hatch and Democratic representative Henry Waxman, this legislation amended the Federal Food, Drug, and Cosmetics Act to encourage the sale of generic drugs. In also changing the rules of ownership of patents for prescription drugs, it had great importance for the drug industry and consumers.

Under U.S. law, a patent lasts 17 years from the issue of the patent or 20 years from the date of the patent's first filing. From the point of view of drug manufacturers, the time taken to develop and gain approval for a drug from the FDA puts them at a disadvantage. It slows the release of a patented drug and means less time for exclusive marketing rights. From the point of view of consumers, the patent period requires users to buy the drugs for a long period and at high prices from the company that filed the patent. Other companies can sell cheaper generic drugs—and save consumers money—only after the patent of a brand-name drug has expired.

As a compromise between the divergent interests of drug companies and consumers, the law aided both groups. On one hand, it gave certain patent holders the right to extend the patent protection period due to delays in the federal approval process. The FDA would work with the Patent Trademark Office to review requests for patent extensions. The extension can last for up to five years and depends on the time spent to approve the product, but the total life of a patent from the product's approval, including the extension, cannot exceed 14 years. By rewarding drugmakers with longer patents, the law encouraged drug companies to develop new and valuable drugs despite the difficulties of the approval process.

On the other hand, generic drug companies gained greater access to the market for prescription drugs. When patents expire, makers of generic drugs need not go through the detailed approval process and sponsor new research studies. Rather, they can rely on the studies used to determine dosage, safety, and effectiveness of the brand-name drug. This saves money for the companies, gets the generic drugs to the public quickly, and keeps prices low. Companies still must meet several other criteria to gain approval from the FDA. A generic drug must

- contain the same active ingredients as the innovator drug (inactive ingredients may vary),
- be identical in strength, dosage form, and route of administration,
- have the same use indications,
- be bioequivalent or absorbed and metabolized by the body in the same ways,
- meet the same batch requirements for identity, strength, purity, and quality, and
- be manufactured under the same strict standards of FDA's good manufacturing practice regulations required for innovator products.

Having met the same standards as the original drugs, generic drugs are be assumed to be both safe and effective, and their lower prices help consumers.

Prescription Drug Marketing Act of 1987

This law amended the Federal Food, Drug, and Cosmetic Act to ensure the safety and quality of prescription drugs by preventing the sale of counterfeit, misbranded, expired, and adulterated products. The preamble to the law stated that, because of the sale of substandard, even counterfeit products, Americans cannot be certain that their drugs are safe and effective. The resale of drugs given out by company representatives as free samples and the sale of drugs reimported back into the United States after being exported elsewhere made it difficult for the government to effectively control the quality of prescription drugs. When sold for lower prices, these drugs unfairly penalized those selling at normal prices. Worse, the diverse sources made it possible for criminals to sell fraudulent drugs under the pretext that they were free samples or reimports. These conditions created unacceptable risks that consumers would get ineffective or diluted drugs.

The law first specifies that a drug manufactured in the United States and exported to another country cannot be imported back into the United States (unless done so by the original manufacturer or required for emergency medical care). The law next specifies that no person may sell, purchase, or trade or offer to sell, purchase, or trade any drug sample (that is, any drug given out for promotion rather than intended for sale). Representatives of drug manufacturers and distributors also cannot sell samples and must keep records of the samples they distribute to health care practitioners.

The Law and Prescription Drugs

With amendments in 1992 and rules set forth by the FDA, the law requires a proof of pedigree for the sale of prescription drugs. The pedigree identifies the origin of the drug and contains a record of each sale, purchase, or trade of the drug. For example, wholesale distributors or authorized distributors for the manufacturer that are involved in interstate commerce must provide the pedigree to the person receiving the drug. With the pedigree, buyers can be sure of the legitimacy and quality of the drugs.

While all agree on the importance of protecting the quality of prescription drugs sold to the public, the law has led to some controversy. Restricting the reimportation of prescription drugs protects the quality but also prevents the purchase of prescription drugs sold at lower prices in other nations. As prescription drug prices rose during the 1990s and 2000s, consumer groups called for a change in this restriction. Americans already traveled to other countries, Canada in particular, to purchase prescription drugs at lower prices. Allowing large-scale reimportation and sale would help others who are unable or unwilling to travel out of the country to also benefit from lower prices. Various efforts of Congress to end this restriction have so far failed, but renewed efforts have emerged in 2009 with a democratic Congress and president.

Prescription Drug User Fee Act (PDUFA) of 1992

Drug companies and potential patients had complained that the long review process for new drugs delayed companies from selling their new products and patients from using and benefiting from them. The Prescription Drug User Fee Act (PDUFA) of 1992 provided a means to fund faster evaluation and approval of new prescription drugs. Before the law, it took an average of 22 months for an application to receive approval. However, the FDA lacked the resources to speed the review process while maintaining quality controls. The PDUFA required the pharmaceutical and biotechnology industry to pay user fees to help cover the FDA costs of drug reviews. By 1997, the FDA estimated it would receive $84 million for the year from the user fees to review new products. In exchange for the user fees, the FDA set up new standards to reduce the approval time for new drugs. The agency hired new staff, implemented computer technology for submitting applications, and streamlined the review process. It aimed to reduce standard review times to 12 months and priority reviews to six months. The user fee scheme remains today.

Several reauthorizations of the PDUFA since 1992, most recently in 2007, have expanded the law. It now gives more attention to using funds for drug safety, reviewing television advertising, and performing more complex and comprehensive reviews.

Prescription Drugs

Food and Drug Administration Modernization Act of 1997

This legislation amended the Federal Food, Drug, and Cosmetic Act to improve the regulation of prescription drugs (as well as medical devices and food). The law notes that the PDUFA of 1992 successfully reduced review times and reauthorized the user fees to expedite the review process. Other provisions aimed to give some patients access to experimental drugs. Beyond that, the law made several other changes.

First, the law allowed the FDA to designate certain products for fast-track review. These products included drugs for life-threatening illnesses and patients with unmet medical needs. The drug company requests fast-track designation for its drug, and the Secretary of Health and Human Services determines if the drug meets the criteria for that designation. If they receive approval for an expedited review, the company must sponsor post-approval studies of safety and effectiveness.

Second, the law requires the National Institutes of Health to establish and maintain a data bank of information on ongoing clinical trials for drugs that treat serious or life-threatening illnesses and conditions. Making the information on drugs under study available to persons suffering from the illnesses and conditions can help the patients gain access to experimental drugs.

Third, the law changes the treatment of off-label use of drugs—that is, drugs used for purposes other than those for which it received approval. According to the FDA,

> *The law abolishes the long-standing prohibition on dissemination by manufacturers of information about unapproved uses of drugs and medical devices. The act allows a firm to disseminate peer-reviewed journal articles about an off-label indication of its product, provided the company commits itself to file, within a specified time frame, a supplemental application based on appropriate research to establish the safety and effectiveness of the unapproved use.*[3]

Supporters of the provision say that patients can now benefit from drugs proven safe for newly discovered conditions. Opponents of the provision say that easing restrictions on the promotion of drugs encourages overuse of drugs and heightens safety risks.

Fourth, the law also addresses some shortcomings in regulations for pediatric medicines. It requires that the FDA identify which drugs should carry special labeling for use by children. For example, children may require special doses, and parents need special warnings about side effects. In return for implementing the new pediatric labeling requirement and developing new research on the effectiveness and safety of adult drugs used by children, companies received another six months of exclusive rights to sell the product. Later, the Best Pharmaceuticals for Children Act of 2002 continued the exclusivity rights for companies carrying out studies on the benefits and side effects of drugs taken by children.

Medicare Prescription Drug Improvement and Modernization Act of 2003

The largest reform in Medicare since its establishment occurred in 2003, when legislation gave new assistance to program participants in buying prescription drugs. The new prescription benefit set up by the Medicare Prescription Drug Improvement and Modernization Act of 2003 began January 1, 2006. Relying on a mix of government funding, cost-sharing from beneficiaries, and service from private insurance companies, the program addressed the problem of rising prices and demand for prescription drugs—but only for the elderly.

The prescription drug plan, called Medicare Part D, allows those eligible for Medicare to enroll voluntarily. Enrollees can select from plans offered by private insurance companies. By dealing with private insurance companies, Medicare participants do not get benefits directly from the government. Instead, insurance companies provide discounts for drugs and receive reimbursement from the government. By having private companies compete for participants, the drug plan aims to keep costs low. The private plans, which vary in the costs they charge and the drugs they cover, also give consumers some choices.

Members of prescription drug plans pay a monthly premium that entitles them to savings of 10 to 25 percent on the drugs they buy. The premium varies depending on the plan and the company but on average costs about $28 a month in 2009. Since costs for drugs also include deductibles and co-payments, the plans lower but do not eliminate out-of-pocket expenses for prescription drugs. Low-income groups get additional subsidies to help with out-of-pocket expenses.

Alternatively, those who belong to Medicare Advantage get prescription drug benefits through their HMO membership rather than Medicare Part D. Still others get drug coverage through employers or unions but must choose between the private and public plans. Retirees who have prescription drug coverage from an employer or union lose these benefits if they join Medicare Part D. To encourage participation of the private sector, employer- and union-sponsored plans receive government subsidies for the prescription-drug discounts they offer to members.

Critics point out some limitations, however. The law does not allow the federal government to negotiate lower prices for drugs with pharmaceutical companies—a condition needed to get bipartisan support for the legislation. The plans vary widely in costs, coverage, and drugs provided, which makes it hard for enrollees to understand the differences and select the best plan.

For example, if the preferred list of drugs used by the plan (called the formulary) does not include a desired drug, participants pay the full cost. More generally, critics say that the reliance on profit-seeking insurance companies and Medicare Advantage HMOs rather than on direct government payments raises costs to elderly consumers.

The Food and Drug Administration Amendments Act of 2007

The most recent legislation affecting prescription drugs consists of a set of amendments that reauthorize and revise existing provisions and adds some new provisions to the Federal Food, Drug, and Cosmetic Act. For example, the Food and Drug Administration Amendments Act of 2007 sets new procedures to deal with safety problems that emerge after approval of a drug. It requires that certain companies have an approved plan for risk evaluation and mitigation strategy. The strategy will help determine whether the benefits of the drug outweigh the risks. Another provision extends the 1997 FDA Modernization Act with new information requirements for the clinical trial database. The additional information submitted to the database (available at www.clincialtrials.gov) can help the public search out new drug treatments.

Most important, the amendments reauthorize the user-fee programs for prescription drugs and enhance the authority of the FDA to ensure the safety of drugs already approved for public use. The reauthorization of the user-fee program, which requires companies requesting approval for drugs to pay for a good part of the approval process, continues the system set up in 1992. According to the amendment, "Congress finds that the fees authorized by the amendments made in this title will be dedicated toward expediting the drug development process and the process for the review of human drug applications, including postmarket drug safety activities."[4] Companies submitting direct-to-consumer (DTC) ads to the FDA for review also must pay fees to help cover the costs. For small companies, the amendments exempt orphan drugs, those designed to treat rare diseases or conditions. The exemption applies to drugs that are owned or licensed and marketed by a company with less than $50 million in gross worldwide revenues during the previous year.

FEDERAL REGULATIONS

Although federal laws set standards and goals to ensure the safety and effectiveness of prescription drugs, the approval depends on rules and regulations set by the FDA. Title 21 of the Code of Federal Regulations has more than 1,400 parts on food and drugs.[5] Although the regulations are extensive, the FDA summarizes them on several topics of special importance, such as advertising, drug safety, generics, and labeling. The guidance documents on many of these topics are technical and detailed, but as an example consider some of the FDA regulations on advertising and labeling.

Federal law requires that advertisements contain a brief summary of side effects, contraindications, and effectiveness. The FDA rules based on this law define the meaning of brief summary. In print locations such as newspapers, magazines, and brochures, ads must list the risks on the product package labeling. In broadcast advertising such as radio and television, the ads must disclose major risks in either the audio or the visual part and make provision to disseminate more detailed information. The potentially diverse audience of a broadcast ad should have reasonably convenient access to a product's full, approved labeling. Access should not depend on use of sophisticated technologies such as the Internet or first require persons to give out personal information. More generally, the regulations require that ads not be false or misleading in any sense, present a fair balance between benefits and risk, and use consumer-friendly language when presenting information.

New regulations from the FDA call for more informative and accessible labeling. They require that prescribing information of new and recently approved products include highlights of key information (to prevent users from being overwhelmed by the wealth of information) and a table of contents (to help find the detailed information of most interest). The rules respond to the increasing length, detail, and complexity of prescribing information for drugs. The changes can help manage the risks of medications and reduce medical errors by health care professionals, who can better communicate risk information to their patients.

Drug companies also must comply with regulations for approval of drugs. The 84-page FDA guidance on this topic provides information on how to report the results from clinical studies of effectiveness, particularly results relating to deaths, adverse events, and patient dropouts. Other reporting topics include laboratory tests, vital signs of the subjects, limitations of the data, and pooling across studies. Although too technical for all but specialists who complete and evaluate the clinical studies, these rules and regulations are crucial to implementing laws for prescription drugs.

STATE LEGISLATION

The role of state legislation relative to federal legislation raises some constitutional issues that have special relevance to prescription drugs. Article VI of the U.S. Constitution states the following:

> *This Constitution, and the Laws of the United States which shall be made in Pursuance thereof; and all Treaties made, or which shall be made, under the Authority of the United States, shall be the supreme Law of the Land; and the Judges in every State shall be bound thereby, any Thing in the Constitution or Laws of any state to the Contrary notwithstanding.*

Federal laws thus take precedence over state laws. Given the key role of the FDA in approving and regulating prescription drugs, states must follow the federal laws. Indeed, the Federal Food, Drug, and Cosmetic Act says that no state may establish requirements for labeling or packaging that differ from requirements of the federal law.

However, state laws have room to address many issues relating to prescription drugs. For example, based on recent court cases, the states have authority to hold drug companies liable for incomplete or misleading warnings. States also have responsibility for licensing pharmacists, setting standards for giving and filling prescriptions, and regulating pharmacy practices. The National Conference of State Legislatures (NCSL) compiles information on state legislation relating to prescription drugs that highlights the importance of several other types of state action.[6]

First, state governments have strong interests in controlling prescription drug costs. With help from the federal government, states pay for Medicaid, a government health program for individuals and families with low incomes and few financial assets. Increased demand for prescription drugs from the poor, many of whom have serious health problems, thereby raises state Medicaid costs. States also pay drug costs under insurance plans for state employees. To control costs for prescription drugs, state laws specify preferred drug lists or formularies for Medicaid patients and state employees, and they require substitution of less expensive generic drugs for brand-name drugs when possible. According to figures from the NCSL, all but seven states have enacted Medicaid preferred drug lists.[7] In addition, many states require manufacturers with drugs on the preferred list to return supplemental rebates—a means to indirectly lower prices. Some states cooperate in multistate rebate agreements with drug companies to lower costs for Medicaid prescription drugs. Similarly, states sometimes pool purchase orders so that they have more power to negotiate with drugmakers. Twelve states (Alaska, Georgia, Hawaii, Kentucky, Michigan, Minnesota, Montana, Nevada, New Hampshire, Rhode Island, New York, and Tennessee plus the District of Columbia) are part of a National Medicaid Pooling Initiative (NMPI).

Second, along with keeping costs of prescription drugs low, state laws help those unable to afford prescription drugs or qualify for Medicaid or Medicare. Those needing help include low-income seniors who cannot afford co-pay and membership costs for Medicare prescription coverage. By 2006, 16 states provided subsidies to these older persons, and six more states have passed laws to begin offering the subsidies. In addition, state laws help with prescription expenses for younger persons who cannot work because of a disability.

Third, states have passed laws to avoid prescription drug errors. The federal government approves drugs and regulates how they are dispensed, but states can do more to ensure local pharmacies minimize mistakes. At least 15 states passed laws in recent years to reduce these errors by calling for increased legibility of prescriptions, electronic prescriptions, and clear labels. For example, Arizona passed a law requiring a continuous quality assurance program to review pharmacy procedures; its goals are to control medication errors. Illinois requires that health care providers set up ways to check the preparation, computer entry, and filling of medication orders, medical devices, and prescriptions. And Massachusetts has proposed a bill to convene a task force for reducing prescription errors.

Fourth, states have an interest in the marketing and advertising of prescription drugs to consumers. They have no control over national advertisements, which the FDA regulates. However, they can address concerns about advertisements that promote use of more expensive products and raise the costs the state pays for prescriptions of Medicaid recipients and state employees. Several innovative strategies focus on the marketing of prescription drugs to physicians. For example, a law in California requires pharmaceutical companies to adopt a Comprehensive Compliance Program that regulates marketing interactions with health care professionals. It also places limits on gifts and incentives to medical or health professionals, including a "specific annual dollar limit on gifts, promotional materials, or items or activities that the pharmaceutical company may give or otherwise provide to an individual medical or health care professional."[8] In Minnesota, a law prohibits any manufacturer or wholesale drug distributor, or any agent thereof, from offering or giving any gift of value over $50 to a practitioner.

Fifth, the states have responsibility for monitoring the prescriptions of drugs, particularly those prone to abuse. Laws in several states prevent abusers from obtaining prescriptions from multiple doctors—usually to feed an addiction. Doctor shopping refers to seeking care from multiple physicians, without informing each physician of the other treatments, in order to get multiple prescriptions. In response, many states have passed laws or regulations to create prescription drug monitoring programs. Under the programs, pharmacies must log each prescription they fill, which are then stored in a state electronic database. Efforts to get an additional prescription will show up in checks of the database. Doctors and pharmacists can check the database for past prescription records to avoid dangerous combinations of drugs as well as to prevent misuse of addictive drugs. In 2007 alone, nine states (Arizona, Colorado, Illinois, Kansas, Kentucky, North Dakota, New Jersey, Nevada, and Tennessee) passed legislation to establish drug-monitoring programs.

Sixth, states have taken another approach to preventing abuse besides monitoring prescription drugs. A few have set up programs to facilitate disposal of unused prescription drugs. Flushing old drugs down the toilet contaminates the water supply with trace amounts of antibiotics, mood stabilizers, and sex hormones, and putting them in the garbage could allow access to illicit users. Leaving prescription drugs in bathroom cabinets allows access and abuse by other family members and visitors. State laws therefore set up provisions for both disposal and reuse of these drugs. These laws must take care not to violate FDA rules prohibiting the redistribution of prescription drugs. Thus, Oklahoma, Louisiana, and Ohio allow for the recovery of unused drugs from nursing homes, long-term care centers, and pharmacies for redistribution to poor patients. Nebraska allows consumers to return unused drugs still in tamper-resistant packaging. Concerning disposal, California has passed legislation to set up programs for the public to return unused prescription drugs for safe and environmentally sound disposal. Iowa has set up a pilot program, and Wisconsin has funded grants for the disposal of unwanted prescription drugs.

More than most states, Maine has passed innovative and comprehensive prescription drug laws and policies. As a result, the state has received national attention. A report from the NCSL summarizes its laws to control the costs of prescription drugs:

> *In 1975 Maine was one of the first two states to create a senior pharmaceutical assistance program. In 1999, Maine's SB 732 mandated the first statewide discount price program. In May 2000, the legislature enacted and the Governor signed a multi-part law that included both discounts and the nation's first state prescription drug price control mechanism. A separate pharmaceutical discount law was enacted in May 2001, and an entirely new law passed in June 2003.[9]*

Court decisions have upheld the Maine price controls, and several states have adopted similar laws.

Maine also added a number of new laws concerning prescription drugs in more recent years. In 2005 alone, several new laws passed the legislature and signed by the governor did the following: set a maximum price for generic drugs; set up a program for persons age 62 and older to obtain drugs from out of the country; prohibited pharmaceutical companies from advertising via television, radio, or print unless the material meets federal guidelines; and required that a committee study the feasibility of importing prescription drugs.

COURT CASES

Court decisions involving prescription drugs cover a wide variety of topics such as advertising as a free speech right, the ability of states to control prices, and the power of the FDA. A review of some major cases follows.

88

Supreme Court Decisions

VIRGINIA STATE BOARD OF PHARMACY V. VIRGINIA CITIZENS CONSUMER COUNCIL
425 U.S. 748 (1976)

Background

Groups representing consumers of prescription drugs, including the Virginia Citizens Consumer Council and the Virginia State AFL-CIO, brought suit in the Eastern District Court against the Virginia State Board of Pharmacy. A Virginia statute defining advertising of drug prices by licensed pharmacists to be unprofessional conduct prevented such advertising. The statute referred to any activity that "publishes, advertises or promotes, directly or indirectly, in any manner whatsoever, any amount, price, fee, premium, discount, rebate or credit terms . . . for any drugs which may be dispensed only by prescription."

This statute was one of many that the state used to regulate a professional practice that affected the health, safety, and welfare of the public. The Virginia State Board of Pharmacy had responsibility to set up by-laws and rules that maintained the integrity and public confidence of the pharmaceutical profession. Of particular importance, the Board had the authority to license those practicing pharmacy and to set up educational and experience requirements. It could revoke the license of pharmacists who violated professional standards by, among other things, engaging in fraud, negligence, or unprofessional conduct. To ensure professional conduct and follow the Virginia statute, the Board prohibited advertising of prescription drug prices. In interpreting the rules, some pharmacists even refused to quote prices over the phone.

The organizations suing the Virginia State Board over its policy on licensing and advertising of prescription drugs had many members using prescription drugs. They claimed that the statute violated the First and Fourteenth Amendments to the Constitution. The district court ruled in favor of the Consumer Council, and the Board appealed the ruling up to the Supreme Court.

Legal Issues

The consumer groups claimed harm from the lack of information on drug prices. Prices varied widely across pharmacies in the state, but without easily obtained information due to the advertising ban, consumers would pay extra for their drugs. Worse, their health might suffer if they could not find the drugs they needed at affordable prices. They believed that consumers had the right to know whatever information pharmacists had about a product.

Prescription Drugs

The legal case made by the Consumer Council relied on the First and Fourteenth Amendments to the Constitution. The First Amendment prohibits Congress from making laws that infringe on the freedom of speech, and the Fourteenth Amendment requires states to provide equal protection under the law to all people within their jurisdiction. The consumer groups argued that the First Amendment protects the flow of information on drug prices and the advertising ban enforced by the Virginia State Board of Pharmacy violated the right of citizens to receive information and ideas. In short, if there is a right to advertise, there is a right to receive the advertisements. The Fourteenth Amendment makes the protection of free speech applicable to the states.

In appealing the district court decision, the Board argued that advertising of prescription drugs was a form of commercial speech. Since previous court decisions provided less protection for commercial speech than political speech, they contended, advertising of drug prices did not warrant protection under the First Amendment. For example, previous decisions had allowed a ban on door-to-door selling of magazine subscriptions. Many believed that the First Amendment protected only speech relating to the marketplace of ideas, to social and political issues. Having little to do with commerce, policies on advertising and professional conduct did not violate the right to free speech, in the Board's view.

The Board further argued that it had a legitimate interest in maintaining the professionalism of licensed pharmacists. If advertising became common and pharmacists competed for customers based on prices, it would lead to unprofessional conduct. Emphasizing prices would downgrade the importance of a pharmacist's expertise, discourage careful and time-consuming treatment of the medications, and reduce the time spent discussing problems and issues with customers. The more diligent and skilled pharmacists would be put at a disadvantage by less skilled and diligent pharmacist advertising their lower prices. Advertising might even detract from the professional image of pharmacists, making them more like salespeople than medical practitioners.

Decision

In a decision written by Justice Harry Blackmun, the Supreme Court rejected the appeal and ruled against the Virginia State Board of Pharmacy. The ruling concluded that commercial speech has some protection under the First Amendment, particularly in relation to the right of citizens to receive information. Because "the individual consumer and society in general may have strong interests in the free flow of commercial information," even commercial speech that has an economic rather than a political or artistic motivation deserves protection. Indeed, such information is crucial to the workings of the free-market economy and to older and poorer individuals who need to get their prescriptions filled inexpensively.

In addition, the state's interest in maintaining professionalism cannot justify the ban on advertising. According to the ruling, the ban does more to promote the ignorance of consumers than maintain the professionalism of pharmacists. Besides, many other regulations related to education, experience, and treatment of customers can weed out unqualified pharmacists without having to limit advertising. If the regulations fail to prevent pharmacists from cutting corners in their professional practice, the advertising ban will do little to change that. To the contrary, access to information on prices would help consumers to make better choices for filling prescriptions.

The ruling thus declared the Virginia statute void and prevented the Board from enforcing it. It did not cover all commercial speech. Laws can ban prescription advertisements that are false and misleading or propose illegal transactions. However, they cannot ban truthful information about lawful economic activity without a stronger justification for the suppression of commercial speech.

Impact

The importance of this case comes generally from its protection of commercial speech by the First Amendment, but it also applies more specifically to advertising for prescription drugs. Previous decades had seen little advertising of prescription drugs to consumers. Ads appeared only in medical journals for professionals. However, by allowing advertising of prescription drug prices, this case set the stage for the expansion of DTC advertising. In the short term, few would take advantage of the opportunity to publicize drug prices. Both professionals and the public viewed the practice with distaste. Another decade or two would follow before DTC became more widely accepted. Yet when acceptance came, the number of ads grew quickly. Those opposed could not pass laws to prevent the ads but instead would focus more on how to regulate the ads so that they provide truthful and complete information.

PHARMACEUTICAL RESEARCH AND MANUFACTURERS OF AMERICA V. WALSH, ACTING COMMISSIONER, MAINE DEPARTMENT OF HUMAN SERVICES NO. 01-188 (2003)

Background

States have responsibility to pay for prescription drugs of Medicaid patients, those persons with too little income and too few resources to pay for their own medical costs. The costs of funding Medicaid have risen greatly in recent decades, in part because of higher prices for prescription drugs. Congress attempted to moderate the problem in 1990 with legislation that required drug companies to pay rebates to states for the purchase of prescription drugs for Medicaid patients. According to the legislation, companies wanting to get their drugs approved for Medicaid payments in essence must return part of the payment they received from purchases by Medicaid patients to the states. These rebates reduced the cost of drugs by amounts ranging from 11.1 to 15.1 percent.

Some states lowered their prices even further by passing their own legislation for supplemental rebates. In 2000, Maine established the Maine Rx Program to reduce prescription drug prices for non-Medicaid residents of the state. The program allowed Maine residents to buy prescription drugs from retail pharmacies at the same discount that Medicaid received for its purchases. Any drug manufacturer selling drugs in Maine through a publicly supported financial assistance program (such as Medicaid) must enter into an agreement with the state. In the agreement, the drug manufacturer pays rebates for non-Medicaid purchases that are at least equal to rebates paid to Medicaid under federal legislation. The state government then distributes the rebates to the retail pharmacies, which can sell the drugs to consumers at discounted prices. The rebates reduce prices for prescription drugs for Maine residents who do not have access to "a comparable or superior prescription drug benefit program" like Medicaid.

If a drug company refuses to participate in this supplemental rebate program, the state can take two kinds of actions. It can discourage purchase of their drugs by publicizing the names and products of the company. More important, it can impose prior authorization requirements on drugs used by the state's Medicaid program. Prior authorization means that the state must give approval for a Medicaid patient to receive a drug made by a company not participating in the supplemental rebate program. Physicians tend not to prescribe drugs that require special rather than automatic approval. According to one executive involved in the case, "Imposition of a prior authorization [(PA)] requirement with respect to a particular drug severely curtails access to the drug for covered patients and sharply reduces the drug's market share and sales, as the PA causes a shift of patients to competing drugs of other manufacturers that are not subject to a PA."

The Pharmaceutical Research and Manufacturers of America (PhRMA), a trade group representing companies that make more than 75 percent of brand-name drugs in the United States, sued the state of Maine over the validity of the Maine Rx Program. It moved for a preliminary injunction to stop implementation of the law until the court could hear its suit. The district court approved the preliminary injunction and later ruled in favor of

The Law and Prescription Drugs

PhRMA and against the state law. A court of appeals reversed the decision, but the Supreme Court agreed to hear an appeal over the injunction because the case raised issues of national importance.

Legal Issues

The suit brought by the manufacturers association argued the Maine law was invalid on two grounds. First, it violated the federal Medicaid act. That act aimed to give Medicaid patients the safest and most effective drug therapy available. However, the prior authorization requirement for Medicaid applied to companies not giving rebates to non-Medicaid patients and illegitimately mixed the programs. The prior authorization had nothing to do with serving Medicaid patients but instead aimed to punish companies not giving discount prices to others. The Maine law therefore created an obstacle to properly administering the Medicaid program and to giving the best treatment to its patients. Prior authorization requirements, put in place because a company failed to cooperate in a non-Medicaid program, made it harder for Medicaid patients to get the drugs they needed.

Second, the manufacturer's association claimed that the law effectively regulated out-of-state commerce. It forced out-of-state companies to accept special prices for their products in the state of Maine. Residents and patients in other states therefore would have to pay higher prices to subsidize the rebates in the state of Maine. The law thus gave the state of Maine authority over commerce elsewhere. The commerce clause of the Constitution (Article 1, Section 8, Clause 3) gives Congress the power to regulate commerce among the several states and prevents states from passing laws that control the commerce in other states. For example, Maine could not pass a law that regulates businesses in Massachusetts. According to the petitioners for the injunction, imposing prior authorization on companies does much the same—it regulates activities of drug companies in other states.

Decision

In a ruling written by Justice John Paul Stevens, the Supreme Court rejected the arguments of PhRMA and the decision of the district court. Agreeing with the appeals court, the Supreme Court overturned the preliminary injunction against the Maine law. In concluding that the probability of success of the suit was not high enough to justify the injunction, the decision in essence ruled against the continuation of the suit.

First, the decision rejected the claim made in the appeal that the Maine law regulated interstate commerce. The law says nothing about the price of drugs in other states, a condition needed to violate the commerce clause. Nor does it impose an undue burden on out-of-state competitors. Since opening a manufacturing site in the state of Maine would not help in avoiding the rebate, the law does not discriminate against out-of-state manufacturers. The rules apply equally to in-state and out-of-state companies. Returning rebates only to in-state drug companies would violate the commerce clause, but the law instead gave the rebates to local pharmacists who do not compete with out-of-state drugmakers.

Second, the decision rejected the claim that federal law preempts the Maine statute. The appeal argued that the statute interfered with delivery of drugs to Medicaid patients for no Medicaid-related purpose; rather it aimed to coerce manufacturers into reducing costs for non-Medicaid patients. However, the decision concluded that the Maine statute in fact did have a purpose related to Medicaid. It provided less expensive drugs to needy persons who do not qualify for Medicaid. Also, providing less expensive drugs to non-needy persons will keep them healthier and help prevent them from needing Medicaid benefits later. By helping to keep people off Medicaid rolls, the Maine program reduces Medicaid costs. Even the prior authorization requirement for some Medicaid drugs can lower costs by encouraging physicians to consider other options for treatment. Even if the motivation for prior authorization lies elsewhere, the requirement brings benefits to the Medicaid program. The federal Medicaid law gives states substantial latitude in setting up its programs, and the Maine law fits within this discretion.

Impact

The unwillingness of the Supreme Court to uphold the preliminary injunction against the Maine law allowed it to go into effect. It also gave manufacturers little hope that they could win a suit should they continue to pursue it. The impact goes well beyond the state of Maine. Its importance relates to the ability of states to control the prices of prescription drugs through supplemental rebate programs. Other states could follow Maine's example by implementing similar cost-control programs. Indeed, all but a few states now have some form of supplemental rebate program. Advocates of the program called it a victory for consumers.

WYETH V. LEVINE
NO. 06–1249 (2008)

Background

Wyeth, a large pharmaceutical company, makes a drug for treating nausea called Phenergan. The drug is given either through an IV-drip method or by injection into a vein, but the injection method brings greater risks and must be administered carefully. If the shot accidentally allows the drug to enter a patient's artery, it causes irreversible gangrene. Diana Levine, a Vermont resident, received two injections of Phenergan on April 7, 2000, to relieve her nausea. In the second injection, the drug entered her artery and later caused gangrene. Doctors had to amputate Levine's hand and then her forearm. Levine settled with the health care center and clinician who gave the shot and then sued the maker of the drug.

Her suit against Wyeth alleged that the company failed to properly instruct users of the drug and therefore was negligent and subject to state laws on product liability. Although the label warned about the dangers of injection and called for extreme care in using the method to give the drug, it should have done something more. The suit argued that the label should have instructed clinicians to use the safer IV-drip method. The risks of the injection method are too great, particularly in relation to the problem of nausea, to warrant its use except in exceptional circumstances. After finding the company negligent and the warnings inadequate, a jury awarded damages of $6.4 million.

The judge in the case addressed a key question relating to the Wyeth's defense: Did approval of the labeling by the federal government preempt (or have precedence over) state laws on liability? The judge concluded that federal approval did not preempt the state law. The instructions to the jury said as much. Wyeth's compliance with FDA requirements for labeling did not establish that the warnings were adequate. The Vermont Supreme Court affirmed the verdict and the judge's decision. The importance of the issues and changing views of the FDA led the Supreme Court to consider the case.

Legal Issues

The legal issues relate to the priority given to federal and state laws in ensuring the safety of prescription drugs. Wyeth argued in favor of the priority for federal law. If the FDA approved a drug as safe and effective and approved the labeling as sufficient to ensure safety and effectiveness, then the company could not be negligent in using the FDA-approved drugs and labels. Over the years, the FDA had requested stronger warning labels about the injection method, and Wyeth had complied with requests. In 1998, the FDA approved the label under dispute, instructing Wyeth to use the wording it had approved. The label provided ample notice about the risk of gangrene with multiple warnings, some in boldfaced capital letters. With these warnings and proper instructions, the FDA had concluded that the injection method was safe and effective. Since Congress entrusted an expert agency, the FDA, to make labeling decisions, the actions of the company could not constitute negligence. To the contrary, the company could not have changed the label without violating federal law. It was impossible to meet both the FDA requirements for labeling and the state demands for stronger wording.

Levine argued in contrast for the priority of the state law and the negligence of the company in the failure to sufficiently warn clinicians and patients about the injection method. If the warning had been stronger, Levine would have received the drug with the safer IV-drip method. That the FDA approved one label did not prevent Wyeth from requesting the FDA to allow a stronger label. Wyeth could have complied with federal standards while also taking appropriate actions to protect patients.

Decision

In a 6-3 decision written by Justice John Paul Stevens, the Supreme Court upheld the earlier decisions of the district judge and Vermont Supreme Court. The decision determined that federal law does not preempt the state suit and let the verdict against Wyeth stand. Under federal law, Wyeth could have made certain changes in the drug's label to strengthen the warning and improve safety. There is no evidence that the FDA would have rejected such a request. The manufacturer rather than the FDA bears ultimate responsibility for the contents of a label, and approval by the FDA does not absolve the company of its responsibility for ensuring the safety of its product. Rather than interfering with a federal agency, requests for label changes increase the agency's effectiveness.

In reaching its decision, the Court concluded that Congress did not intend its federal law for approval of prescription drugs to override state laws based on negligence in the failure to warn of dangers. Had Congress intended to preempt state law, it could have included a clause to that effect. Having included no such explicit statement, the law does not justify overturning the state verdict.

Impact

The decision presented a major setback for businesses wanting to use federal law to protect themselves from injury suits brought under state law. It also was a major setback more particularly for the drug companies. With the decision, they became more liable for unintended side effects of prescription drugs. They must take extra care to warn of possible problems and make clear recommendations of safety, even going beyond the requirements of the FDA. Injured patients can file more suits against drug companies as a result. The drug companies see the decision as allowing state courts to inappropriately second-guess the decisions of doctors and FDA scientists. Consumer groups see the decision as an effective way to prod drug companies to do more than the minimum to protect users of the drugs.

Federal Court

UPJOHN V. FINCH
U.S. COURT OF APPEALS, 422 F.2D 944 (1970)

Background

The Kefauver-Harris Drug Control Act of 1962 required that new drugs approved by the FDA be proven both safe and effective. The law represented a major change from the past, when approval required proof of safety only. It also required the FDA to review drugs approved before 1962 for evidence of safety and effectiveness; absent such evidence, the FDA would remove the drug from the market. To implement the review, the National Research Council established a Drug Efficacy Study Group to evaluate the claims of drug manufacturers about the effectiveness of their products.

In considering the effectiveness of seven antibiotic products made by Upjohn, the experts concluded that no high-quality scientific studies had demonstrated that these drugs did what they claimed. The FDA commissioner published a notice that the agency intended to remove these products from the list of acceptable drugs. The order would take effect on September 16, 1969.

Upjohn filed suit in the U.S. District Court of the Western District of Michigan to stop the FDA from removing the drugs and named Robert H. Finch, secretary of health, education, and welfare, and Herbert L. Ley, commissioner of the FDA, as defendants. With sales of the drugs reaching $30 million a year, Upjohn had a considerable stake in the case. The district judge issued an injunction to prevent the FDA from enforcing its order and then considered the merits of the suit.

Legal Issues

Upjohn argued that physicians had been prescribing its products for 12 years, with millions of patients having taken the drugs. Although the company did not have substantial evidence from well-designed scientific studies, the use of the drugs by patients and the continued prescription of the drugs by physicians offered evidence of effectiveness. The FDA rejected the claim that past usage represented high-quality scientific evidence.

A key source of contention came from the definition of *substantial evidence*, the standard of effectiveness needed to continue to sell a drug. The legislation reads

The term "substantial evidence" means evidence consisting of adequate and well-controlled investigations, including clinical investigations, by experts

qualified by scientific training and experience to evaluate the effectiveness of the drug involved, on the basis of which it could fairly and responsibly be concluded by such experts that the drug will have the effect it purports or is represented to have under the conditions of use prescribed, recommended, or suggested in the labeling or purposed labeling thereof.

Upjohn claimed that documents it submitted, largely testimony from clinicians of the benefits of the drugs, demonstrated substantial evidence. Further, the prescription of the medicines by 23,000 physicians over past years demonstrated effectiveness. If the drugs failed to help in treatment, patients would object and physicians would discontinue the prescriptions. Sales and popularity of the drugs would fall. That widespread use and acceptance of the products thus met the standard of the law.

The FDA argued that the law clearly defined substantial evidence in other terms. Companies must demonstrate effectiveness through randomized controlled studies rather than testimony and usage. Physicians often cannot keep up with the latest scientific findings and rely instead on claims from sales reps of the drug companies. Yet, these claims are often unsubstantiated. Given that possibly misleading information and reliance on past habits influence doctors in making prescriptions, use of drugs cannot demonstrate effectiveness. In fact, several in Congress made statements during debate over the legislation about the inability to rely on past practices to determine a drug's effectiveness.

Decision

In reviewing the justifications for the legislation presented by sponsors in Congress and the plain language of the legislation, the judge ruled against Upjohn. A key conclusion stated: "We hold that the record of commercial success of the drugs in question, and their widespread acceptance by the medical profession, do not, standing alone, meet the standards of substantial evidence." The judge also concluded that Upjohn had sufficient notice to perform the studies needed to present evidence of the drug's effectiveness. The lack of such evidence leads to the conclusion that the drugs do not bring the benefits the company claims.

Impact

The decision cleared the way for the FDA in the 1970s to prevent the sale of ineffective drugs. Besides the drugs that Upjohn included in the suit, other marketed drugs without credible evidence of effectiveness could be, after review and notice, removed from the market. The public could then have more trust in the drugs prescribed and sold. Moreover, the decision confirmed the standards for future drug approval set up by Congress and the FDA. Claims made on behalf of drugs needed strong scientific evidence. Such has been the guiding principle in approval for decades now. The decision and the emphasis on proven effectiveness have not eliminated all problems, however. Prescription drugs sold to the public might have proven effectiveness but do no better than cheaper and older drugs. Some experts suggest that studies of a prescription drug compare its effectiveness to that of existing drugs used for the same kind of treatment. Still, with this decision, effectiveness along with safety has become a key component of prescription drug approval.

BIOTECHNOLOGY INDUSTRY ORGANIZATION AND PHARMACEUTICAL RESEARCH AND MANUFACTURERS OF AMERICA V. DISTRICT OF COLUMBIA 2006–1593 (2007)

Background

The Washington, D.C., city council passed legislation that prohibited any patented drug from being sold in the district for an excessive price. The city council believed that high prescription drug prices threatened the health and welfare of the district's residents, and it took the action to restrain these prices. The wording of the law said that prices more than 30 percent greater than any high-income country (e.g., the United Kingdom, Germany, Canada, Australia) where the product is protected by a patent constitute prima facie evidence of excessive price. Prima facie, or on first appearance, means one can assume such prices are excessive unless evidence to the contrary is shown. It puts the burden on companies charging the prices to prove that they are justified by the costs of invention, development, and distribution.

The legislation went into effect on December 10, 2005, with several provisions for enforcement. Any person in the District of Columbia who is adversely affected by the excessive prices could file suit. Remedies included an injunction to stop sales of the prescription drug, and payment of fines, damages, attorneys' fees, or court costs.

Two trade associations filed suits to invalidate the law. The Pharmaceutical Research and Manufacturers Association and the Biotechnology Industry Organization later joined together in a single case. They argued that the law violated the commerce clause of the Constitution and was preempted by federal law. The district court agreed, ruling with the plaintiffs and against the District of Columbia, found that the law violated the Constitution. The district appealed the decision to the U.S. Court of Appeals for the Federal Circuit.

Prescription Drugs

Legal Issues

As in other cases, the legal issues in this one relate to whether state laws conflict with federal laws. In this case, the federal law at issue concerns patents, and the state or district law concerns prices. The district argued that no major conflict exists between the laws. It has the right as a federal territory to regulate the price of goods sold there. Patent laws give companies the exclusive right to market their own discoveries and prevent other companies from using the discoveries without permission. The law does not violate this right: The district makes no effort to compete with drug companies by producing identical products. However, patent laws do not give companies the right to sell whatever they want at whatever price they want. The district can regulate the prices of drugs, much the way it might regulate prices of other products.

The trade association plaintiffs argued that federal law on patents conflicted with and had priority over the district law. Past court rulings have said that state law must yield to congressional enactments if the state law stands as an obstacle to executing the objectives of Congress. In this case, federal law on patents gave exclusive marketing rights to companies owning the patent, including the right to set their own price. The district law on excessive prices presented a clear obstacle to the goals of the federal law.

Decision

The appeals court ruled in favor of the trade associations and against the District of Columbia. While agreeing that states and territories can regulate prices, the decision noted in this case that the district's laws directly conflicted with—and therefore must yield to—federal law. Congress intended with its law that pharmaceutical companies gain financial benefits from their patents through, among other things, setting prices. That encourages innovation and development that ultimately benefit the public and the nation. The Hatch-Waxman Act says as much in the legislation: "Patents are designed to promote innovation by providing the right to exclude others from making, using, or selling an invention. They enable innovators to obtain greater profits than could have been obtained if direct competition existed. These profits act as incentives for innovative activities." At the same time, federal law balances the rights of patent holders with the needs of the public by limiting the patent period of exclusive rights.

The decision reasoned that the district law presents an obstacle to carrying out the goals of the federal law. By penalizing high prices, the law shifts the balance of patent protection from inventors to consumers. "This may be a worthy undertaking on the part of the district government, but it is contrary to the goals established by Congress in the patent laws." Federal patent law therefore preempts the district law.

Impact

Although states may regulate prescription drug prices, this ruling sets limits on how they can do so. Direct control of prices of patented drugs no long remains an option. Other methods of lowering prices might include rebate programs, negotiation to buy at lower prices, and collecting and publishing retail price information. A Maine supplemental rebate program, found legal by the Supreme Court, offers one model of controlling prescription drug costs. States therefore have developed less direct forms of price controls in recent years.

State Court

ERNST V. MERCK
NO. 14-06-00835-CV (2008)

Background

Vioxx, the brand name of the drug rofecoxib made by Merck, reduces inflammation and offers relief for patients with pain from osteoarthritis, menstruation, and other causes. The FDA approved the drug as safe and effective on May 20, 1999. The next year, a study found that patients taking Vioxx experienced significantly higher cardiovascular thrombotic events (blood clots in the vessels of the heart) than patients taking another type of painkiller. After learning of these findings, Merck examined the results of another ongoing study of Vioxx but found no evidence of increased heart problems. It still proposed a label change to the FDA that noted the increased heart risks from Vioxx and warned against use of the drug in patients with certain types of heart disease. In 2004, another study showed significantly higher heart attacks in patients taking Vioxx compared to those taking a placebo. Merck then voluntarily withdrew the drug from the market.

Bob Ernst began taking Vioxx for pain related to tendinitis on September 15, 2000, and died on May 16, 2001. The autopsy attributed the death to cardiac arrhythmia secondary to coronary atherosclerosis. His widow, Carol A. Ernst, sued Merck in Texas state court, alleging that taking Vioxx triggered a blood clot that caused the death of her husband. The jury agreed, saying that the marketing of Vioxx was defective and that Merck was negligent in not warning of the heart problems. The judgment from the case required Merck to pay Mrs. Ernst $26.1 million in damages. Merck appealed the verdict to the Texas Fourteenth Court of Appeals.

Prescription Drugs

Legal Issues

The central legal issue in the appeal concerned whether Vioxx caused the heart attack of Mr. Ernst. Merck said that the lawyers for Mrs. Ernest failed to present sufficient evidence to prove causation. It noted that the autopsy found no blood clot in Mr. Ernst. Research had found that the deaths caused by Vioxx were the results of a thrombotic cardiovascular event, or a sudden cardiac death triggered by a blood clot. Without evidence of a blood clot in the autopsy, Vioxx could not have caused the death. The lawyers for Mrs. Ernst argued that the heart attack of Mr. Ernst was consistent with a blood clot that Vioxx tends to cause. The blood clot might have disappeared through various means before the autopsy. However, its absence cannot rule out the conclusion that a blood clot triggered the heart attack. No other causes appeared consistent with the death: Mr. Ernst was otherwise fit, had not smoked for 15 years, and had previously shown no evidence of heart disease. According to the case against Merck, Vioxx and an associated blood clot remained the most likely cause of the heart attack and death.

Decision

The appeals court needed to review the scientific research and testimony of medical experts to determine if the evidence met the standard of causation. After review, the court decided that the argument in favor of the blood clot cause was largely conjecture. Although experts testified in its favor, they offered little published evidence to support the claim and relied largely on their well-informed but subjective views. Vioxx increases the risk of blood clots in general, but not every time. The absence of clear evidence of blood clots in this particular case meant the suit failed to prove causation. The ruling thus overturned the district court decision and the damages awarded by the jury.

Impact

Given lack of clear evidence that Vioxx caused the death of Mr. Ernst, the case affected the success of other Vioxx suits. The victory for Merck in the appeal, despite the willingness of an earlier jury to award damages, indicated the difficulty future Vioxx suits would have in winning cases against the company. The decision helped discourage lawyers from pursuing other Vioxx cases. Merck and plaintiff lawyers had already agreed to preliminary terms for a settlement, and the decision pushed plaintiffs to finalize the agreement. The company has set aside $4.58 billion for payments to those who have enrolled in the settlement program. The settlement amounts range from a minimum of $5,000 to several million for those most harmed by the drug.

[1] FDA, "The 1938 Food, Drug, and Cosmetic Act," History of the FDA. Available online. URL: http://www.fda.gov/oc/history/historyoffda/section2.html. Downloaded April 18, 2009.

[2] Syamala Ariyanchira, "BioMarket Trends: Orphan Drug Arena Driven by Biologics," *Genetic Engineering and Biotechnology News*. Available online. URL: http://www.genengnews.com/articles/chitem_print.aspx?aid=2318&chid=0. Posted January 1, 2008.

[3] U.S. Food and Drug Administration, "The FDA Modernization Act of 1997," FDA Backgrounder. Available online. URL: http://www.fda.gov/opacom/backgrounders/modact.htm. Posted November 21, 1997.

[4] 110th Congress, "Public Law 110-85," Government Printing Office. Available online. URL: http://frwebgate.access.gpo.gov/cgi-bin/getdoc.cgi?dbname=110_cong_public_laws&docid=f:publ085.110. Downloaded April 18, 2009.

[5] "Title 21 Database," U.S. Food and Drug Administration. Available online. URL: http://www.accessdata.fda.gov/scripts/cdrh/cfdocs/cfcfr/cfrsearch.cfm. Downloaded April 18, 2009.

[6] National Conference of State Legislatures, "Pharmaceuticals: Facts, Policies, and NCSL Resources," NCSL. Available online. URL: http://www.ncsl.org/programs/health/pharm.htm. Updated April 1, 2009.

[7] National Conference of State Legislatures, "Recent Medicaid Prescription Drug Laws and Strategies, 2001–2009," Health Program. Available online. URL: http://www.ncsl.org/programs/health/medicaidrx.htm. Downloaded April 18, 2009.

[8] National Conference of State Legislatures, "Marketing and Direct-to-Consumer Advertising (DTCA) of Pharmaceuticals," Health Program. Available online. URL: http://www.ncsl.org/programs/health/rxads.htm. Downloaded April 18, 2009.

[9] National Conference of State Legislatures, "Prescription Drug Laws in Maine," Health Program. Available online. URL: http://www.ncsl.org/programs/health/pharm-me.htm#Maine. Downloaded April 18, 2009.

CHAPTER 3

―――――――

CHRONOLOGY

This chapter presents a time line of significant events relating to prescription drugs. It lists passages of laws, important discoveries, developments in regulations, and mergers involving pharmaceutical companies.

1820

- In an effort to reduce the misuse and misrepresentation of drugs, 11 physicians meet in Washington, D.C., to create a U.S. Pharmacopeia that lists available drugs and information on proper ingredients and quality.

1843

- The Beecham Group, a pharmaceutical company founded in England by Thomas Beecham, starts with the sale of Beecham's Pills, a laxative.

1846

- Lewis Caleb Beck calls attention to the misuse of medications and the misleading information about their benefits in *Adulteration of Various Substances Used in Medicine and the Arts.*

1848

- Congress responded to concerns about impurities in drugs by passing an act that requires the U.S. Customs Service to inspect and stop from entry any adulterated drugs imported from overseas.

1849

- Cousins Charles Pfizer and Charles Erhardt found Pfizer in Brooklyn, New York. The company begins with several successful drugs and popular food additives. Some 150 years later, it will have become the world's largest pharmaceutical company.

Chronology

1860

- Reflecting views on the ineffectiveness and dangers of many drugs and patent medicines, the dean of the Harvard Medical School, Oliver Wendell Holmes, Sr., says that if all available drugs "could be sunk to the bottom of the sea, it would be better for mankind, and all the worse for the fishes."

1876

- Eli Lilly founds a pharmaceutical company under his own name that pioneers a gelatin capsule to hold medicine and fruit flavoring for liquid medicine. The company later became successful in the discovery of new drugs and quality control in manufacturing.

1880

- Two Americans, Silas Mainville Burroughs and Henry Solomon Wellcome, found Burroughs Wellcome in London. After more than a century of success, the company will merge with several others to form GlaxoSmithKline.

1884

- Burroughs Wellcome begins selling medicine in tablet form under the trademark name Tabloid. Until then nearly all drugs took the form of powders or liquids.

1886

- Robert Wood Johnson and his brothers found Johnson & Johnson, which begins making sterile products for use in surgery and treatment of wounds and later expands to make a variety of consumer products and prescription drugs.

1896

- Burroughs Wellcome sets up one of the first research labs to develop new drugs, a strategy other companies will come to follow.

1901

- Revealing problems of safety in the drug industry, nine children in Camden, New Jersey, die from tetanus after receiving a commercially produced vaccine for smallpox.

1902

- Poor quality-control standards in drug manufacturing led to the death of 13 children in St. Louis from a contaminated diphtheria antitoxin.

- With the support of President Theodore Roosevelt, Congress passes the Biologics Control Act to require the purity and safety of vaccines and serums.

1903

- Dr. Lyman F. Kebler becomes director of the drug laboratory in the Bureau of Chemistry, a government agency that evaluates the safety and purity of drug products.

1904

- Glaxo is founded in New Zealand, originally to sell baby food, but later becomes a major drug company.

1905

- An exposé of the patent drug industry called "The Great American Fraud" by Samuel Hopkins Adams appears in *Collier's* magazine.
- The American Medical Association sets up a program that requires companies advertising drug products in the association's magazine to submit their drug for a review by experts.

1906

- The Pure Food and Drug Act prohibits interstate commerce in adulterated drugs but requires the government to prove a product is unsafe before removing it from the market.

1911

- In *U.S. v. Johnson*, the Supreme Court rules that the Pure Food and Drug Act did not prohibit false claims about the benefits of a drug, only false claims about the ingredients.
- Dr. Hamilton Wright, the first U.S. opium commissioner, writes, "Of all the nations of the world, the United States consumes most habit-forming drugs per capita. Opium, the most pernicious drug known to humanity, is surrounded, in this country, with far fewer safeguards than any nation in all Europe fences it with."

1912

- In response to the 1911 Supreme Court ruling, Congress passes the Sherley amendment to prohibit labeling of medicines with false claims about therapeutic value that intend to defraud consumers.

Chronology

1914

- Congress passes the Harrison Narcotics Act to control the use of opiates and cocaine for strict medical purposes and deal with the growing problem of addiction.

1927

- The Food, Drug, and Insecticide Administration is created from the Bureau of Chemistry.

1928

- The British bacteriologist Alexander Fleming discovers penicillin, an effective antibiotic that is derived from mold.

1930

- The Food and Drug Administration (FDA) is created from the Food, Drug, and Insecticide Administration.

1937

- Making clear the urgency of passing a new law to protect drug users, 107 persons, mostly children, die from a contaminated medicine used to treat streptococcal infections. The drugmaker had mistakenly used a poisonous chemical to put the drug in liquid form.

1938

- Passage of the Food, Drug, and Cosmetics Act requires companies to demonstrate the safety of their drugs and receive approval from the FDA before marketing them. Further, the law requires that labels give directions for use and warn of any habit-forming properties.

1941

- The FDA receives responsibility for certifying the purity and effectiveness of insulin for treating diabetes.

1942

- Penicillin, a highly effective antibiotic discovered in 1928, begins to be manufactured for sale as a drug.

1945

- The FDA receives responsibility for testing the safety and effectiveness of penicillin products.

Prescription Drugs

1951

- The Durham-Humphrey amendment, known as the prescription drug amendment, sets standards to distinguish prescription drugs that require supervision by a licensed health practitioner from less risky and harmful over-the-counter (OTC) drugs.

1960

- Dr. Frances Kelsey, a newly hired drug reviewer for the FDA, refuses to approve thalidomide, an antinausea sedative drug used for several years by pregnant women in Europe. After she requests more information on side effects of the drug, research emerges to show that thalidomide causes birth defects in children of the pregnant mothers taking the drug.

1962

- Dr. Frances Kelsey receives the president's award for distinguished federal civil service from President Kennedy for blocking approval of thalidomide.
- Congress passes the Kefauver-Harris Drug Control Act, a major change in policy that requires drugs approved by the FDA to be both safe and effective.
- The FDA receives responsibility for regulating the advertising of prescription drugs, while the Federal Trade Commission regulates advertising for OTC drugs.

1964

- Congress creates Medicare, a public health insurance program for elderly persons that covers hospital stays and clinical services but not prescription drugs.

1966

- As required by the Kefauver-Harris Drug Control Act, the FDA begins to review drugs approved as safe from 1938 to 1962 to see if they can demonstrate effectiveness as well as safety.

1968

- Experts conclude that no scientific evidence exists demonstrating the effectiveness of either Panalba, first used in 1957, or several other similar drugs made by Upjohn. The FDA notifies Upjohn that it will no longer allow sales of the drugs.
- For the first time, the FDA requires a patient package insert (PPI) with a medicine. The PPI explains how to use the medication properly, iden-

tifies possible side effects, and tells users to contact their physician if problems result. The medicine, isoproterenol, treats heart problems and asthma with an inhaler device.

- A new agency in the Department of Justice, the Bureau of Narcotics and Dangerous Drugs, merges several organizations previously responsible for control of drugs used unlawfully.

1970

- The Supreme Court rules in *Upjohn v. Finch* that the FDA properly removed Panalba and other similar antibiotic drugs from the market because of a lack of scientific evidence of their effectiveness and that past use by doctors and patients does not demonstrate the drugs work as purported.
- The FDA requires a PPI for birth control pills, first approved for public use in 1960.
- The drug company Ciba-Geigy is formed from a merger of Ciba with J. R. Geigy.
- The Comprehensive Drug Abuse and Control Act gives order to a confusing set of laws about illegal drug use by classifying drugs based on their potential for abuse and setting criminal punishments for five different classes or schedules of drugs.

1973

- An executive order from President Richard Nixon creates the Drug Enforcement Administration, a new federal agency that has responsibility for enforcing drug laws.

1976

- The Supreme Court rules in favor of the Virginia Citizens Consumer Council, which sued the Virginia Board of Pharmacy for prohibiting pharmacists from advertising drug prices. The Court concludes that the public has the right to know price information about prescription drugs.

1980

- The Bayh-Dole Act, or the University and Small Business Patent Procedures Act, gives universities, small businesses, and nonprofit organizations the intellectual ownership of property, including new drugs, that they discover and develop with government funding.

1981

- Ronald Reagan begins his presidency with a mandate for lowering taxes and removing government regulations and restrictions on business. The favorable climate for business and loosening of government regulations will contribute to the success of the drug industry in the next decades.

- Boots Pharmaceuticals, a British company with a subsidiary in the United States, sponsors one of the first direct-to-consumer (DTC) print advertisements for its prescription pain reliever, Rufen.

1983

- The FDA calls for a moratorium on DTC drug ads while it studies the issue. Given the FDA's power to regulate the content of the ads, drug companies follow the voluntary moratorium.
- The Orphan Drug Act encourages companies to develop drugs to help patients with rare disorders by offering tax incentives and exclusive sales rights.

1984

- The Hatch-Waxman Act, or the Drug Price Competition and Patent Term Restoration Act, makes it easier for generic drugs to get approval from the FDA but also allows drug companies to extend their patents when the FDA approval process delays the sales of patented drugs.

1985

- The FDA decides to allow DTC ads if they provide the same information as ads directed at physicians, including a fair balance of facts about the drug and a brief summary of possible side effects and risks.

1987

- The FDA sets up new rules to make it easier for patients with serious diseases to participate in studies on experimental drugs.
- Congress passes the Prescription Drug Marketing Act to safeguard the quality of drugs used by consumers. It bans the sale of drug coupons, restricts the reimportation of prescription drugs, and makes it illegal for American citizens to go to other countries such as Canada and Mexico to buy drugs for use in the United States.

1988

- In a successful ad campaign, Merrill-Dow, the maker of a new antihistamine called Seldane, does not mention the drug by name. The ads merely say that a new drug for allergies is out, it does not make users drowsy, and visit a doctor for more information. By not naming the drug, the ad sidesteps the FDA's requirement to summarize its risks and side effects.

Chronology

1991

- The FDA publishes new regulations to accelerate reviews of drugs for life-threatening diseases.

1992

- Congress passes the Prescription Drug User Fee Act, which requires the pharmaceutical industry to pay user fees to the FDA in return for faster approval time. With the funds, the FDA will hire new workers for the Center for Drug Evaluation and Research and the Center for Biologics Evaluation Research.
- The American Medical Association votes to rescind its opposition to DTC ads.

1993

- The psychiatrist Peter Kramer publishes *Listening to Prozac*, a book about the first SSRI antidepressant that contributes to the popularity of the drug and other SSRIs.

1995

- Drug companies spend $313 million on DTC advertising—26 times greater than the amount spent only six years earlier.
- GlaxoWellcome is formed with the merger of Glaxo with Glaxo Canada and Burroughs Wellcome.

1996

- Novartis is formed from the merger of two Swiss companies, Ciba-Geigy and Sandoz Laboratories.

1997

- The FDA approves the diabetes drug Rezulin for sale, but by the end of the year evidence that Rezulin causes liver failure leads the FDA to recommend that patients taking the drug undergo regular liver enzyme tests to identify any problems.
- An article in the *New England Journal of Medicine* reports that 24 patients taking fen-phen, a combination of two weight-reduction drugs, have an unusual form of heart disease involving abnormalities in the heart valves.
- The FDA approves Baycol, an anticholesterol statin drug made by Bayer. It costs less than competitors but turns out to have a rare but serious side effect that destroys muscle tissue.
- The FDA Modernization Act reauthorizes the Prescription Drug User Fee Act and the system of having drug companies subsidize reviews of

new drugs. It also allows critically ill patients to use promising drugs still undergoing review and not yet approved and allows drug companies to make information available on unapproved, or off-label, uses of drugs.

1999

- The FDA approves Vioxx, an anti-inflammation drug for treatment of osteoarthritis and some other conditions that cause acute pain.
- The FDA finalizes regulations on DTC advertising that require broadcast ads to include a brief summary of both risks and benefits or make provision for distributing FDA-approved information on risks and benefits to consumers.
- Responding to a suit against the FDA by the Washington Legal Foundation, a district court judge rules that the FDA cannot restrict truthful, non-misleading speech in DTC advertising.
- AstraZeneca is formed from the merger of two drug companies, Swedish AB and the British Zeneca Group.

2000

- The FDA requires Warner-Lambert, the maker of the diabetes drug Rezulin, to withdraw the drug from the market after evidence grows that it caused hundreds of users to die from liver failure.
- A study published in the *New England Journal of Medicine* finds that patients taking Vioxx had four times as many heart attacks over 12 months as patients taking Aleve, an OTC pain reliever.
- President Clinton signs a law to allow reimportation of prescription drugs but Secretary of Health and Human Services Donna Shalala concludes that reimportation would not be safe, effectively ending the program before it started.
- Pfizer merges with Warner-Lambert and gains the rights to the highly successful anticholesterol statin drug Lipitor.
- GlaxoSmithKline is formed with the merger of GlaxoWellcome and SmithKline Beecham

2001

- Reflecting the continued fast rate of growth in DTC advertising, drug companies spend $2.38 billion on these kinds of ads.
- *August 8:* Bayer withdraws its statin drug Baycol from the market after analysis of new data shows that 31 patients taking the drug had died from rhabdomyolysis, a rare disease that destroys muscle tissue.

2002

- Congress reauthorizes the Prescription Drug User Fee Act but adds more funds for surveillance of the safety of approved drugs.

- Pfizer merges with Pharmacia, which had earlier merged with Upjohn and G. D. Searle.
- Congress passes the Best Pharmaceuticals for Children Act, which encourages drug companies to carry out more studies on the benefits and side effects of drugs taken by children.
- *April:* The FDA changes the warning labels on Vioxx to highlight increased risks of heart problems.
- *May:* In *Ernst v. Merck,* a Texas woman sues Merck, maker of the pain reliever Vioxx, claiming that the drug caused the fatal heart attack of her husband at age 59.

2003

- The Federal Trade Commission sues Bristol-Myers Squibb for blocking the sale of generic drugs, particularly the cancer drugs Platinol and Taxol and the antianxiety drug BuSpar. In a settlement, the company agrees not to engage in these types of unlawful behaviors.
- Congress passes the Medicare Prescription Drug Improvement and Modernization Act to give new assistance to program participants in buying prescription drugs. The new program relies on a mix of government funding, cost-sharing from beneficiaries, and services from private insurance companies.
- The FDA requires Wyeth to add a new warning to its hormone-replacement drug Prempro about risks of heart attacks, strokes, breast cancer, and blood clots associated with its use.
- The Supreme Court allows a Maine law to go into effect that requires drug companies participating in the state Medicaid program to pay supplemental rebates. The rebates reduce the costs of prescription drugs for non-Medicaid drug users.

2004

- Sanofi-Aventis is formed from the takeover of Aventis by Sanofi-Synthélabo.
- *June 2:* New York attorney general Eliot Spitzer sues the maker of Paxil, GlaxoSmithKline, for fraud in concealing the dangers of the drug for children under age 17 (the suit is settled when the company agrees to publish all its results).
- *September 30:* After obtaining new evidence that Vioxx doubled the risk of heart attack or stroke, Merck voluntarily removes the drug from the market.

2005

- Spending on DTC ads for prescription drugs reaches $4.2 billion.
- A Texas jury awards the widow of a man who died of a heart attack while using Vioxx $253.4 million in damages.

Prescription Drugs

- Responding to criticism over high prices for prescription drugs, a trade organization for the pharmaceutical industry, the Pharmaceutical Research and Manufacturers of America (PhRMA), publishes a booklet that defends the pricing as fair and beneficial for consumers.

2006

- A panel of experts brought together to investigate prescription drug errors in hospitals reports that medication errors harm 1.5 million people each year and increase medical care costs by $3.5 billion.
- Reversing the position it took in 1992, the American Medical Association calls for a moratorium on DTC ads for newly approved drugs and suggests new, stricter guidelines on what ads can say when they are allowed.
- *January 1:* The new Medicare prescription benefit program goes into effect.

2007

- The FDA approves only 19 new prescription drugs, the lowest level in over 20 years.
- *August 1:* A U.S. court of appeals strikes down a Washington, D.C., law to prohibit any patented drug from being sold in the district for an excessive price. The ruling concludes that the law presents an obstacle to federal patent law and therefore is void.
- *September 27:* President George W. Bush signs the Food and Drug Amendments Act, which reauthorizes the payment of fees by drug companies to cover the costs of approving new drugs but adds more fees to review drug advertising.
- *October 8:* Responding to the growth of DTC advertising of prescription drugs, the FDA announces that it will study consumer reactions to drug ads.
- *November 18:* The newborn twins of actor Dennis Quaid nearly die when they mistakenly receive adult rather than infant doses of a blood-thinning drug.

2008

- The FDA approves 24 brand-new medicines, the most in three years, but the new medicines produce lower sales than other new medicines did in the preceding decade.
- Congress introduces the Comparative Effectiveness Research Act to create an institute to present unbiased information to health care practitioners. The proposed institute will review and publicize evidence on how to best treat diseases, disorders, and other health conditions.

114

Chronology

- *January 1–March 31:* The FDA receives nearly 21,000 reports of serious drug reactions, including more than 4,800 deaths.
- *February 19:* The judge on a successful suit brought by three women with breast cancer against Wyeth for its hormone replacement drug Prempro sets final damages at $58 million—$23 million to compensate the women and $35 million in punitive damages.
- *March 3:* In *Warner-Lambert v. Kimberly Kent,* the Supreme Court affirms a lower court decision allowing a Michigan class-action suit to proceed against Pfizer over the diabetes drug Rezulin.
- *April 21:* The FDA sets the number of deaths from contaminated doses of Heparin at 81. The main ingredient of the blood-thinning drug comes from pig intestines processed in China.
- *May:* A committee hearing in the House of Representatives examines what representatives and witnesses describe as misleading ads sponsored by drug companies for their prescription drugs.
- *May 14:* A Texas appeals court overturns the jury verdict of *Ernst v. Merck.* The jury had ruled against Merck, the maker of Vioxx, but the appeals court concludes that the evidence is insufficient to show that the drug caused the death of the husband of the woman who sued.
- *June 19:* Four companies, Johnson & Johnson, Pfizer, Merck, and Schering-Plough, agree to a six-month moratorium on advertising of new drugs and to modify payment of celebrities and experts who endorse their products.
- *September 5:* The FDA names 20 prescription drugs under investigation for safety problems. The agency aims with the list to inform health care providers and patients at an early stage of investigation about possible risks from the drugs.
- *September 25:* The FDA sends five warning letters to drug companies about false, misleading, or incomplete promotional materials relating to use of prescription drugs for children with attention deficit/hyperactivity disorder.

2009

- *January 6:* A government report from the Centers for Medicare and Medicaid Services shows that retail prescription drug spending rose by 4.6 percent in 2007, the lowest pace since 1963. The slower increase in spending results from lower drug prices, reliance on generic drugs, and safety concerns about some drugs.
- *January 26:* Pfizer agrees to buy Wyeth for $68 billion, making the world's largest pharmaceutical company even larger but also resulting in job cuts to improve the performance of the combined company.
- *February 3:* The FDA sues Solvay Pharmaceuticals to block the maker of a brand-name testosterone drug from paying three competitors for not

making and selling cheaper generic versions of the drug. The FDA says that the payments to the competitors violate the Hatch-Waxman Act of 1984, a law that aimed to increase consumer access to generic drugs.

- **March 4:** A Supreme Court decision, *Wyeth v. Levine*, concludes that federal law does not preempt or override a state suit against the drug company Wyeth. The decision leaves the drug company liable under state laws for the harm caused by one of its drug products.
- **March 9:** Merck and Schering-Plough announce a merger, making the combined company one of the largest pharmaceutical companies in the world. Merck pays $41.1 billion for the smaller company.
- **March 12:** Roche agrees to purchase Genentech, a biotech company that developed cancer drugs through genetic engineering, for $48 billion.
- **April 16:** The *Wall Street Journal* reports that the spending on DTC ads by drug companies fell by 8 percent in 2008, the first decline in more than a decade.
- **May 8:** Hackers gain access to prescription drug records of 8 million Virginia patients listed in the state's Drug Monitoring Program and cause concern about the release of private information.
- **May 11:** The deaths of two patients in Delaware prompt review of the blood-thinner drug Heparin, a drug that caused 81 deaths in 2008 when tainted ingredients were imported from China.
- **June 22:** An agreement between President Obama and the pharmaceutical drug industry proposes to reduce the cost of prescription drugs for Medicare beneficiaries by partially covering the "donut hole," or the out-of-pocket expenses paid when purchases cost more than $2,700 and less than $6,154.
- **June 22:** The pharmaceutical industry, represented by its trade group, the Pharmaceutical Research and Manufacturers Association (PhRMA), agrees to spend $80 billion dollars to reduce prescription drug costs.
- **June 25:** The singer Michael Jackson dies from taking a powerful anesthetic called propofol. Jackson had used the drug at home to help him sleep, but experts say the drug should only be used in hospitals under continuous monitoring.
- **June 30:** An expert panel convened by the FDA says that high doses of acetaminophen, the ingredient in Tylenol, are dangerous, sometimes deadly. The panel recommends banning Vicodin and Percocet, analgesic (pain-killing) drugs that combine acetaminophen with opiate-based products.
- **August 5:** The drugmakers Merck and Schering-Plough agree to pay $41.5 million to settle a series of lawsuits over their cholesterol-lowering statin drug Vytorin. The lawsuits claimed the companies withheld evidence that Vytorin was no more effective than older and less expensive drugs.
- **October 26:** A report from the U.S. Government Accountability Office says that the FDA has allowed ineffective drugs to stay on the market.

The drugs, approved under an accelerated evaluation program, were found in subsequent studies to have little benefit, but lack of follow-up from the FDA allowed their sales to continue.

- *November 3:* Reflecting a trend toward reduction and consolidation in the drug industry, the drugmaker Johnson & Johnson announces it will cut 7,000 to 8,200 jobs worldwide.

2010

- *February 4:* The Los Angeles County Coroner rules that prescription drugs probably played a role in the death of actress Brittany Murphy at age 32 on December 20, 2009.
- *February 18:* The FDA warns that popular asthma drugs Advair, Symbicort, Foradil, and Serevent, should be used only when other medications do not work, and even then for the shortest time possilbe. Studies find an increase in adverse events from the drugs.
- *March 23:* President Obama signs a health care bill passed by the House and Senate (formally named the Patient Protection and Affordable Care Act). Among its many provisions to extend health care coverage, the new law will give a rebate to Medicare recipients whose prescription drugs costs have reached a coverage gap called the donut hole. The law will also impose fees on drug companies to help reduce the cost of prescription drugs. The drug industry supported the bill and is expected to benefit from greater government spending on prescription drugs for Medicare recipients and for persons newly covered by health insurance.
- *April 27:* The drug company AstraZeneca agrees to pay $520 million to the federal government and state Medicaid programs for illegal marketing of Seroquel, its high-selling drug for schizophrenia. The government alleges that the company marketed the drug for unapproved or off-label uses, such as the treatment of anxiety, depression, aggression, and Alzheimer's disease. AstraZeneca denies the allegations but agrees to the settlement with the government.

CHAPTER 4

BIOGRAPHICAL LISTING

This chapter contains brief biographical sketches of legislators, activists, government leaders, and scholars who have been involved in issues concerning prescription drugs.

Marcia Angell, physician, former editor in chief of the *New England Journal of Medicine*, and senior lecturer in the department of social medicine at Harvard Medical School. She has been a vocal critic of the pharmaceutical industry, arguing that the companies focus on profits at the expense of health, manipulate scientific research, and deceive the public with their advertising. She has also criticized physicians and researchers for their close ties to the drug industry and potential lack of independence in their research.

Jerry Avorn, professor of medicine at Harvard Medical School and chief of the division of pharmacoepidemiology and pharmacoeconomics at Brigham and Women's Hospital. An expert on how physicians prescribe drugs, he developed a new approach to help give accurate and cost-effective prescriptions that, ironically, is based on the communication strategies of the drug companies. His writings highlight the trade-offs in using drugs to help people while at the same time controlling costs and limiting side effects.

Birch Bayh, Democratic senator from Indiana from 1963 to 1981. With Republican senator Robert Dole, he cosponsored the Bayh-Dole Act of 1980 or the University and Small Business Patent Procedures Act, which gave universities and small businesses ownership of patents resulting from projects funded by the federal government. The major drug companies benefited as well: They can license new drugs from the universities and small businesses that discovered them.

Silas Mainville Burroughs, American pharmacist who founded the highly successful drug company Burroughs Wellcome with Henry Wellcome. The company, established in London in 1880, produced medicine in a compressed form called a Tabloid and eventually a tablet. The invention allowed drugs to be easily taken in standard doses. The company was one of the first to establish a research lab to develop new drugs. In the 1990s and 2000s, the company merged with several others to create Glaxo-SmithKline.

George W. Bush, Republican president of the United States from 2001 to 2009. As president, he signed a major piece of legislation, the Medicare Drug Prescription Act of 2003, that provided new coverage for Medicare participants in purchasing prescription drugs. His administration opposed price controls on prescription drugs, arguing that allowing companies to set their own prices encouraged innovation and the availability of new drugs. It also reaffirmed past decisions not to allow reimportation of prescription drugs from other countries because of concerns over the safety and quality of the drugs.

Walter Campbell, chief of the Food and Drug Administration on its establishment in 1930 to 1940. As chief, he advocated strongly for updated drug regulation laws, and his efforts contributed to the passage of the 1938 Federal Food, Drug, and Cosmetics Act.

Robert Dole, Republican senator from Kansas from 1969 to 1996 and presidential candidate in 1996. With Democratic senator Birch Bayh, he cosponsored the Bayh-Dole Act of 1980 or the University and Small Business Patent Procedures Act, which gave universities and small businesses ownership of patents that resulted from funding by the federal government. The major drug companies benefited as well: They can license new drugs from the universities and small businesses that discovered them.

Charles Erhardt, cofounder with his cousin Charles Pfizer of the pharmaceutical company Pfizer. Erhardt's background in Germany as a confectioner helped in manufacturing pleasant-tasting medicines. The company's first success was to make a palatable form of the drug santonin used to treat parasitic worms, a common problem in the 1800s. Over the next century and a half, the company grew into the world's largest pharmaceutical maker.

Andrew C. von Eschenbach, former director of the National Cancer Institute and FDA commissioner from 2005 to 2009. As commissioner, he played a major role in the 2007 amendments to modernize the agency and improve the process of regulating the safety of drugs. He also faced critics who accused the Bush administration of letting politics influence science policy and failing to do enough to prevent the contamination of drugs made in foreign factories.

Martha Farah, director of the Center for Cognitive Neuroscience Research at the University of Pennsylvania. As a specialist in vision and memory, she joined in a debate over the acceptable uses of prescription drugs by arguing in favor of taking pills to improve brain function. Although concerned about the potential for abuse and harmful side effects, she suggests that people need not have an illness to benefit from prescription drugs.

Brett Favre, future hall of fame NFL quarterback who revealed his addiction to the prescription painkiller Vicodin. In 1996, Favre entered a rehab facility for the addiction, which came from the use of pain pills to deal with numerous football injuries and related surgeries.

Margaret Hamburg, FDA commissioner. She is a graduate of the Harvard Medical School, studied pharmacology at the National Institute of Mental Health, and served formerly as the New York City health commissioner. Hamburg faces several contentious issues in her new position that relate to reimporting prescription drugs, balancing the need to get new drugs to the public with the need to ensure safety, and implementing proposals for national health care. She may also have to deal with proposals from Congress to increase the FDA budget and perhaps even to split the FDA into two agencies—one for food and one for drugs.

Orrin Hatch, Republican senator from Utah since 1977. In an unusual form of cooperation across parties, Hatch cosponsored a bill in 1984 with liberal Democratic representative Henry Waxman called the Drug Price Competition and Patent Restoration Act. The bill helped consumers by making it easier and quicker for less expensive generic drugs to get approval from the FDA. It helped drug companies by allowing their patents to be extended when the development and approval process for the original drugs took a particularly long time.

Oliver Wendell Holmes, Sr., physician at the Harvard Medical School from 1847 to 1882 and opponent of patent drugs. In one quote he said that destroying available drugs would be better for mankind. His views and those of other physicians would lead to reform of drug use for medical purposes.

Hubert Humphrey, Democratic senator from Minnesota from 1949 to 1964, and again from 1971 to 1978, and vice president of the United States from 1965 to 1969. A pharmacist before going into politics, Humphrey cosponsored the 1951 Prescription Drug Amendment that defined the distinction between prescription drugs that required supervision by a physician and OTC drugs. The law remains a key to the system of prescription drugs today.

Michael Jackson, one of the world's most popular singers and performers, who died in 2009 from misuse of a powerful anesthetic to help him sleep. Jackson had a history of abuse of prescription painkillers, caused initially by injuries sustained during a rehearsal accident that set his hair on fire. The inappropriate use of propofol, the drug that killed him, has led authorities to charge Jackson's personal physician with manslaughter.

Robert Wood Johnson, founder with his two brothers of Johnson & Johnson in 1886. The company began making sterile products for use in surgery and treatment of injuries and wounds. The company later became highly successful in making a variety of consumer products and prescription drugs.

Lyman F. Kebler, director of the drug laboratory in the Bureau of Chemistry, one of the first U.S. government agencies dedicated to the safety and purity of drug products. A former chemist at Smith, Kline and French, he became an expert on drug purity and standardization. While leading the drug laboratory, he set up standards to evaluate and improve the quality of drugs, and he played an important role in implementing the 1906 Pure Food and Drug Act.

Estes Kefauver, Democratic senator from Tennessee from 1949 to 1963, and vice presidential candidate in the 1956 election. He was known for his concern about the concentration of economic power among corporations and was an early critic of high prices for prescription drugs and the pharmaceutical industry. He cosponsored the Drug Control Act of 1962, which required that drugs approved by the FDA be proven both safe and effective.

Frances Kelsey, an FDA pharmacologist from 1960 to 2005 who became famous for her work as a drug reviewer. After being hired in 1960, she began to review the safety of the drug thalidomide, a sedative that eased the nausea of pregnant women and became popular in Europe between 1957 and 1961. She withheld approval of the drug and requested further study of side effects. Her caution was vindicated when evidence came from Europe that thalidomide caused severe birth defects. She helped shape the 1962 legislation to improve requirements for safety and effectiveness of prescription drugs.

David Kessler, physician and commissioner of the Food and Drug Administration from 1990 to 1997. While commissioner, he opposed DTC advertising and issued draft regulations for these ads. Later, when serving as dean of Yale Medical School, he came to support advertising of prescription drugs as a way to get information to the public.

Peter Kramer, psychiatrist, faculty member at Brown University, and author of the best-selling book *Listening to Prozac.* The book helped publicize the effectiveness of the SSRI depression medication Prozac, suggesting that it helped change people's personalities as well as deal with their depression. It also contributed to the widespread use (or overuse according to critics) of Prozac and newer SSRI antidepressants.

Michael O. Leavitt, former governor of Utah and secretary of Health and Human Services in the Bush administration from 2005 to 2009. Believing that the free market can do a better job than the government in setting prices, he opposed congressional legislation authorizing the Department of Health and Human Services to negotiate with drug companies to obtain lower prices for Medicare prescription drugs.

Prescription Drugs

Heath Ledger, Australian actor who died at age 28 from a toxic combination of prescription drugs. Discovered unconscious at his New York City apartment on January 22, 2008, Ledger died from an accidental overdose of legitimately prescribed drugs, including oxycodone, hydrocodone, diazepam, temazepam, alprazolam, and doxylamine. While ruling the death accidental, the medical examiner attributed the ultimate cause to abuse of prescription drugs.

Eli Lilly, a pharmacist who founded a company under his own name in 1876. He pioneered two highly successful products: a gelatin capsule to hold medicine and fruit flavoring for liquid medicine. His company devoted resources to discovery and quality control and provided a model for research and development in the drug industry. The company became one of the world's most successful makers of pharmaceuticals.

Rush Limbaugh, highly successful radio host and personality who was addicted for many years to painkillers, particularly OxyContin. A report in 2003 that he was under investigation for illegally obtaining prescription painkillers led him to enter inpatient treatment for the addiction. He said that he became addicted after taking the drugs to deal with back pain. He was later arrested on the charge of doctor shopping—a way to get excess drugs from multiple physicians. The charges were later dropped in a settlement.

Mark McClellan, a physician and economist who led the FDA from 2002 to 2004. As FDA commissioner in the Bush administration, he opposed government regulation of the pharmaceutical industry and criticized European countries for inhibiting drug innovation with price controls.

Richard Nixon, Republican president of the United States from 1969 to 1974. Known as a crusader against the illegal use of drugs, he signed legislation that classified many prescription drugs as controlled substances and regulated their manufacture and distribution. In 1973, he created the Drug Enforcement Administration to enforce the law, and the agency still has responsibility for controlling the illegal sale and use of prescription drugs.

Charles Pfizer, a German chemist who founded the pharmaceutical company Pfizer in 1849. After immigrating to the United States, he and Charles Erhardt borrowed $2,500 to establish their new chemical business in Brooklyn, New York. Their first success was to make a palatable form of the drug santonin used to treat parasitic worms, a common problem in the 1800s. Over the next century and a half, the company grew into the world's largest pharmaceutical maker.

Dennis Quaid, a successful film actor and advocate for drug safety. His 12-day-old twins accidentally received a dosage of the blood thinner Heparin that was 1,000 times stronger than normal for infants. They nearly died, and Quaid sued the maker of the drug for negligence in not making packaging for infant and adults versions of the drug more different. He has testified before Congress on issues of prescription drug safety.

Ronald Reagan, Republican president of the United States from 1981 to 1989. Consistent with his free-market and pro-business ideology and policies, his term coincided with expanding use of prescription drugs and increasing success of pharmaceutical companies. His administration supported DTC advertising and a quicker approval process for new drugs.

Arnold Relman, professor emeritus at Harvard University and former editor of the *New England Journal of Medicine.* As a physician and influential editor of a prestigious medical journal, he became a strong critic of the drug industry. In his view, companies have distorted the medical evidence and scientific studies on drug safety and effectiveness and contributed to widespread overuse of prescription drugs.

Franklin Delano Roosevelt, Democratic president of the United States from 1933 to 1945. Ranked by historians as one of the three greatest presidents, he presided over a major overhaul of U.S. law on prescription drugs with the 1938 Federal Food, Drug, and Cosmetic Act. Although it took several years to pass the law, Roosevelt supported the efforts of the FDA to modernize and improve the control of prescription drugs.

Theodore Roosevelt, Republican president of the United States from 1901 to 1909. Concerned about the impurity and misleading claims of patent medicines, he supported government efforts to improve the safety of drug use with the passage of the 1906 Pure Food and Drug Act. The legislation represented a modest first step but was followed by stronger efforts in decades to follow.

Kathleen Sebelius, former governor of Kansas and secretary of Health and Human Services in the Obama administration. As secretary, she oversees the FDA and the National Institutes of Health and therefore will have an important policy role in dealing with issues relating to the cost, regulation, and advertising of prescription drugs. Her nomination received support from pharmaceutical industry trade groups, but she may be less sympathetic to drug companies than members of the Bush administration.

Donna Shalala, secretary of Health and Human Services in the Clinton administration from 1993 to 2001. Responding to legislation from Congress to allow reimportation of prescription drugs from other countries, she ruled that her agency could not guarantee the safety and quality of the reimported drugs and thereby prevented the law from going into effect.

Joshua Sharfstein, physician, former health commissioner of Baltimore, interim FDA commissioner, and principal deputy to the FDA commissioner. In this role, he will likely have major responsibility for the administration of the prescription drug components of the agency. After the 2008 election, he served as the leader of the Obama transition team for the FDA. He has previously criticized drug companies for their marketing practices and the American Medical Association for making campaign contributions to political candidates.

Henry Waxman, Democratic representative from California since 1975. In an unusual instance of cooperation across parties, Waxman cosponsored a bill in 1984 with conservative Republican senator Orrin Hatch called the Drug Price Competition and Patent Restoration Act. The bill helped consumers by making it easier and faster for less expensive generic drugs to get approval from the FDA. It helped drug companies by allowing their patents to be extended when the development and approval process took a particularly long time.

Henry Solomon Wellcome, American pharmacist who founded the highly successful drug company Burroughs Wellcome with Silas Mainville Burroughs. The company, established in London in 1880, produced medicine in a compressed form called a Tabloid and eventually a tablet. The invention allowed drugs to be easily taken in standard doses. The company was one of the first to establish a research lab to develop new drugs. In the 1990s and 2000s, the company merged with several others to create GlaxoSmithKline.

Sidney Wolfe, physician and director of Public Citizen, a health advocacy group concerned with misuse of prescription drugs. Wolfe edits a book and Web site, *Good Pills, Bad Pills,* that provides guidance to users on safety and effectiveness. He has also campaigned against many drugs he views as dangerous, criticized the drug industry for high prices and hiding facts about unsafe drugs, and pushed the FDA to ban unsafe drugs currently allowed for sale.

Hamilton Wright, appointed U.S. opium commissioner in 1908 and vigorous opponent of use of opium. His efforts and those of many others led to passage of the Harrison Narcotics Act, which allowed use of narcotics for legitimate medical purposes only and greatly reduced abuse of opium products in the United States.

CHAPTER 5

GLOSSARY

This glossary avoids listing drugs and medical conditions. Information on those topics can be found in volumes that aim to give medical advice. It instead concentrates on terms needed to understand debates and issues related to the social, economic, and policy aspects of prescription drugs.

active ingredient   The compound in both brand-name and generic drugs that produces the intended effect on the body.

addictive   Prone to cause a compulsive physiological or psychological need.

adulterated drug   A drug that is compromised by impurities, low strength, poor quality, or inappropriate substances; misrepresented by information on the label; or different in makeup from official standards or requirements.

Adverse Event Reporting System   Procedures used by the FDA to report, collect, and review harmful reactions of patients to prescription drugs.

analgesic   A narcotic or non-narcotic drug used to relieve pain.

antibiotic   A chemical agent or drug that kills microorganisms and cures bacterial infections.

apothecary   An historical name for a person who makes and sells medicines, sometimes used now to refer to a pharmacist.

barbiturate   A drug with limited medical uses that acts as a sedative or central nervous system depressant.

biologic   A medicine such as a vaccine or serum that is obtained from living organisms or products of living organisms, sometimes through genetic engineering.

black-box warning   A warning on the package insert of a prescription drug that is surrounded by black lines and distinguishes serious from more routine warnings in package inserts.

blockbuster drug   A drug with enormous sales, usually defined as $1 billion or more.

brand name The trademarked name of a drug used exclusively by the maker for promotion and sales.

clinical trial A rigorous scientific study of the safety and effectiveness of a drug or medical treatment that usually involves randomization, double-blind procedures, and comparison to a placebo.

commerce clause A statement in the Constitution that the laws of the United States shall be supreme and binding for the states and that gives Congress the power to regulate commerce across states; it proved crucial in court cases involving the preemption of state laws by federal drug laws.

contraindication A condition or factor that makes it inappropriate or dangerous to use a particular drug.

controlled substance A drug or chemical substance whose possession and use is controlled by federal or state laws.

deregulation A lessening of government restrictions or regulations that proved important for the growth of prescription drugs in the 1980s and is a subject of debate today in regard to the pharmaceutical industry.

direct-to-consumer (DTC) ads Advertising of prescription drugs (and other products) directly to the consumer rather than to health care practitioners; once rare, the ads have proliferated on television.

doctor shopping Obtaining care from multiple physicians, without informing each physician of the other treatments, in order to get multiple prescriptions, usually to feed an addiction.

double-blind A term used to describe a clinical trial in which neither the subject nor the researcher knows who receives the placebo and who receives the treatment drug.

DTC Direct to consumers.

formulary A preferred list of prescription drugs that, unless there are exceptional circumstances, a health insurance plan will cover.

generic drug A drug whose patent has expired and can, with FDA approval, be marketed and sold (usually for lower cost) under the chemical or generic name.

generic name The chemical name of the active ingredient in a generic drug (contrasts with the brand name of a drug).

interaction In relation to drugs, the change in the effect of one drug when taken at the same time as another drug.

lifestyle drug A drug for problems such as hair loss, excess weight, poor sleep, or sexual dysfunction that aims to improve enjoyment of life rather than treat a disease.

Medicaid A federal and state partnership to provide health insurance to the needy (or those with low income and assets) that has become the only source of prescription drugs for many.

Glossary

Medicare   A federal health insurance program for people age 65 and older and younger people with disabilities that partially covers hospital, medical, and prescription drug costs.

Medicare Advantage   A Medicare-approved private health care plan, such as a health maintenance network or preferred provider organization, that serves as an alternative to a fee-for-service plan for Medicare participants and partially or totally covers prescription drug costs.

Medicare Part D   The component of Medicare that covers prescription drugs through voluntary enrollment in one of several plans and saves members money on drug purchases.

menopause   A stage of a woman's life marked by shutting down of the reproductive system and sometimes unpleasant symptoms of hot flashes, sleep disturbance, mood swings, and vaginal dryness.

me-too drug   An informal and pejorative name for new drugs that, although different enough to get a patent, treat the same problem and in much the same way as existing drugs and thereby divert resources from discovery and development of altogether new and more valuable drugs.

misbrand   To falsely label the ingredients or strength of a drug.

narcotic   A class of painkilling drugs, many coming from the opium plant, that lead to addiction, are illegal without a prescription, and are controlled by the government.

off label   A term used to describe the use of a prescription drug for purposes other than those approved by the FDA.

opiate   A narcotic drug made or derived from opium such as morphine and codeine that is used medically to eliminate pain.

opioid   A family of natural and synthetic drugs that have the properties of opium products in eliminating pain.

orphan drug   A drug that serves fewer than 200,000 patients in the United States and thereby requires special incentives to encourage drugmakers to develop and produce it.

OTC   Over-the-counter.

out of pocket   Paid for directly by the recipient of goods or services. Out-of-pocket expenses for prescription drugs are those that are not covered by private or public insurance programs and require direct payment by patients.

over-the-counter (OTC) drug   A drug that consumers can buy without a prescription from a medical professional.

patent   Exclusive or monopoly rights granted to the inventor or developer of a product for a fixed period of time in exchange for disclosure of the invention.

patent medicine   A name for medicines used commonly in the 1800s that, because of claims of secret ingredients and excessive benefits, is associated with dishonesty.

patient package insert (PPI)   Information that comes with prescription drugs and describes the drug, its use, and associated warnings.

penicillin   An antibiotic that is produced naturally from mold and able to treat many forms of bacterial infections.

pharmacist   A health professional trained in preparing and dispensing prescription drugs.

pharmacopoeia or **pharmacopeia**   An official or standard list of drugs that includes information on preparation, quality standards, and proper use.

placebo   A harmless substance given to subjects in a clinical trial that may lead them to feel better and can be used for comparisons with the effects of an experimental drug.

PPI   Patient package insert.

prescription   A written order or plan, usually involving the taking of medicines, that a physician or medical practitioner gives to a patient, a pharmacist fills for the patient, and the patient follows in taking the medicine.

prescription drug   A drug that requires physician supervision for use by patients.

prior authorization (PA)   A requirement that drugs prescribed by a physician receive approval from the state or insurance company before a prescription for them can be filled; the requirement tends to reduce use of the drug.

randomization   The random assignment of subjects to experimental and control conditions of a clinical trial. The goal of randomization is to control for any preexisting characteristics of subjects that may affect the outcomes of the trial and the observed effectiveness of a new drug.

reimport   To import goods, often pharmaceutical products, from a country to which they had earlier been exported.

reminder ads   Advertisements that mention the brand name of a prescription drug and encourage viewers to ask their doctors about the drug but do not state its purpose or the condition it treats and thereby are not subject to the same information requirements as other ads for prescription drugs.

selective serotonin reuptake inhibitor (SSRI)   A class of antidepressants that works by affecting the activity of serotonin in the brain.

side effect   A problem resulting from a prescription drug that has undesired consequences beyond the intended therapeutic goal.

smart drug   A drug used to enhance the brain rather than treat a disease, e.g., prescription stimulants such as Ritalin used to improve concentration, focus, and memory.

snake oil   A supposed miracle ingredient of some patent medicines that claimed to treat a variety of ailments (today, the term *snake oil salesman* means a swindler or a fraud).

Glossary

SSRI   Selective serotonin reuptake inhibitor.

statin   A type of drug in pill form that lowers cholesterol in the blood.

stimulant   A drug that induces alertness, nervous activity of the body, and a sense of energy.

sulfa   A class of antibiotics.

supplemental rebate   A program in several states that helps control prescription drug prices by requiring drug companies to pay back some of what the government or the public initially paid.

thalidomide   A sedative drug that eases nausea but, when taken by pregnant women, causes severe birth defects.

toxic   Harmful or poisonous to an exposed organism.

tranquilizer   A sedative drug that depresses the central nervous system to induce calmness, relaxation, or sleepiness and can relieve anxiety.

vaccine   A substance or product given to stimulate the body's antibodies and provide immunity against a disease.

PART II

GUIDE TO FURTHER RESEARCH

CHAPTER 6

HOW TO RESEARCH
PRESCRIPTION DRUGS

The extraordinary presence of prescription drugs in the lives of Americans makes information on the topic easy to find. Media reports regularly discuss the promise of new drugs, concerns over risks of commonly used drugs, and debates over government laws and regulations. Webpages are filled with detailed information about thousands of drugs and opinions on their benefits and dangers. The public rightfully desires such information—they want to know as much as they can about the drugs they currently take or might take in the future. Research on some of these topics, however, is best left to medical experts. Physicians, pharmacists, and health care personnel have proper training to judge the particular needs of individual patients, the suitability of a medicine in treatment of a disease, and the medical effectiveness of a drug.

Researchers interested more in the social, economic, and policy issues revolving around prescription drugs still face an onslaught of information. Consider some of the questions debated in the scholarly literature, popular press, and Internet. Does the FDA adequately protect the public from unsafe drugs, become overzealous in preventing people from choosing the drugs they want, or give in to the demands for approval of powerful pharmaceuticals? Are prescription drug prices fair given the investment companies must make to discover new and highly effective products or does the search for profits among the companies unfairly exploit the medical needs of patients with high prices? Do pharmaceutical companies misleadingly encourage the overuse of drugs with advertising or do they perform a valuable service in informing the public of treatments for conditions they have? How can authorities do more to control the abuse of and addiction to certain prescription drugs without compromising the ability of people with legitimate needs to get access to the drugs? These issues affect the everyday lives of Americans—whether or not they take prescription drugs.

Because these questions are both fascinating and open to opposing answers, the amount of relevant material can be overwhelming. As a help to

133

doing research on the topic, this chapter offers some general suggestions on using bibliographic resources and more specific suggestions on consulting key sources. Even with these suggestions, however, those doing research on prescription drugs will face several challenges.

First, writings on the topic span a variety of fields of study. Even leaving aside issues relating to chemistry, medical diagnosis, and the specifics of drug therapies, the huge literature on other topics concerning prescription drugs covers patent law, government policy, the economics of pricing, the power of corporations, social acceptance of prescription drug use, and criminal misuse of drugs. It further relates to specific knowledge about the FDA, proper evaluation of drug safety and effectiveness in clinical trials, the Food, Drug, and Cosmetics Act of 1938 (plus its many amendments), the Controlled Substances Act, Medicare prescription drug benefits, and the major drug companies. Besides medicine, public health, and pharmacology, these topics encompass fields of study such as law, ethics, economics, political science, sociology, criminology, and biostatistics. Few can master all these specialized fields of study.

Second, the divergent political and economic views of advocates on both sides of debates over prescription drugs can make it hard to separate facts from opinions. Differing viewpoints can lead to widely varying interpretations of the facts and issues. These views come into play, for example, in debates over the proper role of the government in controlling the products and prices of private companies. On one side, supporters of the pharmaceutical industry favor reliance on the market and oppose government controls. They believe that economic freedom allows companies to deliver drugs to consumers at prices that encourage innovation and meet the needs of the public. Government control over prices and products ultimately reduces the incentives for manufacturers and the benefits for patients. They call instead for continued freedom of pricing in the United States and ending policies in other countries that force below-market prices for prescription drugs. On the other side, many see the pharmaceutical industry as unfairly exploiting the needs of people for health care. Unlike other products, prescription drugs are a requirement rather than a choice, and prices do not follow the usual workings of the free market. These critics say that companies mislead through advertising, force people to buy lifesaving drugs at exorbitant prices, pay too little attention to safety and effectiveness, and enjoy excessive profits. The most effective way to eliminate these behaviors is for government to more forcefully regulate drugs and prices. In short, then, underlying assumptions about the value of private enterprise and government control lead to different views on prescription drugs. The often-unstated assumptions in turn shape the interpretation and presentation of facts about prescription drugs that one finds in the literature.

Third, research on prescription drugs frequently includes technically difficult matter. The chemical makeup of prescription drugs, their physiological effect on the body, and the proper drugs and dosages for patients go beyond the understanding of most nonscientists. Only somewhat less problematic, the widespread use of statistical methods in clinical trials can be daunting. In understanding the safety and effectiveness of drugs, the evidence comes not only from the observations of physicians and nurses. It more often comes from the statistical comparison of the benefits and side effects experienced by subjects in clinical trails who, based on random assignment, received the experimental drug or received a placebo. Issues of randomness of samples, validity of measurements, and appropriateness of statistical techniques that come into play relate more to the skills of specialists than general researchers. Readers of studies thus run across intimidating terms such as double-blind, relative risk ratios, statistical significance, and confidence intervals. Similarly, the legal and economic complexities involved in debates over patents, the workings of government health programs and private insurance programs, and the pricing of drugs challenge nonspecialists.

TIPS FOR RESEARCHING PRESCRIPTION DRUGS

How can researchers overcome these challenges? Here are some tips.

- **Define the topic and questions carefully.** Rather than researching prescription drugs, pick topics that allow for more focused and in-depth research. More narrowly defined topics might include early history of drug laws, requirements for approval of a new drug, the cost of research and development in the pharmaceutical industry, the Medicare Prescription Drug Program, ways to reduce prescription drug costs, the use of prescription stimulants by children, and the growth of addiction to Oxy-Contin. With so many choices available, making the research manageable requires care and precision in selecting topics. A precise topic can help a researcher avoid feeling overwhelmed by the material and allow for in-depth treatment.

- **Consider the underlying perspectives.** Relying on a variety of sources will help make sense of the differing values and beliefs that shape views on prescription drugs. Toward that end, the annotated bibliography in the next chapter includes a wide selection of readings that represent diverse perspectives. In addition, however, it helps to consider the background and potential biases of the authors. Given the heated disputes

135

over the costs of prescription drugs and the profits of pharmaceutical companies, information on the expertise and underlying perspectives of authors can help separate opinions and emotion from facts and reason.

- **Evaluate your sources.** In reviewing books and articles, check the date of publication to make sure the information is recent, check the qualifications of the author and the citation of sources to make sure the information is reliable, and check for the presentation of alternative views to make sure the information is presented fairly. Books and articles often differ in their readership, with some more focused on nonexpert audiences and some more focused on scholarly audiences. Both popular information and scholarly information are useful, but it helps to recognize how they differ in the depth of information, citation of sources, and recentness of publication. In reviewing Internet sources, use even more care. Nearly anyone can post documents, and many webpages lack checks on the reliability of their information. Evaluate the qualifications of the author, the legitimacy of the sponsoring organization, and the potential for bias.

- **Master the basic facts and terms.** Few can make sense of the material on prescription drugs without having some familiarity with common terms, names, and acronyms. Try to learn the basic terminology; careful and precise usage lends authority to research.

- **Search for balance.** Since complex questions about prescription drugs seldom have simple answers, do not accept claims at face value. It is easy to assign blame for problems involving prescription drugs, and the government and pharmaceutical industry get much criticsm. To avoid simple solutions, however, search for balanced presentations based on evidence—even if highly technical—and careful weighing of the alternatives. Researchers should seek to understand the complexity that underlies the topic and treat all sides of the debates fairly.

The rest of this chapter reviews various types of research resources. It considers online, print, and legal resources.

ONLINE RESOURCES

GENERAL SITES

Given its ease in providing information, the Internet offers a good place to begin doing research on prescription drugs. It contains a wide variety of research, reference, and opinion pieces on the topic that can be easily accessed with an Internet connection. One can find useful facts and perspectives on nearly any aspect of prescription drugs by patiently working through even a small portion of available webpages. Finding one suitable site suggests links to others, which in turn leads in new directions. Innovative ideas and fresh information emerge in this process. Indeed, many web documents are updated or created anew to keep up with recent events and the latest information.

However, the extraordinary wealth of information that the Internet makes available to researchers can be overwhelming. Most searches return an impressive but dauntingly large number of hits. The advice to define narrow research topics applies particularly to using the Internet. Otherwise, combing through all the Web sites listed by searches can result in wasted effort. In addition, the information obtained does not always meet high standards of reliability and balance. Unlike books and articles, web documents generally do not go through a process of review and editing before publication. With the increasing presence of blogs, many pages offer little more than the opinions of strangers.

Users must take care in relying on materials obtained from Web sites and inquire into the background of the site. Take note of who sponsors the webpage. Is the organization reputable; does the author have expertise? Does the webpage aim for objectivity? Is it written well and based on careful thinking? Those webpages where one can answer these questions affirmatively will be the ones to rely on the most. With these qualifications in mind, Internet research can proceed in several ways.

Popular and general search engines such as Google (URL: http://www. google.com), Yahoo! (URL: http://www.yahoo.com), Alta Vista (URL: http://www.altavista.com), Excite (URL: http://www.excite.com), Lycos (URL: http://www.lycos.com), Ask (URL: http://www.ask.com), and many others can find webpages with information on prescription drugs. A new search engine, Bing (www.Bing.com), has recently been put online by Microsoft. Effectively using these search engines requires thoughtful selection of search terms and patient effort but can lead to unexpected and intriguing discoveries. Broad searches that focus on prescription and drugs will work less well than narrower searches on prescription drug costs, prescription drug abuse, pharmaceutical companies, and prescription drug overuse. Even with narrower searches, most pages returned offer little of value, and researchers need to search for the few documents of most use.

Wikipedia, a free web-based encyclopedia (URL: http://en.wikipedia. org/wiki/Main_Page), has entries for most prescription drugs, pharmaceutical companies, and relevant federal laws. Created in 2001, Wikipedia allows readers to collaboratively make and revise entries, which is particularly helpful in keeping up-to-date with current events. Critics point out that the entries lack an authority or known author to ensure reliability, and many schools prohibit use of Wikipedia as a source for student papers. Sometimes the objectivity of writers and editors is disputed. While recognizing these limitations, the entries for topics on prescription rights can be useful to researchers when consulted in combination with other sources. If nothing else, the entries typically include external links to primary information sources.

ORGANIZATION SITES

Knowledge of key organizations—government, business, advocacy, and professional—is crucial for researching prescription drugs. Chapter 8 lists a variety of such organizations, but consulting the home pages of a few of them can help in getting started in doing research.

The key federal government agency for prescription drugs, the Food and Drug Administration (FDA), has a useful home page (URL: http://www.fda.gov). Highlight the menu item on "Drugs" to obtain a list of links to pages on news, drug approvals, consumer resources, and safety. Then clicking on "More information on drugs" produces a full page of links. Searching through these links can be helpful. The home page also contains a menu item on vaccines, blood, and biologics. The webpage of the Center for Drug Evaluation and Research (URL: http://www.fda.gov/AboutFDA/Centers Offices/CDER), the FDA division responsible for the safety and effectiveness of prescription and OTC drugs, has information on how the division evaluates and regulates drugs.

Among private organizations, two offer competing views on prescription drugs. The Pharmaceutical Research and Manufacturers of American (PhRMA) has a webpage (URL: http://www.phrma.org) that presents views supportive of the industry. It lists facts on the costs of bringing new drugs to market and describes its goals for reforming health care and keeping America healthy. The Health Research Group of Public Citizen (URL: http://www.citizen.org/hrg), headed by Sidney Wolfe, has been a longtime critic of the pharmaceutical industry and the FDA. The webpage lists Dr. Wolfe's advice on the best and worst pills (details require a subscription), news on drug safety, and expert views on reforming health care.

SITES ON PRESCRIPTION DRUG TOPICS

Along with getting resources from broad—and perhaps overwhelming—general searches and from organizations with wide-ranging goals, it helps to begin a search from particular sites. Here are some recommendations organized by the major topics on prescription drugs.

General Treatments. The Kaiser Family Foundation supports a wide variety of health-related projects, including many related to prescription drugs. Its webpage on prescription drugs (URL: http://www.kff.org/rxdrugs/index.cfm) lists dozens of relevant documents, many relating to costs and prescription drug coverage by Medicare and Medicaid. A related page (URL: http://facts.kff.org) lists key facts on health and prescription drugs. Although the documents are better suited for those familiar with prescription drug policies than for those new to the topic, they present information fairly and clearly.

Policy and Regulation. The *Frontline* television series has a webpage (URL: http://www.pbs.org/wgbh/pages/frontline/shows/prescription) on its 2003 show, "Dangerous Prescription." Although dated, the material maintains its value. Interviews with experts on drug safety offer competing views on how well the FDA does in protecting the safety of prescription drug users.

Prices and Access. In "An Update on Americans' Access to Prescription Drugs" (URL: http://www.hschange.org/CONTENT/738), the Center for Studying Health System Change describes the facts on prescription drug access. The nonpartisan organization does not take positions but uses a variety of survey sources to make information available to policy makers. Researchers can benefit from the information as well. The numbers point to a serious problem that is expected to get worse. For more practical advice, see a February 2009 piece, "Strategies for Saving on Prescription Drugs" by Lesley Alderman on the *New York Times* webpage (URL: http://www.nytimes.com/2009/02/07/health/06patient.html?_r=1&scp=2&sq=prescription%20drugs&st=cse).

The Pharmaceutical Industry. Yahoo! Finance reports pharmaceutical industry news (URL: http://biz.yahoo.com/n/y/y0022.html) and reviews economic performance of pharmaceutical companies (go to http://finance.yahoo.com, type in a company name, and click "Get Quotes"). On pages for particular companies, the webpage links give a profile of the company and recent news related to company performance. Another source of objective information on the pharmaceutical industry, with particular attention to employment opportunities, comes from IMDiversity.com (URL: http://www.imdiversity.com/Villages/Channels/pharmaceutical/Articles/pharma_overview.asp). Although not focused directly on drug companies, "Prescription Drug Trends" by the Kaiser Family Foundation (http://www.kff.org/rxdrugs/upload/3057_07.pdf) describes trends in prices, profits, and advertising.

Use, Overuse, and Advertising. Webpages critical of drug advertising and excess use of prescription drugs are easy to find with web searches. More useful background comes from the FDA. It summarizes its role in regulating advertising in "Prescription Drug Advertising: Questions and Answers" (URL: http://www.fda.gov/Drugs/ResourcesForYou/Consumers/PrescriptionDrugAdvertising/UCM 076768.htm). The Kaiser Family Foundation supplies some facts on the issue in "Impact of Direct-to-Consumer Advertising on Prescription Drug Spending" (URL: http://www.kff.org/rxdrugs/6084-index.cfm).

Risks, Dangers, Side Effects. *Consumer Reports* has a webpage entitled "Drug Risks the System Missed" (URL: http://www.consumerreports. org/health/healthy-living/health-safety/common-drugs-hidden-dangers-106/highrisk-drugs/index.htm). The webpage lists relatively common drugs that the magazine's experts identified as having known or suspected serious risks that were undetected or underestimated when the FDA approved the drugs. Popular but high-risk drugs such as Celebrex for pain and inflammation, estrogen for hormone therapy, and Crestor for high cholesterol make the list. The webpage does not oppose use of these drugs but suggests that patients fully discuss the risks and benefits with a physician before taking them and use the lowest does possible. For a general overview of the risks of addiction, see the Office of National Drug Control Policy ("Prescription for Danger," URL: http://www.theantidrug. com/pdfs/prescription_report.pdf).

PRINT SOURCES

Despite the ease of obtaining sources from the Internet, books and articles available from conventional and electronic libraries and bookstores remain essential sources of information. Good books integrate material that is otherwise scattered, present information in a logical and understandable format, and allow for a comprehensive approach to the issues. Edited volumes (anthologies) provide multiple perspectives on a topic but usually within a common framework, while other books present a single but in-depth viewpoint—both of which have advantages. Exploiting these advantages requires use of catalogs, indexes, bibliographies, and other guides.

BIBLIOGRAPHIC RESOURCES

Besides using catalogs at a city or university library, researchers can consult the comprehensive bibliographic resource of the Library of Congress (URL: http://catalog.loc.gov). To browse holdings by subject, click Basic Search, then type in keywords. Typing "prescription drugs" will return more than 600 sources, but narrowing the search to include terms such as *prices, risks,* or *abuse* will limit the number of sources. Clicking the button on "Add Limits to Search Results" allows selection of publications in more recent years. The Library of Congress webpage has a variety of other hints to narrow searches.

A listing of catalogs for specific libraries appears on a Yahoo! webpage (URL: dir.Yahoo.com/Reference/Libraries). The numerous libraries allow users to browse catalogs outside their local library and discover new references. Each library will have its own search procedures, but the general rule of searching for more specific keywords is the best approach for finding relevant materials.

Bookstore catalogs not only allow for searches of books currently in print on any variety of topics but also have another advantage. They often include summaries and reader reviews of books that can help determine their relevance and value. In some cases, one can browse through an electronic version of parts of a book. At the same time, bookstore catalogs will not have as many books, compared with libraries, that are out of print but still valuable. Overall, electronic bookstores such as Amazon.com (URL: http://www.amazon.com) and Barnes & Noble (URL: http://www.barnesandnoble.com) are good bibliographic resources.

Most libraries give their users access to periodical indexes used to search for print articles. *OCLC First Search* contains an electronic version of *Reader's Guide to Periodical Literature* that lists titles and abstracts from a large number of magazines (and sometimes allows access to the full text). However, users generally need access to a subscribing library for this database. *InfoTrac* also has dozens of databases to search but again requires library privileges. *Ingenta Connect* (URL: http://www.ingentaconnect.com) allows a search of scholarly works from more than 4 million articles and reports and from more than 13,000 publications. Searching *Ingenta* is free but delivery of an article sometimes requires a fee. Magazines such as *Time* (URL: http://www.time.com/time) often have a webpage that allows users to search for articles.

Libraries usually subscribe to catalogs of newspaper articles. In addition, many newspapers maintain an archive of past articles. The *New York Times*, for example, allows searches of its stories (and presents the day's major news) at its webpage (URL: http://www.nytimes.com). A search on "prescription drugs" produces a compilation of articles back to 1981 that can be accessed without cost. The *Washington Post* also provides a webpage with a search option (URL: http://www.washingtonpost.com). Otherwise, Yahoo! (URL: http://dir.yahoo.com/News_and_Media/Newspapers) lists links to many newspapers that can be accessed via the Internet. However, local libraries offer a better source for finding past articles without a fee. For all these sources, a search on "prescription drugs" will typically return too many stories to sort through, and narrower searches will provide more useful information.

SPECIFIC BOOKS AND ARTICLES ON PRESCRIPTION DRUGS

In using general bibliographic resources for print materials and the annotated bibliography in chapter 7, it helps first to have a few books and articles to get started. Here are some recommendations organized by the major topics of prescription drugs.

Prescription Drugs

General Treatments. Two books, one by a physician and one by a journalist, offer excellent treatments of the issues relating to the growing use of prescription drugs. *Powerful Medicines: The Benefits, Risks, and Costs of Prescription Drugs* by Dr. Jerry Avorn of Harvard University (New York: Alfred A. Knopf, 2004) nicely describes the dilemmas physicians face in prescribing many drugs and the costs and benefits to society of higher rates of prescription. *Generation Rx: How Prescription Drugs Are Altering American Lives, Minds, and Bodies* by Greg Critser (Boston: Houghton Mifflin, 2005) is less academic and more entertaining than Avorn's book but also is filled with useful facts and stories. Both these books contain some history of drug use and the drug industry, but for a more detailed account of life before effective prescription drugs, see "What It Was Like to Be Sick in 1884" by Charles E. Rosenberg (*American Heritage* [35] October/November 1984: 22–27).

Policy and Regulation. An excellent and comprehensive resource on policy and regulation comes from a volume put together to help pharmacy students understand the social, political, and legal context of prescription drugs, *Handbook of Pharmaceutical Public Policy* (New York: Pharmaceutical Products Press, 2007), edited by Thomas R. Fulda and Albert I. Wertheimer. Each of the 30 chapters covers an issue of current debate. The book is long, but picking chapters of most interest can help researchers enormously. For something on the most current policy and regulation issues, see "Stronger Research Just One Item on Drug Agency's Wish List" by Jennifer Couzin (*Science* 323 [March 20, 2009]: 1,549).

Prices and Access. Although many dispute its claims, a short book put out by PhRMA, the drug industry trade group in Washington, D.C., explains why prescription drugs cost so much. *What Goes into the Cost of Prescription Drugs?* (Washington, D.C.: Pharmaceutical Research and Manufacturers of America, 2005). It also gives some insight into the nature of drug development today. An article published in the open-access journal *PLoS Medicine* says that the drug industry spends less on research and more on marketing than it claims. For those willing to work through the detailed estimates, consult "The Cost of Pushing Pills: A New Estimate of Pharmaceutical Promotion Expenditures in the United States" by Marc-André Gagnon and Joel Lexchin (*PLoS Medicine* 5, no. 1 [2008]: e1). URL: http://medicine.plosjournals.org/perlserv/ ?request=get-document&doi=10.1371/journal.pmed.0050001&ct=1).

The Pharmaceutical Industry. For general treatments, sometimes positive but often negative, several books and articles can help researchers understand the industry. On the negative side, *The Truth about the Drug Companies: How They Deceive Us and What to Do About It* by Marcia Angell (New York: Random House, 2004) makes a strong case against the pharmaceutical industry. She has the authority of a Harvard professorship and writes well. One can find some half-dozen books equally critical of the industry. A book for industry professionals, *Understanding Pharma: The Professional's Guide to How Pharmaceutical and Biotech Companies Really Work* by John J. Campbell (second edition, Raleigh, N.C.: Pharmaceutical Institute, 2008), offers more description and less criticism. An article by John E. Calfee, "The Indispensable Industry" (*The American* 2, no. 3 [May/June 2008]: pp. 41–47), presents a clearly positive view of the industry.

Use, Overuse, and Advertising. Books and articles on this topic also tend to view the pharmaceutical industry negatively. Although critical of the drug industry and its advertising, Melody Peterson in *Our Daily Meds: How the Pharmaceutical Companies Transformed Themselves into Slick Marketing Machines and Hooked the Nation on Prescription Drugs* (New York: Sarah Crichton Books, 2008) also emphasizes the acceptance of greater use of prescription drugs by the public. If the drug industry is a villain in pushing excess drug use on the public, the public is often a willing accomplice. As discussed by Jason Kirby in "Going to Work on Smart Drugs" (*Maclean's* 121, no. 40 [October 13, 2008]: pp. 94–95), the trend may accelerate as people come to use drugs to improve their brains rather than treat disease.

Risks, Side Effects, and Abuse. Key sources on this topic often relate to particular kinds of drugs—those causing the most adverse effects or leading to the most abuse. Chapter 7 contains books and articles on use and misuse of tranquilizers, painkillers, and antidepressants. A more general treatment of abuse of prescription drugs, a problem of increasing concern to policy makers, can be found in a Senate hearing. Expert witnesses lay out the problems and recommend legislative changes to deal with them in *Generation Rx: The Abuse of Prescription and Over-the-Counter Drugs: Hearing before the Subcommittee on the Constitution of the Committee on the Judiciary, United States Senate, One Hundred Tenth Congress, Second Session, March 12, 2008* (Washington, D.C.: U.S. Government Printing Office, 2009, URL: http://frwebgate.access.gpo.gov/cgi-bin/getdoc.cgi?dbname=110_senate_hearings&d ocid=f:47336.pdf). A shorter document from the National Institute of Drug Abuse, *Prescription Drugs: Abuse and Addiction* (Bethesda, Md.: National Institute on Drug Abuse, 2005, URL: http://www.nida.nih.gov/ResearchReports/Prescription/prescription.html) nicely summarizes key facts about abuse of prescription drugs.

LEGAL RESEARCH

The Federal Food, Drug, and Cosmetics Act, the key legislation that guides regulation of prescription drugs in the United States today, has been amended many times since its first passage in 1938. A webpage sponsored by the FDA contains the full law and all its details. (URL: http://www.fda.gov/RegulatoryInformation/Legislation/FederalFoodDrugandCosmetic

Prescription Drugs

ActFDCAct/default.htm). One can find many other federal laws on prescription drugs through a search for legislation. For example, a search for the Medicare Modernization Act of 2003 returns a page with the full bill (URL: http://frwebgate.access.gpo.gov/cgi-bin/getdoc.cgi?dbname=108_cong_bills&docid=f:h1enr.txt.pdf).

For more detail—and more complexity—a search of the U.S. Code will locate a variety of specific laws on other topics relating to prescription drugs. The U.S. Code is a compilation and systematic arrangement of permanent federal laws of the United States. Go to the Cornell Law School search webpage (URL: http://www4.law.cornell.edu/uscode/search/index.html) and type "prescription drugs." Then scroll through the 115-plus separate listings of the code to find those of most interest. Finding the codes for individual states or cities requires separate searches. A FindLaw webpage helps in the searches by listing links to each state (URL: http://www.findlaw.com/11stategov/indexcode.html). Searching state webpages for statutes on prescription drugs is difficult but might produce special details on illegal drug laws, licensing, and price controls.

Court decisions on prescription drugs involve disputes over drug injuries, advertising, and price controls (see the material in chapter 2). Information on the suits, jury decisions, awards, appeals, and final judgments can be found through searches of newspapers such as the *New York Times* (URL: http://www.nytimes.com) and general search engines such as Google, Yahoo!, and Ask. To obtain the written decisions for specific cases, electronic law libraries such as Westlaw (URL: http://www.westlaw.com) and Lexis-Nexis (URL: http://www.lexisnexis.com) include court opinions but require a subscription. Opinions of the Supreme Court can be obtained from the Legal Information Institute (URL: http://www.law.cornell.edu).

CHAPTER 7

ANNOTATED BIBLIOGRAPHY

The following annotated bibliography on prescription drugs contains six sections:

- history and background,
- policy and regulation,
- prices and access,
- the pharmaceutical industry,
- use, overuse, and advertising,
- risks, side effects, and abuse.

Within each of these sections, the citations are divided into subsections on books, articles, and web documents. The topics and citations include technical and nontechnical works, in-depth and short treatments, and research and opinion pieces (see chapter 6 for an overview on how to most effectively use these materials).

HISTORY AND BACKGROUND

BOOKS

Avorn, Jerry. *Powerful Medicines: The Benefits, Risks, and Costs of Prescription Drugs.* New York: Alfred A. Knopf, 2004. A physician at Harvard University and specialist on how physicians prescribe drugs presents nuanced and insightful arguments on the modern medical uses of prescription drugs. He provides considerable history and background, gives numerous examples of the difficult decisions physicians face in prescribing drugs, and packs the chapters with fascinating details. The book is long and comprehensive, making it hard to summarize, but the wealth of ideas and facts makes it a crucial resource.

Prescription Drugs

Critser, Greg. *Generation Rx: How Prescription Drugs Are Altering American Lives, Minds, and Bodies.* Boston: Houghton Mifflin, 2005. This well-written book gives the background and history behind the widespread growth of prescription drug use. Freeing drug companies from past restrictions on the approval, sale, and marketing of prescription drugs greatly increased the supply, while the enthusiastic acceptance of prescription drugs as a means to deal with life's problems increased the demand. Critser says that "today the expectation is that pills can and will do everything." The examples and facts he presents in support of that view are fascinating and insightful.

National Center for Health Statistics. *Chartbook on Trends in the Health of Americans.* Hyattsville, Md.: National Center for Health Statistics, 2007. Also available online. URL: http://www.cdc.gov/nchs/data/hus/hus07.pdf. Posted in November 2007. This book consists of tables with statistics on a variety of health-related topics. The absence of any text to go with the figures makes the information overwhelming, but Table 96 contains interesting statistics on prescription drug use. Skimming through other tables might reveal more interesting and useful figures.

Tone, Andrea. *The Age of Anxiety: A History of America's Turbulent Affair with Tranquilizers.* New York: Basic Books, 2009. This book traces the history of drugs to treat anxiety from the first tranquilizer sold in 1955 to the billions of antianxiety drugs sold today. Although tranquilizers like Valium fell out of favor because of their addictiveness, the use of selective serotonin reuptake inhibitor (SSRI) antidepressants have become widely popular treatments for anxiety. The book places the popularity of these types of drugs within the larger context of what Tone calls the tranquilizer culture.

Walker, Bingham, A. *The Snake-Oil Syndrome: Patent Medicine Advertising.* Hanover, Mass.: Christopher Publishing House, 1994. With reprints of the words and images from patent medicine ads, this book illustrates the excessive claims made by merchants, marketers, and manufacturers during the 1800s and early 1900s.

Williams, Simon J., Jonathan Gabe, and Peter Davis, eds. *Pharmaceuticals and Society: Critical Discourses and Debates.* Hoboken, N.J.: Wiley-Blackwell, 2009. This recent book marks the development of a sociological approach to pharmaceuticals. It includes theory on the medicalization of society (turning social and personal problems into medical ones) and the pharmaceuticalization of daily life (the use of drugs to deal with social and personal problems). In addition, it includes chapters on specific drugs such as modafinil for sleep disorders, HPV vaccine for cervical cancer, antidepressant medications, and antiretroviral drugs for HIV/AIDS. Although written mostly for academics, the chapters address social issues that are crucial to understanding people's attraction to and reliance on prescription drugs.

Annotated Bibliography

ARTICLES

"America's Best Drugstores." *Consumer Reports* 73, no. 6 (June 2008): 12–17. A survey of this magazine's readers about drugstores gives advice on buying prescription drugs. For example, fewer consumers than in a 2000 survey are asking pharmacists questions about their prescriptions, a trend that may hurt consumers. The article reviews other results from the survey that relate to effective and inexpensive use of drugstores.

Bren, Linda. "Frances Oldham Kelsey: FDA Medical Reviewer Leaves Her Mark on History." *FDA Consumer* 35, no. 2 (March/April 2001): 24–29. This article tells the story behind Kelsey's actions to block the approval of thalidomide and prevent the epidemic of birth defects that occurred in Europe from playing out in the United States. When working for the FDA, she demanded better studies of the drug's long-term safety, after which evidence of harm from Europe emerged and justified her careful approach.

Lichtenberg, Frank R. "The Impact of New Drugs on U.S. Longevity and Medical Expenditure, 1990–2003: Evidence from Longitudinal, Disease-Level Data." *American Economic Review* 97, no. 2 (May 2007): 438–443. Estimating the impact of prescription drug use on health is difficult, but this economic study tries. It finds that new drugs allowed Americans under age 65 to live 1.56 million years longer than they would have otherwise, and that new drugs reduced hospital expenditures in 2003 by $58 billion and nursing home expenditures by $9.5 billion. Experts can dispute the methods used to get these numbers, but the estimated size of the effects is impressive.

Marks, Harry M. "Revisiting the Origins of Compulsory Drug Prescriptions." *American Journal of Public Health* 85 (January 1995): 109–115. This history of the 1938 regulations on prescription drugs considers debates in the 1930s over the relative roles of the FDA and drug industry in passing the legislation.

Musto, David. "America's Forgotten Drug War: Early Use of Cocaine." *Reader's Digest* 136 (April 1990): 147–150. As this article describes, many in the 1880s viewed cocaine as a medicine that effectively treated a variety of ailments. In fact, Coca-Cola once contained cocaine. The growing evidence of addiction, however, led to new state laws in the early 1900s and a federal law in 1914 that required a doctor's prescription for use of the drug. The change represented an early effort to require a medical prescription for use of certain dangerous drugs.

Pollan, Michael. "A Very Fine Line: Boundary between Licit and Illicit Drugs." *New York Times Magazine* (September 12, 1999): 27–28. A historical review in this article shows that many illicit drugs have become legal and many legal drugs have become illicit. A recent example concerns marijuana, which is approved for medical uses in many states. The author sees inconsistency in the strong belief of Americans in prescription drugs and their strong opposition to illegal drugs.

Rosenberg, Charles E. "What It Was Like to Be Sick in 1884." *American Heritage* 35 (October/November 1984): 22–27. No distinction existed in 1884 between prescription drugs and OTC drugs, and pharmacists dispensed most drugs without prescriptions from doctors. The picture of medical care more than a century ago contrasts starkly with use of prescription drugs today.

"Take as Directed: Risks of Stopping Medicines Too Soon." *Reader's Digest* 173 (September 2008): 140–145. In giving advice to prescription drug users, the article offers several examples of the harm caused by stopping medications too soon. Part of the problem may come from a sudden withdrawal. The article also contains other advice on using prescription drugs wisely.

WEB DOCUMENTS

Drugs.com. "Drug Information Online." Available online. URL: http://www.drugs.com. Downloaded June 16, 2009. Self-identified as a free, accurate, and independent source of information on 24,000 prescription drugs, OTC medicines, and natural products, this Web site does indeed contain an enormous amount of information on prescription drugs. The descriptions of drugs are clearly written and detailed, and daily medical news stories and pharmaceutical industry news offer added information. Without a specific topic or question of interest, however, the sheer amount of information makes the material overwhelming.

FDA Consumer. "The Story of the Laws behind the Labels. Part II: 1938—The Federal Food, Drug, and Cosmetic Act." Available online. URL: http://www.foodsafety.gov/~lrd/histor1a.html. Updated July 27, 2006. Although amended many times, this 1938 act defines the legal basis for federal regulations on prescription drugs in the United States today. This webpage reviews the circumstances that led to passage of the legislation and the amendments that followed.

Hagley Museum and Library. "Patent Medicine." Available online. URL: http://www.hagley.org/library/exhibits/patentmed/index.html. Downloaded June 19, 2009. The text on this webpage is short and to the point, but the exhibits on advertising, trade catalogs, and manuscripts that the library owns help to make the history real. Browsing the exhibits gives insights into the history of patent medicines that other treatments often miss.

Kaiser Family Foundation. "USA Today/Kaiser Family Foundation/Harvard School of Public Health Survey: The Public on Prescription Drugs

and Pharmaceutical Companies." Available online. URL: http://www.kff.
org/kaiserpolls/pomr030408pkg.cfm. Posted March 4, 2009. The 2008
survey finds that the public greatly values prescription drugs and recognizes the benefits they provide to themselves and family members. However, they also say that drugs cost too much and they have trouble paying
for the drugs they need. Besides reporting these results in more detail,
this webpage summarizes public views on issues of prescription drug advertising, government drug research, and prescription drug safety. The
report describes the results clearly and without bias.

Kaiser Public Opinion Spotlight. "Views on Prescription Drugs and the
Pharmaceutical Industry." Available online. URL: http://www.kff.org/
spotlight/rxdrugs/upload/Rx_Drugs.pdf. Updated April 2008. The wealth
of figures reported here covers most aspects of the public's opinions on
prescription drugs and the pharmaceutical industry. People hold much
more positive views about the former than the latter, and the text reviews
the responses fairly, letting readers reach their own opinion. A link on the
webpage reports figures on the views of the public and physicians on
OTC advertising. Although based on the same survey as the USA/Kaiser/
Harvard survey described above, this page provides more detailed charts
and tables.

U.S. Food and Drug Administration. "Drugs@FDA." Available online.
URL: http://www.accessdata.fda.gov/Scripts/cder/DrugsatFDA. Downloaded June 16, 2009. One can select the name of a drug to obtain documents on its history of approval by the FDA or a month and year to see
drug approval reports. Although technical and specialized, the information comes directly from the FDA rather than outside sources.

———. "History." Available online. URL: http://www.fda.gov/AboutFDA/
WhatWeDo/History/default.htm. Updated June 3, 2009. The FDA gives
a brief (and generally positive) overview of its history. Links listed on this
webpage cover origins, important milestones, and leaders and deputies.
Other links include some oral histories of the FDA and research tools.
Although a bit superficial, the material outlines the development of the
FDA.

POLICY AND REGULATION

BOOKS

Baciu, Alina, Kathleen Stratton, and Sheila P. Burke, eds. *The Future of Drug
Safety: Promoting and Protecting the Health of the Public.* Washington, D.C.:
National Academies Press, 2007. The FDA asked the Institute of Medi-
cine to evaluate the drug safety system. This report comes from the panel

of experts who did the evaluation. It is hard to summarize all the information contained in the volume, but the experts identified a host of problems in ensuring the safety of drugs: lack of clear regulatory authority, poor funding, organizational problems, and a scarcity of data on post-approval risks and benefits of drugs. The recommendations for change include reorganizing the FDA and improving the system for reporting adverse events.

Ceccoli, Stephen J. *Pill Politics: Drugs and the FDA*. Boulder, Colo.: Lynne Rienner, 2003. This overview of FDA regulations sees a new pattern emerging in recent years. Cutting review times for new drugs, permitting DTC advertising, and allowing off-label drug use signals a new period of consumer dominance. The author suggests that the new approach, while having important benefits, has created some problems in protecting users from the dangers of prescription drugs and recommends that the FDA do more to resolve these problems.

Daemmrich, Arthur A. *Pharmacopolitics: Drug Regulation in the United States and Germany*. Chapel Hill: University of North Carolina Press, 2004. Germany and the United States have developed surprisingly different systems for the approval and monitoring of prescription drugs. The United States has a more centralized system in which one agency makes decisions based on statistical evidence of safety and effectiveness. In Germany, doctors have more say over approval and rely more often on their own experiences than clinical trials. The broad treatment of the topic looks for underlying differences in the cultures and histories of the two countries that led to the different approaches.

Erlen, Jonathon, and Joseph F. Spillane, eds. *Federal Drug Control: The Evolution of Policy and Practice*. Binghamton, N.Y.: Pharmaceutical Products Press, 2004. This volume focuses on drug control more generally but several chapters cover prescription drugs (e.g., "FDA and the Practice of Pharmacy: Prescription Drug Regulation before 1968" by Rebecca Carroll). The chapters begin with a study of the Harrison Narcotic Control Act of 1914 and move to changes in drug laws through 2001. The historical perspective of the book helps readers to understand current policies and regulations.

Fulda, Thomas R., and Albert I. Wertheimer, eds. *Handbook of Pharmaceutical Public Policy*. New York: Pharmaceutical Products Press, 2007. The articles in this volume examine the influence of economics and politics on prescription drug policies. The chapters cover topics such as prescription drug coverage by Medicare, the drug approval process, innovative state drug practices, importation and reimportation of drugs, abuse of prescription drugs, and health care systems in Europe. Designed to help pharmacy students understand drug polices and pharmaceutical companies, this comprehensive volume is an excellent resource.

Annotated Bibliography

Hawthorne, Fran. *Inside the FDA: The Business and Politics Behind the Drugs We Take and the Food We Eat.* Hoboken, N.J.: John Wiley, 2005. The FDA's importance in regulating prescription drugs and protecting the public cannot be overemphasized. It must foster the development of new drugs but also make sure that they are both safe and effective. The author is an expert on the health care business, and she offers an overview of how the agency works and the pressures it faces. Among the questions it examines: How did dangerous drugs like Vioxx get past the FDA's safety measures; why did the FDA let drug ads on TV; and why is the FDA's role moving beyond science and into public policy?

Hilts, Philip J. *Protecting America's Health: The FDA, Business, and One Hundred Years of Regulation.* New York: Alfred A. Knopf, 2003. This highly praised history of the FDA, perhaps the nation's most important regulatory agency, covers much more than prescription drugs. However, its theme of the battle of the FDA to overcome aggressive industry lobbying and opposition to regulation certainly fits prescription drugs. It gives many examples of the persistent efforts to sell ineffective drugs and the FDA's counteractions. The FDA has generally done well, according to the author, in protecting the public's health and deserves more support and better funding than it gets.

Parrish, Richard Henry, II. *Defining Drugs: How Government Became the Arbiter of Pharmaceutical Fact.* New Brunswick, N.J.: Transaction Publishers, 2003. The author believes that the government more than physicians and pharmacists has taken the power to decide what prescription drug treatments are suitable for patients. He presents much historical detail on the evolution of policy and criticizes the loss of physician and patient choice in treatments.

Pisano, Douglas J., and David S. Mantus, eds. *FDA Regulatory Affairs: A Guide for Prescription Drugs, Medical Devices, and Biologics.* New York: Informa Healthcare USA, 2008. This book describes what it calls the maze of regulations governing drugs and other products that the FDA oversees. It aims to help those having to deal with the FDA, including organizations that must comply with FDA regulations. In addition, its clear exposition can help those wanting general information on how the process of drug approval works. Chapters cover topics such as submitting new drug applications, the development of orphan drugs, and drug laws.

Richards, Byron J. *Fight for Your Health: Exposing the FDA's Betrayal of America.* Minneapolis, Minn.: Wellness Resources, 2006. The harsh criticism of the FDA in this book contrasts with the more balanced tone of the book by Fran Hawthorne. A clinical nutritionist and advocate of natural health options, Richards says the FDA covers up adverse reactions of dangerous yet popular drugs and prohibits many natural health options. He views the search for profits by drug companies as the source of many prescription drug problems and says the FDA works primarily on behalf of the drug companies.

Schweitzer, Stuart O. *Pharmaceutical Economics and Policy.* Oxford: Oxford University Press, 2007. The author, a professor at UCLA, provides an economic overview of the drug industry and the policies that regulate it. Unlike many books critical of the drug industry, he presents balanced coverage of the issues and recognizes the complexities that drug companies face in producing and selling drugs and meeting conflicting demands.

United States Congress, House Committee on Energy and Commerce, Subcommittee on Health. *Reauthorization of the Prescription Drug User Fee Act: Hearing before the Subcommittee on Health of the Committee on Energy and Commerce, House of Representatives, One Hundred Tenth Congress, First Session, April 17, 2007.* Washington, D.C.: U.S. Government Printing Office, 2008. Also available online. URL: http://frwebgate.access.gpo.gov/cgi-bin/getdoc.cgi?dbname=110_house_hearings&d ocid=f:40159.pdf. Downloaded June 4, 2009. Before Congress reauthorized the Prescription Drug User Fee Act in 2007, this hearing described problems in how past legislation worked. For example, the drug review process sometimes occurred too quickly, and postapproval safety received too little attention. The many witnesses in the hearing describe both strengths and weaknesses of the Prescription Drug User Fee Act and the need for changes.

ARTICLES

Armstrong, Drew. "Detail of the FDA Overhaul." *CQ Weekly* 65, no. 46 (December 3, 2007): 3,605–3,606. This article describes 2007 legislation to change how the FDA regulates advertising and safety of drugs.

Benderly, Beryl Lieff. "Experimental Drugs on Trial." *Scientific American* 297, no. 4 (October 2007): 92–99. The FDA often finds itself in caught between two contradictory sets of demands. On one hand, many want the agency to protect the safety of prescription drugs users by not approving drugs in the absence of rigorous evidence on their safety. On the other hand, some patients with serious illnesses want access to experimental drugs that, although not yet proven safe, may save their lives. This article describes the dilemma the agency faces in the context of a lawsuit by patients who want quicker access to anticancer drugs. The FDA has come down on the side of safety and delayed access, but the issue is a difficult one.

Couzin, Jennifer. "Stronger Research Just One Item on Drug Agency's Wish List." *Science* 323 (March 20, 2009): 1,549. The new leaders of the FDA in the Obama administration, Margaret Hamburg and Joshua Sharfstein, face many problems. This short article describes these problems, giving particular attention to the need for stronger research skills among the staff who evaluate new drugs based on stem-cell and genetic research. Other problems mentioned in the article include an antiquated computer system and difficulty regulating overseas production of drugs.

Drazen, Jeffrey M. "Getting All the Facts on Drugs: Clinical-Trial Registries." *Newsweek* 145, no. 26A (Summer 2005): 72. The federal government created a registry of clinical trials so the public can get full information on the safety and effectiveness of any prescription drugs they might use. This article notes, however, that companies can still report selective results that highlight benefits and minimize risks. Many major medical journals have attempted to make the data more widely available by refusing to publish results from a clinical study that has not been registered. This article describes regulatory efforts to make sure information on prescription drugs is fully and accurately released.

"Evolution of Current Law." *Congressional Digest* 82, no. 9 (November 2003): 260–261. This chronology through 2000 presents milestones in the history of prescription drug laws.

Gottlieb, Scott. "Medicine by Mandarins: FDA's Rigid Drug Testing Regulations." *American Spectator* 35, no. 6 (November/December 2002): 22–23. Most articles criticize the FDA for not doing enough to ensure the safety of prescription drugs. This article provides a contrast. It says that greater FDA control of drug approval has led to vagueness, unpredictability, and delay, and it calls for more transparency and consistency in decision making at the agency.

Jetter, Alexis. "Strong Medicine: FDA Problems." *Reader's Digest* 172 (April 2008): 118–131. According to this story, the FDA is woefully underfunded and understaffed to regulate the billions of prescription drugs used today. The approval of Vioxx and the slow reaction to evidence that the new painkiller caused heart problems hurt the reputation of the agency, and morale has worsened. The article suggests some potential solutions to these and other problems.

Lewis, Carol. "The 'Poison Squad' and the Advent of Food and Drug Regulation." *FDA Consumer* 36, no. 6 (November/December 2002): 12–15. One early form of clinical trial came from a study in 1902 that fed volunteers several poisons commonly used in small amounts as food preservatives. The volunteers, called the poison squad, did not appear to suffer long-term harm from the poisoning, but short-term sickness led the scientists in charge to conclude that accumulation of poisons, even when taken in small amounts, presented dangers to the public. The study led to banning of these preservatives, better government regulation of food additives, and, more generally, called for testing prescription drugs.

Mandavilli, Apoorva. "Rx for the FDA." *Discover* 29, no. 1 (January 2008): 24. This article describes some of the changes in the FDA legislated by 2007 amendments. The changes increase the agency's budget and give it

new powers to ensure safety. They also require the FDA to create a surveillance system that will identify drug safety problems earlier.

Meadows, Michelle. "The FDA's Drug Review Process: Ensuring Drugs
Are Safe and Effective." *FDA Consumer* 36, no. 4 (July/August 2002):
19–24. The FDA's magazine describes the 12-step process of a drug review in terms that consumers can easily understand. The theme is that the
careful review process protects the safety of prescription drug users.

Pear, Robert. "Senate Approves Tighter Policing of Drug Makers." *New
York Times* (May 10, 2007): A1, A30. This description of 2007 legislation
shows the efforts of Congress to strengthen the regulation of prescription
drugs and protect consumers. The law requires the FDA to monitor drug
safety after as well as before approval and reauthorizes payments from
drug companies to cover the additional costs of the safety monitoring.

Walters, Jonathan. "Pills of Protest." *Governing* 20, no. 10 (July 2007): 24.
The federal government finds itself in the middle of a battle over reimporting prescription drugs at lower prices than sold in the United States.
According to this article, state governments favor ways to reduce prices
for their health programs and meet the needs of their citizens; pharmaceutical companies remain opposed to reimportation. Although the legislation described by the article failed to pass the Senate, the goal of
lowering prices will likely lead to new bills to allow reimportation.

WEB DOCUMENTS

AARP. "International Forum on Prescription Drug Policy." Available online. URL: http://www.aarp.org/research/health/drugs/a2003-05-09-
drugsummary.html. Posted June 10, 2003. The presentations listed on
this page come from a conference that examines how Canada, Australia,
and countries of Europe have dealt with the problem of providing prescription drug access to citizens at reasonable cost. Key facts about systems in other countries highlight the contrast with the United States.
Changes have occurred since 2003 in all countries, but the national differences remain large.

AARP. "Rx Drug Smarts." Available online. URL: http://www.aarp.org/
health/conditions/rxdrugs. Downloaded July 8, 2009. This organization
for the elderly and retired offers diverse and detailed information on use
of prescription drugs. The webpage covers topics on drug safety, price,
and effectiveness.

Almanac of Policy Issues. "Prescription Drugs: Accessibility and Prices."
Available online. URL: http://www.policyalmanac.org/health/archive/
prescription_drugs.shtml. Downloaded June 17, 2009. This excerpt from
a 2000 report sponsored by the Department of Health and Human Services describes several problems that patients face in gaining access to

needed prescription drugs. Legislation in 2003 to create the Medicare Prescription Drug Program addressed several of the problems for seniors, but other groups still lack access to the drugs they need. This document describes both past and continuing problems.

CMS Legislative Summary. "Medicare Prescription Drug, Improvement, and Modernization Act of 2003, Public Law 108-173." Available online. URL: http://www.cms.hhs.gov/MMAUpdate/downloads/PL108-173 summary.pdf. Posted April 2004. At 148 pages, this summary from the Centers for Medicare and Medicaid Services, the federal agency that administers these two programs, includes considerable detail on the legislation. Not all the details will matter for most researchers, but the document describes problems older persons faced in paying for the prescription drugs and how this federal legislation dealt with the problems.

Crowley, Jeffrey S., Deb Ashner, and Linda Elam. "State Medicaid Outpatient Prescription Drug Policies: Findings from a National Survey, 2005 Update." Kaiser Commission on Medicaid and the Uninsured. Available online. URL: http://www.kff.org/medicaid/upload/State-Medicaid-Outpatient-Prescription-Drug-Policies-Findings-from-a-National-Survey-2005-Update-report.pdf. Posted October 2005. The results of this survey of 36 states describe how they control Medicaid costs for prescription drugs. Some states put limits on the number of prescriptions or refills that beneficiaries may receive, but others are developing policies that do not deny benefits. They instead require clinical justification for the additional drugs. This report discusses these and other policies in some detail.

Frontline. "Dangerous Prescription." Public Broadcasting Service (PBS). Available online. URL: http://www.pbs.org/wgbh/pages/frontline/shows/prescription. Posted November 13, 2003. This investigation of the drug safety system in the United States begins with the fact that, from 1997 to 2001, more than a dozen previously approved drugs had been pulled from the market for the damage they caused to patients. This leads to the question of how effectively the FDA meets its goal of protecting the public from dangerous drugs. The crux of the story comes from interviews with experts. The interviews cover contentious issues involving the FDA, pharmaceutical companies, and the dangerous drugs themselves.

Gokhale, Jagadeesh. "An Evaluation of Medicare's Prescription Drug Policy." Cato Institute. Available online. URL: http://www.cato.org/testimony/ct-jg092005.html. Posted September 22, 2005. This senior fellow at the Cato Institute, an organization supporting free markets, calls for scaling back the Medicare prescription drug benefit passed by Congress in 2003. Supported by detailed statistics and charts, the author argues that the policy is shortsighted and based on bad economics. The statement was made before the Committee on Homeland Security and Government Affairs but represents a minority view of this popular program.

Medicare. "Prescription Drug Coverage." Available online. URL: http://
www.medicare.gov/pdphome.asp. Downloaded June 18. 2009. This government webpage on obtaining prescription drug coverage for Medicare
beneficiaries covers questions such as who is eligible, what prescription
drug plans exist, and how to enroll. In addition, the webpage contains
background publications and press releases on how the program works.

U.S. Food and Drug Administration. "Prescription Drug User Fee Act
(PDUFA)." Available online. URL: http://www.fda.gov/ForIndustry/
UserFees/PrescriptionDrugUserFee/default.htm. Updated May 22,
2009. The background information and reports on this webpage describe
a crucial component of the drug evaluation system. The Prescription
Drug User Fee Act, first passed in 1992 and renewed three times, autho-
rizes the FDA to collect fees from companies that have developed new
drugs to pay for the review of the drugs. The fees help the FDA employ
the staff needed to carry out the reviews with due speed.

PRICES AND ACCESS

BOOKS

Congressional Budget Office. *Prescription Drug Pricing in the Private Sector.*
Washington, D.C.: Congress of the U.S., Congressional Budget Office,
2007. Also available online. URL: http://purl.access.gpo.gov/GPO/
LPS77539. Downloaded June 4, 2009. The supply chain through which
drugs go from manufacturers to consumers is remarkably complex, and
this report written for members of Congress tries to explain this chain and
its influences on prices. In turn, the chain by which payments flow back
from consumers to manufacturers adds even more complexity. Wholesalers, retail pharmacies, hospitals, HMOs, nursing homes, insurance companies, government programs, and consumers all have a role in prescription
drug pricing. Although not easy to summarize, the information in this
report supplies a unique overview of the drug pricing system.

Dicken, John E. *Prescription Drugs: Oversight of Drug Pricing in Federal Programs: Testimony before the Committee on Oversight and Government Reform,
House of Representatives.* Washington, D.C.: U.S. Government Accountability Office, 2007. Also available online. URL: http://purl.access.gpo.
gov/GPO/LPS78826. Downloaded June 4, 2009. Since federal and state
governments spend large sums on prescription drugs through Medicare
and Medicaid, Congress wanted to know more about how governments
can make sure they get the best prices. This report identifies some instances where companies charged the government more than they should
for Medicaid and Medicare drugs. It suggests some steps needed to

ensure that the prices reported and charged by private organizations are accurate. These steps do not directly affect consumers, but they affect taxes and the costs to the government of prescription drugs.

———. *Prescription Drugs: An Overview of Approaches to Negotiate Drug Prices Used by Other Countries and U.S. Private Payers and Federal Programs: Testimony before the Committee on Finance, U.S. Senate.* Washington, D.C.: U.S. Government Accountability Office, 2007. Also available online. URL: http://purl.access.gpo.gov/GPO/LPS78520. Downloaded June 5, 2009. The Medicare Prescription Drug Act prevents the U.S. government from negotiating for lower prescription drug prices with pharmaceutical companies. In considering amendments to this part of the legislation, Congress asked the Government Accountability Office to describe how negotiations over prescription drug prices might work. In considering negotiations in other countries, private health plans in the United States, and other federal programs, the report finds a wide range of approaches that the government might use and offers insights into the nature of pricing and purchasing for prescription drugs.

———. *Prescription Drugs: Trends in Usual and Customary Prices for Drugs Frequently Used by Medicare and Non-Medicare Health Insurance Enrollees.* Washington, D.C.: U.S. Government Accountability Office, 2007. Also available online. URL: http://purl.access.gpo.gov/GPO/LPS87653. Downloaded June 4, 2009. Given the payments the federal government makes for Medicare prescription drugs, it has a stake in rising prices. This report describes price changes from January 2004 through January 2007 using information from New York and Pennsylvania. The figures reveal that brand-name drug prices rose faster than the rate of inflation, but generic drug prices decreased.

Goozner, Merrill. *The $800 Million Pill: The Truth behind the Cost of New Drugs.* Berkeley: University of California Press, 2004. The $800 million figure refers to the cost of developing a new prescription drug according to the drug industry (now estimated to be considerably higher). In examining the process of developing a new drug and what it really costs, Goozner disputes this claim. Breakthrough drugs come from dedicated and passionate scientists who often work at universities and government institutes rather than drug companies. Going beyond this general point, the book contains stories and details about drug discovery.

Harrison, Christopher Scott. *The Politics of the International Pricing of Prescription Drugs.* Westport, Conn.: Praeger, 2004. In response to concerns that drug prices in America are too high in comparison to other countries, some American government officials have pushed for other countries to raise their prices to similar levels. Others call for the United States to lower its prices to levels in other nations. The debate raises issues of intellectual property in the context of world trade. A lawyer and political scientist with a Texas law firm, Harrison discusses many complex issues of patent law and international relations.

Jardini, Edward. *How to Save on Prescription Drugs: 20 Cost-Saving Methods.* Berkeley, Calif.: Celestial Arts, 2008. Described as a way to fight back against outrageous prescription drug costs, this book offers practical advice to consumers. The physician author suggests ways to eliminate unnecessary drugs, substitute less expensive drugs, and buy medicines at a discount. The book also discusses how to save money with the Medicare prescription drug benefit program.

PhRMA. *What Goes into the Cost of Prescription Drugs?* Washington, D.C.: Pharmaceutical Research and Manufacturers of America, 2005. Also available online. URL: http://www.phrma.org/files/Cost_of_Prescription_Drugs.pdf. Downloaded April 4, 2009. This document authored by the major pharmaceutical industry trade group defends the industry with clear and well-presented arguments. Critics strenuously dispute the claims made here, but the material is an excellent overview of what the industry says about the benefits of its products and the reasons for the high costs of the drugs companies sell.

Robinson, Ira Charles. *Prescriptions, Patients, Profits, Perils and Pro-People Choices: Be Drug Smart, Slash Costs, Be Safer, Be Healthier.* Lincoln, Neb.: iUniverse, 2007. While giving much attention to how consumers can save costs in purchasing medications, this book offers more general advice on the effective use of prescription drugs. It gives background on the drug development process, drug safety regulation, and the potential for drug abuse. Like many other books, it criticizes the drug industry for high prices and focus on profits.

United States Congress, House Committee on Government Reform, Subcommittee on Human Rights and Wellness. *The Economic Aspects of the Pharmaceutical Industry in the United States: Hearing before the Subcommittee on Human Rights and Wellness of the Committee on Government Reform, House of Representatives, One Hundred Eighth Congress, First Session, June 25, 2003.* Washington, D.C.: U.S. Government Printing Office, 2003. Also available online. URL: http://frwebgate.access.gpo.gov/cgi-bin/getdoc.cgi?dbname=108_house_hearings&d ocid=f:89849.pdf. Downloaded June 4, 2009. This hearing examines the problem of high prescription drug prices. Although dated, many examples illustrate the much higher drug prices in the United States than other countries and the effort of many Americans to go to Canada to purchase prescription drugs. The representatives at the hearing strongly criticize the drug industry for the high prices, but one witness defends the drug industry and argues that drug prices are reasonable given the health benefits they bring.

———. *International Prescription Drug Parity: Are Americans Being Protected or Gouged? Hearing before the Subcommittee on Human Rights and Wellness of the*

Annotated Bibliography

Committee on Government Reform, House of Representatives, One Hundred Eighth Congress, First Session, April 3, 2003. Washington, D.C.: U.S. Government Printing Office, 2003. Also available online. URL: http://frwebgate.access.gpo.gov/cgi-bin/getdoc.cgi?dbname=108_house_hearings&d ocid=f:87228.pdf. Downloaded June 4, 2009. With a focus on lower drug prices in Canada, this hearing considers both sides of debates over the benefits of allowing Americans to purchase drugs in other countries. Higher prices in the United States, as some witnesses note, encourage innovation by the drug companies. Others suggest, however, that the high prices exploit American consumers. Most congressional representatives at the hearing favor greater access of Americans to drugs in other countries.

United States Congress, Senate Special Committee on Aging. *The Effects of Escalating Drug Costs on the Elderly: Hearing before the Special Committee on Aging, United States Senate, One Hundred Second Congress, Second Session: Morning Session, Macon, GA, April 22, 1992.* Washington, D.C.: U.S. Government Printing Office, 1992. As illustrated by this 1992 hearing, concern about prescription drugs prices dates back several decades. The hearing gives some background on a problem that would escalate until the 2003 passage of the Medicare Prescription Drug Act.

———. *The Impact of Direct-to-Consumer Drug Advertising on Seniors' Health and Health Care Costs: Hearing before the Special Committee on Aging, United States Senate, One Hundred Ninth Congress, First Session, Washington, DC, September 29, 2005.* Washington, D.C.: U.S. Government Printing Office, 2006. Also available online. URL: http://frwebgate.access.gpo.gov/cgi-bin/getdoc.cgi?dbname=109_senate_hearings&docid=f:25879.pdf. Downloaded June 8, 2009. Senators have worried that DTC ads increase the costs that the government pays for prescription drugs under Medicare Part D. The witnesses in this hearing present multiple viewpoints on how the ads affect physicians and health care consumers. For example, a representative from the FDA points out that the ads clearly get to consumers—81 percent of those responding to a survey had been exposed to prescription drug ads. However, most discount the message: "60 percent of patients and physicians believe that direct-to-consumer advertisements overstate the benefits of the product and almost as many believe that the ads understate the risks."

ARTICLES

Anderson, Jessica L. "Save Big on Prescriptions." *Kiplinger's Personal Finance* 62, no. 5 (May 2008): 71–72. Among the pieces of advice given by this article on how to lower prescription drug costs are to buy generics, use mail-order programs, and participate in spending accounts for health-related expenses.

Prescription Drugs

Barlett, Donald L., and James B. Steele. "Why We Pay So Much for Drugs." *Time* 163, no. 5, February 2, 2004, pp. 44–52. This cover story contrasts the regulation of prescription drug prices in other nations with the limited regulation in the United States. According to the authors, Americans have a general distaste for price controls on any good, and drug-company lobbying makes it particularly difficult to set prescription drug prices by legislation. However, the article predicts that growing resistance to higher prices at the state level will lead to changes.

Beran, Mary Sue, Marianne Laouri, and Marika Suttorp. "Brief Reports: Medication Costs: The Role Physicians Play with Their Senior Patients." *Journal of the American Geriatrics Society* 55, no. 1 (January 2007): 102–107. How often do physicians discuss costs when choosing medications for senior patients? A survey of 678 doctors found that they rarely discussed prices and, when they did, patients usually initiated the topic. The discussion typically results in recommending generic drugs and offering free samples.

Buntin, John. "Minding the Detailers: State Challenges to Drug Companies." *Governing* 22, no. 5 (February 2009): 28–33. This story describes various state efforts to restrict or regulate direct-to-physician sales efforts of drug companies. Since states pay for the prescription drug costs of Medicaid patients and state employees, they have interests in controlling prices. According to the article, drug company sales representatives (known as detailers) have undue influence, often encouraging prescription of expensive patented drugs when cheaper generics would work. States hope that limiting this influence can lead to considerable cost savings.

Capretta, James C., and Peter Wehner. "A Bush Success (Not That He Gets Credit)." *Weekly Standard* 13, no. 31 (April 28, 2008): 18–19. According to this article in a conservative magazine, the Medicare prescription drug benefit passed and implemented during the George W. Bush administration has been a huge success. Patients benefit from the discounted costs of drugs and report high satisfaction with the program. Further, competition among private plans that enroll Medicare beneficiaries seems to have worked well, keeping monthly premiums for beneficiaries well below what was expected.

"Cholesterol Drugs: Lipitor Battles Generics." *Consumer Reports* 73, no. 3 (March 2008): 48–49. This article says that generic statin drugs work just as well as brand-name statin drugs like Lipitor but cost only half as much; however, drug company ads wrongly imply superiority of their brand-name products over generics. The article gives advice about generic versions of statins to those needing to take an anticholesterol drug.

Cunningham, Peter J. "Medicaid Cost Containment and Access to Prescription Drugs." *Health Affairs* 24, no. 3 (2005): 780–789. States have attempted to control the costs they must pay for Medicaid by limiting benefits for prescription drugs. This study reports on the ability of Medicaid enrollees to get the drugs they need. According to reports of the enrollees, policies such as prior authorization and mandatory generic substitution have created problems in access to prescription drugs.

Enserink, Martin. "Malaria Drugs, the Coca-Cola Way." *Science* 322 (November 21, 2008): 1,174. High prices make it difficult for patients in wealthy nations like the United States to buy certain drugs, but the developing world confronts even greater problems. The inability of poor families to purchase medications gives companies little incentive to develop products for diseases common in the developing world. This article describes one plan to get new antimalaria drugs to low-income people who need them. The essence of the plan is for donor agencies to subsidize the production costs of the drugs so companies can sell them inexpensively. The article also describes some potential obstacles faced by the plan.

Frakt, Austin B., Steven D. Pizer, Ann M. Hendricks. "Controlling Prescription Drug Costs: Regulation and the Role of Interest Groups in Medicare and the Veterans Health Administration." *Journal of Health Politics, Policy and Law* 33, no. 6 (December 2008): 1,079–1,106. By comparing drug programs for Medicare (which prohibits negotiation of prices with drug companies) and the Veteran's Administration (which allows the negotiation), the authors make recommendations on how Medicare can reduce the prices it pays for prescription drugs. However, such efforts will need to overcome protests of the pharmaceutical industry.

Gagnon, Marc-André, and Joel Lexchin. "The Cost of Pushing Pills: A New Estimate of Pharmaceutical Promotion Expenditures in the United States." *PLOS Medicine* 5, no. 1 (2008): e1. Available online. URL: http://medicine. plosjournals.org/perlserv/?request=get-document&doi=10.1371/journal. pmed.0050001&ct=1. Downloaded April 6, 2008. The authors attempt to estimate the costs of developing and selling drugs. They find that much more goes to marketing and less to research and development than drug companies typically claim.

Harris, Gardiner. "British Balance Benefit vs. Cost of Latest Drugs." *New York Times* (December 3, 2008): A1, A18. The British government holds down the costs of prescription drugs by relying on the National Institute for Health and Clinical Excellence (NICE) to set guidelines on what drugs and treatments are worth the cost. Complaints among Britons have risen just as other nations have started to look at the model for dealing with their own cost problems. In reviewing the controversy, the article tells the story of a British cancer patient who was refused payment by the government for an expensive cancer drug. Because of protests involving cases like this, the British government is reconsidering its payment policies for certain drugs.

Huber, Peter. "Who Pays for a Cancer Drug?" *Forbes* 183, no. 1 (January 12, 2009): 72. The author argues in favor of protecting the patents of drug companies so that market incentives encourage innovation. He notes that most of the costs for prescription drugs fall on a small group. Wealthy Americans pay high prices while the patent lasts, but Americans with less income and residents of other nations that control prescription drug prices pay less. Those paying lower prices are subsidized by those paying more.

"Importing Prescription Drugs." *Congressional Digest* 82, no. 9 (November 2003): 257–288. This article covers the debate over importing drugs back into the United States from other countries that rely on government controls to keep prices low. It describes varied legislative proposals to make such importation legal. Although none of the proposals has passed, the issues remain and similar legislation is being proposed today in Congress.

Laliberte, Richard. "The Great Drug Switcheroo: Therapeutic Substitution." *Prevention* 61, no. 5 (May 2009): 117–121. In some cases, pharmacists can fill prescriptions with other drugs that are similar or identical without the doctor or patient knowing. This article describes some cases in which the substitution drug caused problems. The substitution aims to reduce costs, but more care is needed to make sure that treatment is not compromised.

Ornes, Lynne, and Thomas J. Hendrix. "Prescription Drug Re-importation: A Balanced Look." *Journal of Gerontological Nursing* 32, no. 8 (August 2006): 15–19. This article discusses price and safety concerns about reimporting drugs from other countries or buying drugs from other countries via foreign mail-order sites. It presents helpful facts and a history of the contentious debate over reimportation.

Postrel, Virginia. "My Drug Problem: Refusal of New Zealand Government to Pay for Herceptin Treatments." *Atlantic Monthly* 303, no. 2 (March 2009): 32–34. The author describes how, at the cost of $60,000 to her insurer, the drug Herceptin successfully treated her breast cancer. She argues that a more centralized U.S. health care system will need to limit costs for expensive drugs like this. Already, the New Zealand government has refused to pay for treatment by Herceptin.

Reinhardt, Erika. "Access to Medicines." *UN Chronicle* 43, no. 3 (September/November 2006): 56–57. The UN offers a way to increase access to desperately needed medications among poor people throughout the world. Countries can take advantage of flexibility built into international patent and trade agreements to buy high-priority medicines for HIV/AIDS. However, the article criticizes national trademark laws than hinder these types of public health efforts in developing nations.

Santerre, Rexford E., John A. Vernon, and Carmelo Giacotto. "The Impact of Indirect Government Controls on U.S. Drug Prices and R&D." *Cato*

Journal 26, no. 1 (Winter 2006): 143–158. This article in a journal supportive of the free market presents data on the costs of government controls on drug prices. It concludes that government actions to keep prices low obstruct development of new drugs, cost drug companies millions that would have gone toward research, and ultimately slow increases in longevity among the public. The figures presented are complex and no doubt controversial.

Saul, Stephanie. "In Sour Economy, Some Scale Back on Medications." *New York Times* (October 21, 2008): A1. Also available online. URL: http://www.nytimes.com/2008/10/22/business/22drug.html?scp=10&sq=prescription%20drugs&st=cse. Downloaded May 18, 2009. During the recent recession, many individuals and families faced tough decisions about whether to cut living expenses by reducing prescription drug use. This article gives several examples of patients who stopped taking expensive medications or lowered their dosage. If drugs are being overprescribed, the cutback may not cause much harm. However, it could also result in increased medical expenses later. In any case, the inability to afford needed products puts the drug companies on the defensive for charging high prices for brand-name drugs.

Spring, Tom. "Online Drugs: Mostly Legal, Maybe Lethal." *PC World* 27, no. 3 (March 2009): 12–14. On the plus side, the availability of prescription drugs via the Internet has made difficult-to-find drugs more accessible. However, some of the sales may be illegal, and the Drug Enforcement Agency is cracking down on illegal Internet drug purchases.

Volland, Adam. "Shopping for a Drug Plan." *U.S. News & World Report* 143, no. 18 (November 19, 2007): 79–80. Medicare participants need to select their prescription drug plans carefully. As reported in this article, costs can vary widely across plan providers and even across years for the same provider. The author gives advice on making effective choices and on keeping costs for prescription drugs low.

WEB DOCUMENTS

Alderman, Lesley. "Strategies for Saving on Prescription Drugs." *New York Times.* Available online. URL: http://www.nytimes.com/2009/02/07/health/06patient.html?_r=1&scp=2&sq=prescription%20drugs&st=cse. Posted February 6, 2009. The first sentence of this news story, "Drugs have never been so expensive—or so cheap," summarizes the complexity of issues surrounding prescription drugs. Costs for brand-name drugs averaged about $120 in 2007, compared to $34 for generic drugs (and only $4 per 30-day supply at Wal-Mart or Target). Besides buying generics, consumers can do other things to find cheap drug prices, such as taking advantage of private health insurance coverage, talking to a doctor about cheaper alternatives, and comparing costs at retail outlets. Those with few resources can also get aid from organizations listed in the story.

Associated Press. "States Consider Cutting Drug Help for Seniors: But Some Say Those Who Stop Taking Meds May End Up Needing Pricier Care." MSNBC Health/Health Care. Available online. URL: http://www.msnbc.msn.com/id/30966094. Posted May 27, 2009. Although Medicare Part D pays for part of the cost of prescription drugs for eligible older and disabled persons, some states help cover addition out-of-pocket expenses for those using particularly expensive drugs. Yet, according to this news story, financial problems of the states may lead them to cut this benefit and the access of some older persons to the drugs they need. It describes, for example, the plans of Rhode Island to reduce the prescription benefits it provides and the problems the reduction will cause for some patients.

ConsumerReportsHealth.org. "Generic Drugs: Your Questions Answered." Available online. URL: http://www.consumerreports.org/health/prescription-drugs/generic-drugs-your-questions-answered-4-07/overview/0704_generic-drugs-your-questions-answered_ov.htm. Posted April 2007. The questions and answers can help prescription drug users who may worry about replacing brand-name drugs with generic drugs. The answers are reassuring—generics cost much less but meet the same manufacturing standards as brand-name drugs. The text does emphasize the need to talk to the prescribing doctor about substituting generics, however.

Democratic Leadership Council. "Restraining Prescription Drug Costs." Available online. URL: http://www.dlc.org/ndol_ci.cfm?contentid=253949&kaid=139&subid=275. Posted June 30, 2008. This liberal advocacy group takes state programs that have had some success in controlling prescription drugs prices as models for what the nation can do. Among the recommendations are to increase use of generic drugs, allow consumers to obtain information on price comparisons so they can shop at pharmacies with the best prices, and give doctors more information on safety warnings of prescription drugs.

Espo, David. "Baucus, White House in Deal with Drug Industry." SFGate: Home of the *San Francisco Chronicle*. Available online. URL: http://www.sfgate.com/cgi-bin/article.cgi?f=/n/a/2009/06/20/national/w002129D31.DTL&tsp=1. Posted June 20, 2009. As part of new health care reforms, President Obama and allies in Congress are putting pressure on drug companies to keep down the costs of prescription drugs. As reported in this news story from the Associated Press, pharmaceutical companies have agreed to help. They will spend $80 billion over the next decade to improve Medicare drug benefits for seniors. More generally, they agreed to cooperate in reducing health care costs in the future.

Annotated Bibliography

FoxNews.com. "Price of Generic Prescription Drugs Gets Cheaper." Available online. URL: http://www.foxnews.com/story/0,2933,465366,00. html. Posted December 11, 2008. In contrast to rising prices for brand-name drugs, prices for generic drugs have declined in recent years and likely will continue to do so. This story attributes a good part of the decline to low prices offered by discount stores such as Wal-Mart. Also, intense competition among generic manufacturers for popular drugs leads to lower prices. As the patents on several top-selling drugs such as Lipitor run out in the next few yeas, it will further increase competition for sales and reduce prices.

Gladwell, Malcolm. "High Prices: How to Think about Prescription Drugs." *New Yorker* (October 2005). Available online. URL: http://www. newyorker.com/archive/2004/10/25/041025crat_atlarge. Downloaded April 4, 2009. This popular writer of several best-selling books such as *The Tipping Point*, argues that prescription drug prices in the United States are not that much higher than in other countries. Rather, prices of brand-name drugs are more expensive and prices of generic drugs are cheaper.

Goldstein, Jacob. "Shift to Pills Can Leave Cancer Patients on the Hook." Wall Street Journal Health Blog. Available online. URL: http://blogs.wsj. com/health/2009/04/15/shift-to-pills-can-leave-cancer-patients-on-the-hook/. Posted April 15, 2009. The complexity of health insurance rules for paying for prescription drugs shows in ways of treating cancer. The same drug given as an injection in a doctor's office is covered more often than taking pills bought from a pharmacist. As reported in this story, pills are easier to take and allow for treatment at home but may cost thousands of dollars more.

———. "More Prescriptions for Generics, Fewer for Branded Drugs." Wall Street Journal Health Blog. Available online. URL: http://blogs.wsj.com/ health/2009/04/07/more-prescriptions-for-generics-fewer-for-branded-drugs. Posted April 7, 2009. The author reports a 12 percent increase in purchase of generic drugs from 2004 to 2008 and a 6 percent decrease in brand-name drugs. By 2008, generics had become more common, selling 2.4 billion prescriptions compared to 1.4 billion prescriptions for brand-name drugs. The recent loss of patents for many popular drugs and the efforts of consumers to cut costs contribute to the trend, which will likely continue.

Maryland's People's Law Library. "Special Reduced and Free Prescription Drug Programs." Available online. URL: http://www.peoples-law.org/ health/charity-care/special_drug.htm. Posted November 10, 2008. Many public and private organizations offer prescription drugs for free or at reduced prices. Among the public organizations are state governments and foundations, and among the private organizations are drug manufacturers. The webpage gives details or links on how to access these benefits.

More generally, it gives a sense of some ways to deal with problems faced by many in paying for prescription drugs.

Prescription Access Litigation. "Final Settlement of Two Conspiracy Lawsuits Rolls Back Prices on Hundreds of Drugs, Saving Billions in Future Prescription Drug Costs." Available online. URL: http://www. prescriptionaccess.org/press/pressreleases?id=0049. Posted March 19, 2009. This press release illustrates one strategy to control drug prices. It reports on efforts to use litigation against drug companies, and in particular the settlement of two class-action suits against publishers of prescription drug prices who were accused of inflating prices.

Prescription Policy Choices. "Best Practices Fast Facts: Drug Prices and Spending on Prescription Drugs." Available online. URL: http://www. policychoices.org/documents/DrugCostsAccess_FastFacts.pdf. Updated April 2008. This short but helpful list of facts shows that drug prices and spending continue to rise unabated, particularly for specialized drugs. The document concludes that high drug prices are a major limitation in access to health care.

Public Citizen. "Rx R&D Myths: The Case against the Drug Industry's R&D 'Scare Card.'" Available online. URL: http://www.citizen.org/ publications/release.cfm?ID=7065. Downloaded April 6, 2009. An organization that is highly critical of the pharmaceutical industry disputes claims that research and development costs justify high prescription drug prices. This page contains the summary of the arguments made by the organization as well as a link to the full report and more detailed evidence.

Reed, Marie C. "An Update on Americans' Access to Prescription Drugs." Center for Studying Health System Change. Available online. URL: http:// www.hschange.org/CONTENT/738. Posted May 2005. According to this study, 14 million Americans with chronic conditions in 2003 could not afford the prescription drugs they needed. The Medicare Prescription Drug Program has made progress for the elderly, but cost problems remain for younger groups. This report examines the role of insurance, income, and race in problems of affording prescription drugs and suggests that the problem will get worse without substantial policy changes.

THE PHARMACEUTICAL INDUSTRY

BOOKS

Angell, Marcia. *The Truth about the Drug Companies: How They Deceive Us and What to Do about It.* New York: Random House, 2004. Of the numerous books critical of the drug companies, this one has received the most attention and makes a persuasive if one-sided case. The author, a physician at Harvard University and former editor of the prestigious *New England Journal of Medicine*, has the credentials to criticize the medical profession as well as the drug industry. She writes clearly and vigorously and includes detailed source material. Her indictment covers topics ranging from profits and patents to lobbying and leads to specific recommendations for change.

Blackett, Tom, and Rebecca Robins, eds. *Brand Medicine: The Role of Branding in the Pharmaceutical Industry*. Basingstoke, U.K.: Palgrave, 2001. This book begins with the premise that branding—giving names and identities to products that distinguish them from other similar products—has become crucial to the success of pharmaceutical products. This requires drug companies to create direct relationships with consumers and consumers to have information and freedom of choice. The chapters in the volume on DTC branding and the role of advertising in branding give insights into the strategies used by drug companies to sell their products.

Campbell, John J. *Understanding Pharma: The Professional's Guide to How Pharmaceutical and Biotech Companies Really Work*. 2nd edition. Raleigh, N.C.: Pharmaceutical Institute, 2008. Written to help workers in the pharmaceutical industry understand how their companies work, this book contains helpful background information for researchers. Chapters cover topics such as supply and demand for drugs, drug development, marketing and brand management, and the importance of sales. While most treatments of the drug industry are critical, this more supportive one aims to help workers succeed within the industry rather than to change it.

Chandler, Alfred D., Jr. *Shaping the Industrial Century: The Remarkable Story of the Evolution of the Modern Chemical and Pharmaceutical Industries*. Cambridge, Mass.: Harvard University Press, 2005. Chapter 7, on American pharmaceutical companies, focuses on growth through prescription drug sales; chapter 8 focuses on sales of over-the-counter products; and chapter 10 focuses on the growing importance of biotechnology. One other chapter compares American and European drug companies.

Cohen, Jillian Clare, Patricia Illingworth, and Udo Schüklenk, eds. *The Power of Pills: Social, Ethical and Legal Issues in Drug Development, Marketing, and Pricing*. London: Pluto Press, 2006. Chapters in this edited volume address issues concerning the ethics of developing and distributing drugs. The first section examines the pharmaceutical industry and the pursuit of profit relative to its obligations to help poor countries of the developing world. Other chapters consider diseases that the pharmaceutical industry neglects because of the low potential for profits or of the high prices of developing and producing some drugs.

Congressional Budget Office. *Research and Development in the Pharmaceutical Industry*. Washington, D.C.: Congressional Budget Office, 2006. Also available online. URL: http://www.cbo.gov/ftpdocs/76xx/doc7615/

10-02-DrugR-D.pdf. Downloaded June 3, 2009. In response to a request from the Senate majority leader, the Congressional Budget Office aimed to makes sense of competing facts about research and development in the pharmaceutical industry. This resulting report presents basic facts on the cost of developing drugs, recent declines in the drug industry's performance, and the profitability of drug companies. The CBO remains nonpartisan and offers an impartial analysis without recommendations about changing drug laws and policies. This balanced report represents an exception to the one-sided views either for or against the drug industry.

Gassmann, Oliver, Gerrit Reepmeyer, and Maximilian von Zedtwitz. *Leading Pharmaceutical Innovation: Trends and Drivers for Growth in the Pharmaceutical Industry.* 2nd edition. Berlin: Springer, 2008. This technical work is filled with tables and figures of most interest to specialists in the field of pharmaceutical research. Still, it addresses an interesting question before getting to the details of science, technology, and management: Why has innovation recently slowed in the drug industry despite increases in investment in research and development? Part of the answer has to do with the enormous complexity of the industry. The last chapter on future trends and directions considers some possible outcomes of the growing complexity.

Greider, Katharine. *The Big Fix: How the Pharmaceutical Industry Rips Off American Consumers.* New York: Public Affairs, 2003. This book on the drug industry compares to *The Truth about Drug Companies* by Marcia Angell in its harsh criticisms. It focuses on the high prices of prescription drugs, the extent of advertising for blockbuster drugs, and the lack of attention to getting consumers the safest and most effective drugs available.

Handen, Jeffrey S., ed. *Industrialization of Drug Discovery: From Target Selection through Lead Optimization.* Boca Raton, Fla.: CRC Press, 2005. Part history and part current problems, this book traces how three steps have led in the past to drug discovery and development and can help improve current performance. These steps are understanding the science, unraveling the story, and intelligently applying the technology. While the principles sound simple, the details covered in the chapters are complex. Examples from the history of drug discovery, however, help make the material more accessible and readable.

Hawthorne, Fran. *The Merck Druggernaut: The Inside Story of a Pharmaceutical Giant.* Hoboken, N.J.: Wiley, 2003. The author, a business journalist, has praise for this pharmaceutical company. It has a reputation for ethical practices and devotion to research and development. However, the author also describes the problems of declining profits, intense competition, and the complexity of discovering new drugs that the company and the drug industry must face.

Law, Jacky. *Big Pharma: Exposing the Global Healthcare Agenda*. New York: Carroll & Graf, 2006. Law argues that a conflict exists between the goals of corporate wealth for drug companies and the health of the public. The goal of profit increasingly wins according to the book, which gives many examples of expensive drugs with little benefit or harmful side effects. The author also criticizes the medical profession for not doing more to protect the public. The book contains little information not available elsewhere but aims to pull together facts that warrant criticism of large pharmaceutical companies.

Ng, Rick. *Drugs: From Discovery to Approval*. Hoboken, N.J.: Wiley-Liss, 2004. Written for professionals in the industry, this book covers the research and development process step by step. It will have too much technical detail for most researchers, but chapter 8, on regulations, can be helpful. Also, an appendix on the history of the drug industry is less technical than other chapters.

Petryna, Adriana, Andrew Lakoff, and Arthur Kleinman, eds. *Global Pharmaceuticals: Ethics, Markets, Practices*. Durham, N.C.: Duke University Press, 2006. The articles in this volume offer several case studies on the use of prescription drugs across the world and the influence of the global pharmaceutical industry on that use. For example, chapters examine the adoption of SSRIs in Japan, high-dose synthetic opiates in France, and AIDS treatment in Uganda. The book goes far afield from common concerns with drug marketing and sales in the United States but also gives a unique worldwide perspective on international growth of the pharmaceutical trade.

Reidy, Jamie. *Hard Sell: The Evolution of a Viagra Salesman*. Kansas City, Mo.: Andrews McMeel Pub., 2005. A former drug representative of Pfizer, the maker of Viagra and the world's largest drug company, tells of his experiences. They are not positive. He describes, for example, questionable practices used by salespeople in dealing with nurses and doctors. Based on personal experiences and meant to entertain, the book does not present an evenhanded evaluation, but it does include real-life specifics about drug marketing that few other sources have.

Richmond, Lesley, Julie Stevenson and Alison Turton, eds. *The Pharmaceutical Industry: A Guide to Historical Records*. Aldershot, Hampshire, England: Ashgate, 2003. This guide facilitates the study of the pharmaceutical industry in Britain by providing information on the location of archives and company records. Few will want to examine the archives, but the book also includes brief histories of some companies, a chronology of pharmaceutical legislation, and essays by experts on the history of the industry. The material on Britain shows both similarities and differences to the history of the pharmaceutical industry in the United States.

Rodengen, Jeffrey L. *The Legend of Pfizer.* Ft. Lauderdale, Fla.: Write Stuff Syndicate, 1999. This history of the first 150 years of the world's largest drug company describes the sources of the company's success. The 1999 publication means it misses more recent and less positive experiences during a period of general underperformance by drug companies. Still, it contains much detail on expansion of Pfizer from its founding in 1849 to its 1999 award from *Forbes* as company of the year.

Rost, Peter. *The Whistleblower: Confessions of a Healthcare Hitman.* Brooklyn, N.Y.: Soft Skull Publishers, 2006. Dr. Rost, a former senior executive at Pfizer, one of the world's largest pharmaceutical companies, gives an insider's view of the drug industry in this exposé. He describes illegal marketing practices, misleading accounting practices, and efforts to silence his criticisms while he still worked for the company. His claims have generated controversy, but the book's readability comes from the personal story of his battle with the company. Although he could not be fired for his whistle-blowing, he slowly lost his executive responsibilities and duties at the company.

Santoro, Michael A., and Thomas M. Gorrie. *Ethics and the Pharmaceutical Industry.* Cambridge, Mass.: Cambridge University Press, 2005. A variety of ethical issues face the pharmaceutical industry—whom to allow to participate in clinical trials, how to market and advertise products, whether to promote medicines for uses not approved by the government, how to balance the goals of profit with the health needs of the public, and how much to cooperate with the government in meeting public health needs. Chapters in the book cover these and other topics. Of particular interest are the chapters by Thomas Abrams on direct-to-consumer advertising and by Charles L. Bardes on regulating promotion of prescription drugs.

Shah, Sonia. *Body Hunters: How the Drug Industry Tests Its Products on the World's Poorest Patients.* New York: New Press, 2006. The growth of new drugs and the requirements for clinical trials to get new drugs approved creates a problem for drug companies. They need to find sufficient numbers of subjects for studies of their drugs. The author considers several ethical issues relating to the use of humans in these medical and scientific experiments. She views instances of using the impoverished and sick in drug trials as particularly unethical.

Smith, Mickey C., ed. *Studies in Pharmaceutical Economics.* New York: Haworth Press, 1996. Although a bit dated, the issues addressed here generally apply today. For example, chapters on Medicaid drug cost containment, insurance coverage and physician prescribing, and the economics of prescription drug advertising continue to have relevance. The technical nature of the material makes it of most interests to scholars and academics, however.

United States Congress, Senate Special Committee on Aging. *Paid to Prescribe? Exploring the Relationship between Doctors and the Drug Industry:*

Annotated Bibliography

Hearing before the Special Committee on Aging, United States Senate, One Hundred Tenth Congress, First Session, Washington, DC, June 27, 2007. Washington, D.C.: U.S. Government Printing Office, 2008. Also available online. URL: http://frwebgate.access.gpo.gov/cgi-bin/getdoc. cgi?dbname=110_senate_hearings&docid=f:39865.pdf. Downloaded June 4, 2009. Since physicians are allowed to take money from companies whose products they prescribe, there is potential for conflicts of interest. The hearing notes that the gifts and meals physicians receive from drug companies are modest but can contribute to prescribing of higher cost drugs that rely on extensive marketing. Witnesses further testify of strengthening financial ties of doctors to drug companies. However, drug company witnesses argue that they have ethical guidelines that limit the potential for abuse. The hearing overall provides a summary of the debate over the influence of drug companies on doctors.

Veatch, Robert M., and Amy Haddad. *Case Studies in Pharmacy Ethics.* Oxford: Oxford University Press, 2008. The ethical issues relate to difficult decisions faced by pharmacists (rather than pharmaceutical companies). Examples of the topics covered in this book include assisted suicide, conscientious refusal, pain management, equitable distribution of drug resources within institutions and managed care plans, confidentiality, and alternative and nontraditional therapies. Another ethical issue concerns weighing costs and benefits in helping consumers choose drugs.

Voet, Martin A. *The Generic Challenge: Understanding Patents, FDA and Pharmaceutical Life-Cycle Management.* Boca Raton, Fla.: Brown Walker Press, 2005. A former legal counsel for a large pharmaceutical company who was involved in litigation with generic companies over patent rights gives advice to leaders and workers in the pharmaceutical industry. The product description nicely summarizes the book: "It explains clearly and understandably the role of patents, FDA regulation of generic drugs and the Hatch-Waxman Act on drug development today and how improvements in innovative drug products provide enhanced benefits to patients while extending the commercial lives of the drugs." The book presents perspectives of drug companies on patents and generics that contrast with perspectives of drug company critics.

White, Bruce D. *Drugs, Ethics, and Quality of Life: Cases and Materials on Ethical, Legal, and Public Policy Dilemmas in Medicine and Pharmacy Practice.* New York: Pharmaceutical Products Press, 2007. Among the case studies of drug ethics are several relating to drug research.

ARTICLES

Antos, Joseph R. "Ensuring Access to Affordable Drug Coverage in Medicare." *Health Care Financing Review* 27, no. 2 (Winter 2005/2006): 103–112.

171

Prescription Drugs

The Medicare Prescription Drug Program aims to keep prices low by having private companies compete for participants. Critics say the government should intervene directly by setting price controls rather than relying on the market. This article discusses the pros and cons of both approaches.

Arnst, Catherine. "Cancer's Cruel Economics." *Business Week* 4,086 (June 2, 2008): 58–62. The approval process of new drugs by the FDA may be slowing progress against cancer, according to reports cited in this article. The FDA has attempted to implement some added requirements for testing new drugs that have the potential for quickly identifying effectiveness, but concerns over approving another drug like Vioxx, which ended up killing many users, have slowed the process. The article describes some additional recommendations for improving the drug approval process.

Azar, Alex M., II. "Generic Medicines: Address to the Annual Mentor Dinner, Harris School of Public Policy Studies, University of Chicago." *Vital Speeches of the Day* 74, no. 12 (December 2008): 559–563. This speech given by the senior vice president of corporate affairs and communication at Eli Lilly highlights the important role of generic drugs in making health care less expensive and more accessible. Although drugmakers like Eli Lilly have traditionally viewed generics as competition for their brand-name drugs, Mr. Azar believes that reasonable patent protections for companies lead to more generic drugs and to more help for patients throughout the world.

Bender, A. Douglas. "The Coming of the Baby Boomers: Implications for the Pharmaceutical Industry." *Generations* 28, no. 4 (Winter 2004/2005): 26–31. As the baby-boom generation moves into old age and increases the size of the elderly population in the United States and other countries of the world, it will increase opportunities for the drug industry. High usage rates of prescription drugs by older persons means higher sales in aging populations. However, this article notes that improvements in the health of the elderly and changes in the the drug industry may make it hard for companies to take advantage of this opportunity.

Calfee, John E. "The Indispensable Industry." *The American* 2, no. 3 (May/June 2008): 41–47. This defense of the pharmaceutical industry argues that a key component of the success has been the ability of companies to withstand the many failures of new products. For the few successful products to make it through the difficult process of development and distribution, the industry must have the financial resources to withstand failure. Because of the high degree of risk involved in drug development, the government and taxpayers or nonprofit and donor organizations are unable to replace profit-based drug companies.

Couzin, Jennifer. "The Brains behind Blockbusters." *Science* 309 (July 29, 2005): 728–730. Interviews with inventors of top-selling drugs, many of whom are at or near retirement, offer insights into drug discovery. Many believe that the environment of drug discovery has changed for the worse in some ways. Although technology for discovery has improved, scientists working for drug companies now have less freedom to explore novel ideas.

Curtis, Patricia. "Exciting New Drugs." *Reader's Digest* 170 (March 2007): 114. The past success of prescription drugs gives reasons for hope about exciting benefits of new drugs. This article discusses new drugs that treat diseases such as cervical cancer, shingles, whooping cough, cancer, diabetes, heart conditions, and nicotine addiction.

Engardio, Pete, and Arlene Weintraub. "Outsourcing the Drug Industry." *Business Week* 4,099 (September 15, 2008): 48–52. The global nature of the pharmaceutical industry shows in a trend described in this article—the collaboration of Western companies with Indian companies. India has advantages of well-trained scientists and lower costs for labor and production. Work being done in India focuses on both developing and testing new drugs.

Garnier, Jean-Pierre. "Rebuilding the R&D Engine in Big Pharma." *Harvard Business Review* 86, no. 5 (May 2008): 68–76. An analysis of recent declines in stock prices of pharmaceutical companies identifies one major source of the problem—declining productivity in research and development of new drugs. The author recommends reorganization of the research divisions to become more flexible and decentralized and to better exploit the enthusiasm of scientists.

Gelfand, Alexander. "Selective Testing: Pharmacogenetic Testing." *The Walrus* 5, no. 9 (December 2008): 25–28. New tests aim to match appropriate pharmaceutical medicines with genetic characteristics of patients. Proper knowledge of genetic traits can prevent the damage drugs do to some people and target drugs for people who will most benefit. However, the research needed to develop these medicines is complex, and scientific understanding of genetics remains rudimentary. This article describes the economic benefits of these kinds of tests to pharmaceutical companies and the pressures to develop them for widespread use.

Heller, Michael. "Where Are the Cures?" *Forbes* 182, no. 2 (August 11, 2008): 30. The author suggests that to deal with the slowdown in newly patented drugs pharmaceutical companies need a different approach. Rather than putting efforts into defending or extending the patents of existing drugs, which creates gridlock in getting new drugs improved, companies can support modest changes to the patent system that make it easier to develop innovative new drugs.

Herper, Matthew. "Valuing Pharma Like Metal Benders." *Forbes* 181, no. 12 (June 16, 2008): 72–73. This article for investors makes the case that pharmaceutical companies remain a valuable investment. Although the companies have performed less well in recent years than in the past, they still have much potential for rising sales, profits, and stock prices.

Huber, Peter W. "Of Pills and Profits: In Defense of Big Pharma." *Commentary* 122, no. 1 (July/August 2006): 21–28. The author describes the special economic circumstances of the drug industry, the high risks in developing new drugs, and the enormous investment required for new drugs. These circumstances help explain high prices for patented drugs and the tendency for companies to focus on products with large sales. He suggests that streamlining regulation and eliminating controls on prices will help most to generate new drug products.

Malakoff, David. "Spiraling Costs Threaten Gridlock." *Science* 322 (October 10, 2008): 210–213. The spiraling costs refer to expenses required to run clinical trials for new drugs. The author cites figures that the cost of testing a new drug in the United States has reached $400 million. Efforts to improve the quality of clinical trails have in particular made them more expensive and difficult to complete. The resulting slowdown in testing and approval has led some companies to move clinical trials to other countries.

Miller, Henry I., and David R. Henderson. "The FDA's Risky Risk-Aversion." *Policy Review* 145 (October/November 2007): 3–27. The authors argue that government regulation relating to the financing of research, protection of intellectual property, imposition of price controls, and pre-market approval needs reform. Despite the inefficiencies created by regulations, no groups other than pharmaceutical companies are calling for changes in policies. The authors recommend an approach to regulation that is less averse to risk and more focused on benefits of prescription drugs.

Mooney, Pat. "Making Well People 'Better.'" *World Watch* 15, no. 4 (July/August 2002): 13–16. The author sees much potential for pharmaceutical companies to benefit from genetic engineering. They can make human performance drugs to improve sleep or enhance memory that are designed for the particular genetic makeup of an individual. These drugs have an enormous market, but according to the author, would give too much power to pharmaceutical companies and make the public too dependent on what the companies provide.

Nocera, Joe. "Generic Drugs: The Window Has Loopholes." *New York Times* (July 1, 2006): C1. Also available online. URL: http://query. nytimes.com/gst/fullpage.html?res=9403E4DC1530F932A35754C0A9609 C8B63&sec=&spon=&pagewanted=all. Downloaded May 18, 2009. As illustrated in this story on the end of the patent for the anticholesterol statin drug Zocor, pharmaceutical companies in recent years have adopted new strategies in competing with generic drugs. Rather than allowing generic companies to sell the drug unimpeded, Merck has licensed an "authorized generic" version of Zocor to another company, which allows

Merck to obtain some of the profit from generic versions of its drug. Prices will still be much lower for the generic version but makers of successful drugs that lose their patents can still keep part of the profits. Critics worry that the strategy will keep prices higher than if the drugs were left to generic companies.

Peterson, Iver. "Smaller Firms Gain Foothold as Big Drug Makers Shrink." *New York Times* (May 15, 2009). Also available online. URL: http://www. nytimes.com/2009/05/17/nyregion/new-jersey/17pharmanj.html. Downloaded May 18, 2009. Focusing on changes taking place in pharmaceutical companies located in New Jersey, a center of nearly 38,000 industry jobs in 2007, this news story describes a shift in the industry. While the large companies are doing less well and moving many jobs to states and countries with lower labor costs and taxes, smaller innovative companies that specialize in biomedical research are doing better. The trend in New Jersey reflects larger changes occurring across in the country in the pharmaceutical industry.

"The Pharmaceutical Industry: Beyond the Pill." *The Economist* 385 (October 27, 2007): 76. This article suggests that the pharmaceutical industry will need to change its business model in the coming decade. In the past, companies discovered, developed, marketed, and sold their drugs, but the lack of big-selling new drugs in recent years has disrupted the model. Some companies have already started to outsource some of their business, and other changes to reduce costs and increase sales may also be needed.

"Pharmaceuticals: Heartburn." *The Economist* 380 (August 19, 2006): 52–53. This article illustrates the nature of competition between brand-name drugs and generics. The makers of a highly successful drug to prevent heart attacks and strokes, Plavix, enjoyed sales of $6 billion in 2005 and have a patent that lasts until 2012. However, a Canadian drug company believes that the patent has some flaws and has launched a generic version of the drug at a much lower price; the companies later reached a settlement. The loss of the patent would hurt the maker of the brand-name drug, Sanofi-Aventis.

Pressman, Aaron. "How to Play It: Drugmakers." *Business Week* 4,117 (Jan./ Feb. 2009). This analysis of the financial prospects of drug companies and their stocks notes positive and negative signals for the future. On one hand, health care reforms under the Obama administration will likely allow government agencies to negotiate prices when purchasing drugs for Medicare. That may lower prices and keep profits down. On the other hand, health care reforms should increase the sales of generic drugs.

Ridgeway, James. "Medicare's Poison Pill." *Mother Jones* 33, no. 5 (September/October 2008): 53–57, 106–107. The author criticizes the health care initiative under President George W. Bush that created a prescription drug benefit for seniors. He says that the drug companies had too much power in designing the legislation, which eventually limited the access of seniors to the drugs they need.

Rockoff, Jonathan D. "Drug CEOs Switch Tactics on Reform: Pharmaceutical Companies Join Health-Care Overhaul, Hoping to Influence Where Costs Are Cut." *Wall Street Journal* (May 27, 2009): A6. Also available online. URL: http://online.wsj.com/article/SB124338375682356635.html. Downloaded May 27, 2009. As described in this news story, drug companies are participating rather than opposing efforts to overhaul the U.S. health care system. Drug companies hope that their participation will help prevent steep cuts in prescription drug prices and encourage better prescription drug benefits for patients.

———. "Merck to Buy Rival for $41 Billion." *Wall Street Journal* (March 10, 2009): A1. Also available online. URL: http://online.wsj.com/article/SB123659326420569463.html. Downloaded May 19, 2009. The details of the purchase described in this news story reflect a trend toward consolidation in the drug industry. Companies hope that by increasing in size they can better manage downturns in the economy while continuing to produce new drugs.

Simons, John. "The Fortune 500: From Scandal to Stardom: How Merck Healed Itself." *Fortune* 157, no. 3 (February 18, 2008): 94–96, 98. This article reviews the recent downs and ups of one major drug company. Since 2006, Merck has received approval for many new and promising drugs, won important court cases involving its drug Vioxx, and enjoyed increases in stock prices.

———. "The $10 Billion Pill: Lipitor." *Fortune* 147, no. 1 (January 20, 2003): 58–62, 66, 68. Invented by Bruce Roth in the late 1980s and now sold by Pfizer, the anticholesterol drug Lipitor became the world's best-selling drug. This article tells the story of the drug's development and success.

Wallace-Wells, Ben. "Bitter Pill: Eli Lilly and the Ethics of Olanzapine." *Rolling Stone* 1,071 (February 5, 2009): 56–63, 74–76. This exposé argues that drug companies have made billions on a type of drug that appears to cause diabetes and other fatal diseases. Olanzapine is one of a new generation of antipsychotic drugs that Eli Lilly markets under the name Zyprexa for treatment of schizophrenia. The author alleges that the new class of antipsychotic drugs works no better than earlier medications and has worse side effects.

Wayne, Alex. "Drugmakers' Sour Image Gets a Spoonful of Sugar." *CQ Weekly* 66, no. 39 (October 13, 2008): 2,755–2,756. This report on a speech made by the chief executive of Eli Lilly notes that drug companies plan to change the negative images they have with the public. More consumer-friendly policies and better dealings with congressional Democrats might help reduce the unpopularity of drugmakers.

Weintraub, Arlene. "Can Pfizer Prime the Pipeline?" *Business Week* 4,065 (December 31, 2007/January 7, 2008): 90–91. The new president of research and development at Pfizer, Martin Mackay, hopes to improve the company's recent poor performance in developing new drugs. For example, many new promising drugs developed by the company have failed when undergoing large-scale tests. The article describes some of Mackay's plans to deal with such problems.

WEB DOCUMENTS

Davidson, Larry, and Gennadiy Greblov. "The Pharmaceutical Industry in the Global Economy." Indiana University Kelley School of Business. Available online. URL: http://www.bus.indiana.edu/davidso/lifesciences/ lsresearchpapers/pharmaceutical%20industryaug12.doc. Posted summer 2005. This paper by two business professors aims to acquaint the public with recent developments in the pharmaceutical industry, including challenges and prospects it faces. Although a few years old, it offers a helpful overview of the major companies and important trends.

Federal Trade Commission. "The Pharmaceutical Industry: A Discussion of Competitive and Antitrust Issues in an Environment of Change." Available online. URL: http://www.ftc.gov/reports/pharmaceutical/drugexsum. shtm. Updated June 25, 2007. The Federal Trade Commission has no control over drug approval, but it does have authority to limit antitrust or monopoly activity. This summary of a longer report identifies several concerns about such activity in the pharmaceutical industry. For example, information technology may allow companies to coordinate price information when they negotiate with HMOs and hospitals. The webpage also gives access to the full report.

Herper, Matthew. "The Value of New Drugs Is Dropping." Forbes.com. Available online. URL: http://www.forbes.com/2009/01/07/pharmaceuticals-sales-biz-healthcare-cx_mh_0108drugssales.html?partner=alerts. Posted January 8, 2009. Although the pharmaceutical industry is in many ways stronger economically than other industries, it does face a problem: The development of new drugs, particularly drugs that turn out to be blockbusters, has slowed. As this article describes, low sales of new drugs combined with the end of patents on older drugs foretell coming problems for drug companies.

IMDiversity.com. "Overview: The Pharmaceutical Industry." Available online. URL: http://www.imdiversity.com/Villages/Channels/pharmaceutical/ Articles/pharma_overview.asp. Downloaded June 22, 2009. This webpage gives basic information without addressing controversial issues about costs, prices, and profits. The material on job growth, opportunities for employment, and earnings of workers in the industry is informative and encouraging for those interested in pharmaceutical careers.

Kaiser Family Foundation. "Prescription Drug Trends." Available online. URL: http://www.kff.org/rxdrugs/upload/3057_07.pdf. Posted September 2008. While focused on trends in use of prescription drugs, this document reports numerous statistics on the market for pharmaceutical products. For example, sections review trends in the prices charged, the advertising used, and the profits made by the pharmaceutical industry. The reported figures suggest that spending on prescription drugs will increase but other forces will restrain industry profits.

Pharmaceutical Business Review. "Opportunity Knocks for Big Pharmaceutical Companies in the Credit Crunch." Available online. URL: http://www.pharmaceutical-business-review.com/article_feature.asp?guid=99C88B49-D9FA-412B-A7D9-8A665404A8A7. Posted October 9, 2008. This short piece assesses the economic circumstances of the pharmaceutical industry during the fall 2008 meltdown of the stock market and credit shortage. It concludes that the industry is better prepared to withstand the problems than most other industries, including the biotechnology industry. Pharmaceuticals generally have low debt and can use their cash for mergers and acquisitions and to improve their profits. The review concludes that opportunities for the industry are not as good as in the recent past, but the economics still look positive.

Pharmaceutical Research and Manufacturers of America. "New Report Shows Record Number of Medicines in Development to Treat Leading Causes of Cancer." Available online. URL: http://www.phrma.org/news_room/press_releases/new_report_shows_record_number_of_medicines_in_development_to_treat_leading_causes_of_cancer. Posted April 1, 2009. This press release and the report associated with it come from an industry trade group that can be expected to accentuate the positive. The ability of new drugs to make progress against cancer remains unknown, but the document emphasizes the effort drug companies are devoting to anticancer drugs. Indeed, the document says that companies have 122 drugs for lung cancer, 107 for breast cancer, 70 for colorectal cancer, and 103 for prostate cancer under development.

———. "Pharmaceutical Industry Profile 2008." Available online. URL: http://www.phrma.org/files/2008%20Profile.pdf. Posted March 2008. An industry's description of itself, this document contains interesting facts and responses to criticisms. It presents arguments that the costs of drug development are enormous, drug costs are only a small part of all health care costs, and medicines contribute enormously to the health and well-being of the population. The first few pages on key facts summarize these claims in a compressed format.

Waxman, Henry A. "Pharmaceutical Industry Profits Increase by over $8 Billion after Medicare Drug Plan Goes into Effect." Committee on Government Reform. Available online. URL: http://oversight.house.gov/documents/20060919115623-70677.pdf. Posted September 2006. This document from Democratic representative Waxman criticizes the drug industry for high prices and excessive profits. Beyond the criticisms, however, the document contains data on increases in the profits of major drug companies after the start of the Medicare Prescription Drug Program on January 1, 2006. It concludes that "the privatized structure of the program and the ban on federal negotiations with drug manufacturers for price discounts" benefit drug companies and make the program more expensive.

USE, OVERUSE, AND ADVERTISING

BOOKS

Abramson, John. *Overdosed America: The Broken Promise of American Medicine.* New York: HarperCollins, 2004. The overmedication of Americans described by Abramson refers to the use of unnecessary and expensive drugs. The cause of overmedication is the commercialization of medicine or the search for profits by drug companies. These forces create pressures on doctors and patients to use drugs to deal with health conditions. The author's review of the evidence for many drugs suggests that they are less effective than claimed and sometimes harmful. He calls for a new model of medical care, one where the search for profits does not compromise the relationship between doctor and patient.

Barber, Charles. *Comfortably Numb: How Psychiatry Is Medicating a Nation.* New York: Pantheon Books, 2008. The prescription of 230 million antidepressants each year greatly concerns the author. He argues that pharmaceutical companies first created the need for these drugs and then rushed in to fill the need. Drugs remain crucial for treatment of severe mental illness but now are used to treat the normal sorrows and problems of life. Further, the excess reliance on prescription drugs to treat emotional difficulties displaces the use of nonpharmaceutical or traditional therapies.

Breggin, Peter. *Medication Madness: A Psychiatrist Exposes the Dangers of Mood-Altering Medications.* New York: St. Martin's Press, 2008. The psychiatrist author describes how psychiatric medicines can cause suicide, violence, crime, and emotional breakdowns. He argues that the FDA, pharmaceutical industry, and medical establishment encourage overuse of psychiatric drugs and fail to adequately protect the consumer. Breggin has written several other books critical of SSRI antidepressants, Ritalin and stimulants for ADHD, and other drugs. Although many dispute his claims, the warnings about the widespread use of psychiatric drugs deserve a hearing.

Brody, Howard. *Hooked: Ethics, the Medical Profession, and the Pharmaceutical Industry*. Lanham, Md.: Rowman & Littlefield, 2007. A professor at the University of Texas Medical Branch at Galveston, Brody argues that medicine is hooked in two ways: It depends greatly on gifts and rewards from the pharmaceutical industry, and it depends on the discoveries and manufacturing of the industry to give patients the best treatment possible. While recognizing the enormous benefits of prescription drugs, the book criticizes the close ties between the pharmaceutical industry and the medical profession and offers several solutions to deal with the problem.

Brownlee, Shannon. *Overtreated: Why Too Much Medicine Is Making Us Sicker and Poorer*. New York: Bloomsbury, 2007. The author argues that up to a third of what Americans spend on medical care does nothing to improve their health. The excess cost not only wastes money but leads to medical errors and health problems. While focused more broadly on medical care, the book makes the same case for prescription drugs. The title of chapter 8, "Money, Drugs, and Lies," gives a sense of the author's criticisms of drug company promotions and the unnecessarily high rates of prescription. The book has less on prescription drugs than others devoted more completely to the topic but places the issues within the larger context of the medical care system.

Conrad, Peter. *The Medicalization of Society: On the Transformation of Human Conditions into Treatable Disorders*. Baltimore, Md.: Johns Hopkins Press, 2007. Medicalization refers to the process of change that treats problems once thought to have personal or social causes as having medical or biological causes. Examples include menopause, alcoholism, anxiety, obesity, and erectile dysfunction. The general trend expands the domain of medicine, and as the domain of medicine expands, so does the reliance on prescription drugs. Conrad argues that the pharmaceutical industry has played an growing role in the process of medicalization in recent years.

Crosse, Marcia. *Prescription Drugs: Trends in FDA's Oversight of Direct-to-Consumer Advertising: Testimony before the Subcommittee on Oversight and Investigations, Committee on Energy and Commerce, House of Representatives*. Washington, D.C.: U.S. Government Accountability Office, 2008. Also available online. URL: http://purl.access.gpo.gov/GPO/LPS94931. Downloaded May 29, 2009. In 2002, the Government Accountability Office criticized the FDA for its oversight of advertising of prescription drugs. This 2008 report follows up on the previous one by considering trends in FDA oversight and action against violators of advertising regulations. It finds that the FDA has had limited success in halting ads for prescription drugs. For example, by the time the FDA sent letters objecting to ads, companies had already discontinued many of them. The report gives a sense of the difficulties, despite efforts of the FDA, in controlling advertising of prescription drugs.

Davis, Peter, ed. *Contested Ground: Public Purpose and Private Interest in the Regulation of Prescription Drugs*. New York: Oxford University Press, 1996. The contributors to this volume include international experts in the social sciences, medicine, pharmacy, and public policy. Of particular interest are several chapters that compare regulation of prescription drugs across countries.

Elliott, Carl, and Tod Chambers, eds. *Prozac as a Way of Life*. Chapel Hill: University of North Carolina Press, 2004. Most of the essays in this volume address ethical issues over the use of SSRI antidepressants for self-improvement. The title mentions Prozac, the first successful SSRI antidepressant, but the book considers similar drugs that have become widely popular for purposes other than treating clinical depression. However, the authors note the difficulty of living up to the high expectations people have for these drugs. Titles of the chapters highlight their academic nature: "Passion, Activity, and Care of the Self: Foucault and Heidegger in the Precincts of Prozac" and "Pursued by Happiness and Beaten Senseless: Prozac and the American Dream."

Greene, Jeremy A. *Prescribing by Numbers: Drugs and the Definition of Disease*. Baltimore, Md.: Johns Hopkins University Press, 2007. The author, a professor at Harvard University, argues that a new model of chronic disease has emerged in the last 50 years. The model calls for treatment before clear symptoms of the disease emerge, is based on measures of risk, and aims for prevention. Expanding definitions of cardiovascular disease to include hypertension, diabetes, and high cholesterol illustrate the changing perception of disease. Drugs have played a crucial role in the emergence of this model. Marketing by pharmaceutical companies responded to public health priorities, thus increasing prescriptions and sales of drugs for hypertension, diabetes, and high cholesterol. This highly praised book helps readers to understand the social conditions and public health goals behind expanded use of prescription drugs.

Healy, David. *Let Them Eat Prozac: The Unhealthy Relationship between the Pharmaceutical Industry and Depression*. New York: New York University Press, 2004. The psychiatrist author prescribed Prozac when it first came out but found that many patients who took it became agitated and a few attempted suicide. His book reviews the history of Prozac and similar antidepressants, describes the controversies over the drugs, and ultimately criticizes the pharmaceutical industry for overstating the benefits and minimizing—or hiding—the risks.

181

Prescription Drugs

Jain, Shaili. *Understanding Physician-Pharmaceutical Industry Interactions: A Concise Guide*. Cambridge: Cambridge University Press, 2007. The physician author notes that the medical school curriculum fails to prepare physicians for the dealings most will have with the pharmaceutical industry. Yet these interactions raise a host of ethical issues related to receiving gifts, dealing with sales reps, and participating in academic partnerships with the industry. Although written for doctors, the book is clear and nontechnical in its writing, has many concrete examples, and offers useful information to nonphysicians. Even the chapters on improving medical education have broader implications for understanding the influence of the pharmaceutical industry on medical decisions.

Kassirer, Jerome P. *On the Take: How Medicine's Complicity with Big Business Can Endanger Your Health*. New York: Oxford University Press, 2005. A physician himself and former editor of the *New England Journal of Medicine*, Kassirer is highly critical of his profession. Too often doctors have conflicts of interest in which ties to the drug industry compromise their treatment of patients. He lauds those who stay free of such ties and are fully devoted to patient care, but the title, suggesting that medicine is on the take, presents a harsh indictment.

Kramer, Peter. *Listening to Prozac*. New York: Viking, 1993. This influential book argued that Prozac, the first popular SSRI to treat depression, did more than deal with emotional problems—it also changed the personalities of many who took the drug. This led Kramer to speculate in his book about the nature of personality and self, but most took from the book that SSRIs could have amazing results and might benefit those without serious depression. The book both created controversy and contributed to the success of Prozac and other SSRIs.

Lane, Christopher. *Shyness: How Normal Behavior Became a Sickness*. New Haven: Yale University Press, 2007. Lane writes, "Before you sell a drug, you have to sell the disease. And never was this truer than for social anxiety disorder." Criticizing both drug companies and psychiatrists, his history describes the influence of the pharmaceutical industry in the creation over the last several decades of new classifications of mental disorders related to shyness and social anxiety. The book also describes the marketing techniques used to sell drugs for these conditions. A key theme is that making shyness into a pathology leads to overdiagnosis and pressures on shy children and teens to change their personalities.

Moynihan, Ray, and Alan Cassels. *Selling Sickness: How the World's Biggest Pharmaceutical Companies Are Turning Us All into Patients*. New York: Nation Books, 2005. The book describes a basic strategy used by drug companies to make a successful prescription drug: Redefine problems as diseases or redefine a disease to include a wider part of the population. Unlike most other books critical of the drug industry, this one focuses on

182

specific conditions and the strategies used to sell drugs to treat the conditions. Thus, chapters cover how drug companies expanded the needs for drugs to treat high cholesterol, depression, menopause, high blood pressure, attention deficit disorder, social anxiety, irritable bowel syndrome, osteoporosis, and female sexual dysfunction.

Peterson, Melody. *Our Daily Meds: How the Pharmaceutical Companies Transformed Themselves into Slick Marketing Machines and Hooked the Nation on Prescription Drugs.* New York: Sarah Crichton Books, 2008. Although the title sounds overly sensational, the author, a former *New York Times* reporter, clearly lays out the facts on the modern marketing of prescription drugs. Her theme is that drug companies and advertisers have come to create diseases rather than meet the needs of existing diseases. Many other books criticize drug companies, but this one tells the stories of executives who developed the marketing approach and medication users who accepted the philosophy of a drug for every problem. Thoroughly researched and detailed, this book provides a wealth of concrete examples that make debates on excess use of prescription drugs real.

Tone, Andrea, and Elizabeth Watkins, eds. *Medicating Modern America: Prescription Drugs in History.* New York: NYU Press, 2007. This history of medicine in America covers eight of the most influential and important drugs: antibiotics, mood stabilizers, hormone replacement therapy, oral contraceptives, tranquilizers, stimulants, statins, and Viagra. Each chapter describes how the drugs become such an essential part of medical care and change the way Americans think about disease.

United States Congress, Senate Special Committee on Aging. *Direct-to-Consumer Advertising of Prescription Drugs: What Are the Consequences? Hearing before the Special Committee on Aging, United States Senate, One Hundred Eighth Congress, First Session, Washington, D.C., July 22, 2003.* Washington, D.C.: U.S. Government Printing Office, 2003. Also available online. URL: http://frwebgate.access.gpo.gov/cgi-bin/getdoc. cgi?dbname=108_senate_hearings&docid=f:90049.pdf. Downloaded May 29, 2009. This hearing addresses numerous questions about consumer advertising for prescription drugs: Does it drive up prices? Does it lead to inappropriate prescribing? Does it provide useful information to consumers? And ultimately, does DTC advertising of prescription drugs benefit or harm the health care system and seniors in most need of prescription drugs? The committee chairman says that legislators hear about these questions quite often. The witnesses are generally critical of the ads but also recognize the benefits of acquainting people with treatments for their conditions.

Weber, Leonard J. *Profits before People? Ethical Standards and the Marketing of Prescription Drugs.* Bloomington: Indiana University Press, 2006. This book examines ethical issues raised by commercial interests in selling

Prescription Drugs

prescription drugs. The author, a former professor, argues for placing limits on drug companies and discusses topics such as scientific integrity, marketing to health professionals, and DTC advertising. Although written more for academics than the public, it clearly presents key ethical debates and makes a case for the adoption of new ethical standards by the pharmaceutical industry.

ARTICLES

Angell, Marcia. "Drug Companies and Doctors: A Story of Corruption." *New York Review of Books* 56, no. 1 (January 15, 2009): 8, 10, 12. A vigorous and well-qualified critic of the drug industry reviews several books on the dependence of the medical profession on the drug industry. Angell describes how money and gifts provided by drug companies to doctors in a variety of forms influence research and prescription decisions. The review compares and evaluates several recent books on the topic.

Armstrong, David. "Children's Use of Psychiatric Drugs Begins to Decelerate." *Wall Street Journal* (May 18, 2009): B1. A trend to prescribe antipsychotic drugs to children has slowed because of concerns from the government, courts, and psychiatrists. Few antipsychotic drugs, which are used for severe forms of mental illness, have received approval for use in children, but the practice of prescribing them to children has grown in recent years, often with funding from Medicaid. This article describes the reversal of this trend: State Medicaid programs started to question the prescriptions; companies settled suits over use of the drugs for children; and harmful side effects have concerned doctors.

Arnst, Catherine. "Where Are the Wonder Drugs?" *Business Week* 4,056 (October 29, 2007): 84. The wonder drugs refer to antibiotics. The problem described by the article relates to the spread of a drug-resistant strain of bacteria. Yet companies have not discovered new drugs to deal with the pathogens. The lack of development of antibiotics, despite the need, relates to the economics of the pharmaceutical industry. While developing a new antibiotic is enormously expensive, only a small number of patients will use the drug and then only for a short time. The small return in sales on the investment in development discourages research and development.

Binns, Corey. "Medicating Rover." *Popular Science* 271, no. 5 (November 2007): 36. The popularity of prescription drugs shows not just in high use by humans but also by their pets. Drugs for animals, although not prescribed as they are for humans, cost almost $10 billion a year and treat problems like nausea, separation anxiety, depression, obesity, and dry eyes.

Caplan, Paula J. "Pathologizing Your Period: Classification of Premenstrual Syndrome in Diagnostic and Statistical Manual of Mental Disorders." *Ms.* 18, no. 3 (Summer 2008): 63–64. Feminists criticize psychiatrists for including the diagnosis of extreme premenstrual distress in their manual of disorders. The author argues that the change penalizes women for mood changes when there is little evidence that their problems are worse than for men without menstruation. Perhaps the ability of drug companies to market antidepressants for the problems contributes to the willingness of experts to classify normal feelings as a psychiatric condition.

Carmichael, Mary. "An Rx to Push Generic Drugs." *Newsweek* 152, no. 12 (September 22, 2008): 18. This article tells of how drug companies are moving beyond regular advertisements to acquaint consumers with their products. For example, product placements put drugs in television shows, making them seem an accepted part of daily life. The same strategy applied to generic drugs could help gain the trust of viewers. If doctors on television shows encouraged use of generic rather than brand-name drugs, it could change prescription drug preferences.

"Celebrex: New Ad, with Questionable Claims." *Consumer Reports* 72, no. 8 (August 2007): 52–53. This article illustrates the kind of misleading claims that often appear in DTC drug ads. It examines claims made in an ad that Celebrex poses no more risks than other prescription pain relievers.

Conrad, Peter, and Valerie Leiter. "Medicalization, Markets and Consumers." *Journal of Health and Social Behavior* 45, Extra Issue (2004): 158–176. The authors examine changing views of four drugs—Viagra, Paxil, human growth hormone, and in vitro fertilization—to show how people increasingly have come to view the problems underlying use of these drugs as medical or physiological ones. Advertising, insurance coverage, and changes in advertising regulations contribute to these changing views.

DeLorme, Denise E., Jisu Huh, and Leonard N. Reid. "'Others Are Influenced, but Not Me': Older Adults' Perceptions of DTC Prescription Drug Advertising Effects." *Journal of Aging Studies* 21, no. 2 (April 2007): 135–151. Although they notice DTC ads of prescription drugs and believe the ads influence consumers, older persons in this study deny being influenced themselves. Although finding the ads to be annoying, they favor the general ideal of advertising prescription drugs to consumers. This article suggests some reasons for the inconsistent views.

Donohue, Julie. "A History of Drug Advertising: The Evolving Roles of Consumers and Consumer Protection." *Milbank Quarterly* 84, no. 4 (2006): 659–699. DTC ads for prescription drugs have been controversial for many years. This article describes the ethical debates over the ads and emphasizes the role played by activist patient and consumer organizations in the public's growing acceptance of the ads. These groups see access to information on medications, through advertising or other sources, as crucial to the health of the population.

Donohue, Julie M., Marisa Cevasco, and Meredith B. Rosenthal. "A Decade of Direct-to-Consumer Advertising of Prescription Drugs." *New*

England Journal of Medicine 357, no. 7 (August 16, 2007): 673–681. This study demonstrates the rise in spending on DTC advertising by pharmaceutical companies over the last decade. Despite much criticism of the ads, the pace of spending has increased rather than slowed. The study also notes that the number of warning letters sent by the FDA to manufacturers about violations of regulations fell dramatically during the period.

Flora, Stephen Ray, and Sarah Elizabeth Bobby. "The Bipolar Bamboozle: Part of a Special Section: Questionable Medical Treatments." *Skeptical Inquirer* 32, no. 5 (September/October 2008): 41–45. The authors say that an increasing trend among psychiatrists to diagnose bipolar disorder has been accompanied by aggressive marketing of drugs to treat the condition. They question the validity of the new diagnoses and say that, as a result, millions are being prescribed unnecessary but powerful antipsychotic medications.

Fox, Nick J., and Katie J. Ward. "Pharma in the Bedroom . . . and the Kitchen. . . . The Pharmaceuticalisation of Daily Life." *Sociology of Health and Illness* 30, no. 6 (September 2008): 856–868. The authors use two terms to describe the growing use of prescription drugs. The first term, domestication of pharmaceutical use, refers to use of drugs for private, domestic activities such as sex. The second term, pharmaceuticalization of daily life, refers to the use of drug to deal with everyday problems. The authors see these changes as closely connected to the economics and politics of the pharmaceutical industry.

Fugh-Berman, A., and S. Ahari. "Following the Script: How Drug Reps Make Friends and Influence Doctors." *PLoS Medicine* 4, no. 4 (April 4, 2007): e150. Available online. URL: http://www.plosmedicine.org/article/info:doi/10.1371/journal.pmed.0040150. Downloaded on June 23, 2009. Based in part on conversations with a drug company sales representative, the physician authors describe the strategies used to influence the prescriptions doctors give. It lists techniques that work best for different kinds of doctors and discusses the role of gifts.

Gibson, Ellen. "Mental Pick-Me-Ups: The Coming Boom." *Business Week* 4,114 (December 29, 2008/January 5, 2009): 84–85. The use of drugs to improve cognitive skills raises several ethical issues discussed in this article. Drugs such as Adderall and Ritalin for attention deficit/hyperactivity disorder are used by students to study and professionals to keep up with work demands. Since people use them to deal with daily problems rather than diseases, these so-called "smart drugs" are profitable and several companies are developing new versions. However, the side effects create problems and the risks for overuse are high.

Howley, Kerry. "Dying for Lifesaving Drugs." *Reason* 39, no. 4 (August/September 2007): 24–33. This article reviews debates over access of patients to experimental drugs. Some patient groups believe that, under certain circumstances, doctors and patients should have the choice to use drugs under investigation but not yet approved as safe and effective. The groups believe that withholding the drugs from patients with life-threatening illnesses denies them a last chance at survival. The FDA and others believe that giving easy access to experimental drugs would counteract the scientific approach to approving drugs for public use.

Huh, Jisu, Denise E. DeLorme, and Leonard N. Reid. "The Information Utility of DTC Prescription Drug Advertising." *Journalism and Mass Communication Quarterly* 81, no. 4 (Winter 2004): 788–806. To help understand the influence of DTC ads for prescription drugs, this article reports on the perceptions of consumers. Older consumers tend to hold less negative views about the ads than younger consumers, and consumers who value the information contained in the ads tend to act on that information in asking questions to their doctors.

Kirby, Jason. "Going to Work on Smart Drugs." *Maclean's* 121, no. 40 (October 13, 2008): 94–95. Smart drugs refer to pharmaceuticals used to enhance the brain rather than treat a disease. Long a practice among students needing to study and complete projects, the use of prescription stimulants such as Ritalin to improve concentration, focus, and memory has spread to scientists, academics, and office workers according to the article. The article also discusses a related ethical concern: Bosses wanting to improve worker productivity may pressure workers to take the drugs.

Klein, Daniel B., and Alexander Tabarrok. "Do Off-Label Drug Practices Argue against FDA Efficacy Requirements? A Critical Analysis of Physicians' Argumentation for Initial Efficacy Requirements." *American Journal of Economics and Sociology* 67, no. 5 (November 2008): 743–775. Off-label practices refer to the use of a drug for purposes other than those approved for by the FDA. This study of physicians' views finds that most approve of off-label practices, even though the FDA has provided no evidence that the practices are effective. It notes that the physicians believe the FDA should have evidence of effectiveness for initial uses of drugs. That they also do not want requirements for evidence of effectiveness of off-label uses presents something of a contradiction.

McHenry, Leemon. "On the Origin of Great Ideas: Science in the Age of Big Pharma." *Hastings Center Report* 35, no. 6 (November/December 2005): 17–19. This article reports on a practice that, according to many, threatens the integrity of pharmaceutical science. The practice involves clinical trials of drugs run by pharmaceutical companies, which write up the results to emphasize the positive and minimize the negative. The companies then pay people with academic qualifications to put their names on the study and submit it for publication. This form of ghostwriting represents a way for drug companies to get attention for their drugs but lacks scholarly controls on the quality of the work.

"Medicine's Magic Bullets?" *Discover* 29, no. 7 (July 2008): 46–52. According to this article, many so-called miracle drugs are less safe and effective than claimed. The media contribute to the problem by exaggerating study results, as do drug companies with their DTC ads. The article suggests some reforms of the FDA to prevent excessive claims made on behalf of drugs.

Pinto, Sharrel L., Earlene Lipowski, Richard Segal, Carole Kimberlin, and James Algina. "Physicians' Intent to Comply with the American Medical Association's Guidelines on Gifts from the Pharmaceutical Industry." *Journal of Medical Ethics* 33, no. 6 (June 2007): 313–319. The American Medical Association has ethical guidelines for accepting gifts from pharmaceutical companies. This report on a survey of Florida physicians obtains opinions on the ethical guidelines and the respondents' willingness to follow them. Most know of the guidelines and about half believe that following the guidelines would increase the credibility of physicians.

Renkl, Margaret. "Are We Overmedicating Our Kids?" *Parenting* 21, no. 10 (November 2007): 150–154. Presenting both sides of the debate over this question, the author suggests that cultural changes have made taking prescription medications at young ages much more acceptable today than in the past. Stories of parents who overcome resistance to use of drugs as a necessary way to deal with severe behavioral problems of their children offer another side of the debate.

Saul, Stephanie. "For Jarvik Heart Pioneer, Drug Ads Raise Profile and Questions." *New York Times* (February 7, 2008): A1, A21. Ads for the statin drug Lipitor that featured Dr. Robert Jarvik, inventor of an artificial heart, raised concerns. Although Jarvik is not a practicing physician, he appears to give medical advice in the ad. In criticizing these ads, members of Congress express more general concerns about prescription drug advertising and the difficulties in regulating it.

Shorter, Edward. "How Prozac Slew Freud." *American Heritage* 49, no. 5 (September 1998): 42–44. In this brief history of psychiatry, the author examines remarkable changes in the treatment of mental illness. Rather than treating problems with drawn-out therapy, psychiatrists most often end a patient visit with a prescription to antidepressant drugs like Prozac. The article illustrates the wide-ranging impact over the last several decades of new prescription drugs.

Singer, Natasha. "No Lipitor Mug? Drug Makers Cut Out Goodies for Doctors." *New York Times* (December 31, 2008): A1, A18. For decades now, drug company sales reps have given small gifts to doctors. It's hard to know if these gifts have any influence, but drug companies have responded to criticisms by agreeing to a moratorium on free merchandise for doctors. The article describes the nature of the gifts and the concerns of some that companies will find other ways to encourage doctors to prescribe their drugs.

Stange, Kurt C. "Time to Ban Direct-to-Consumer Prescription Drug Marketing." *Annals of Family Medicine* 5, no. 2 (March/April 2007): 101–104. Also available online. URL: http://www.annfammed.org/cgi/reprint/5/2/101. Downloaded June 23, 2009. This editorial argues that the system in place to monitor the accuracy of ads has failed and that the best solution is to ban the ads altogether. With many references to scientific works, the editorial makes a strong case for its view.

Underwood, Anne. "Thanks, But No Thanks: Drug Company Promotions." *Newsweek* 150, no. 18 (October 29, 2007): 49. This article gives several examples of medical groups that turn down promotions and refuse to see pharmaceutical sales representatives. These groups claim that drug companies focus on selling expensive drugs that sometimes work no better than older, less expensive drugs.

Weintraub, Arlene. "Lifestyle Drug Binge." *Business Week* 4,041 (July 2, 2007): 40–41. The most popular lifestyle drugs treat four types of problems: excess weight, hair loss, poor sleep, and sexual dysfunction. Although lifestyle drugs generally do not treat serious disease conditions, they generate high sales. This article says that the demand by consumers for these drugs, despite the risks they bring, has led drug companies to focus even more on developing products to treat lifestyle problems.

———. "Teaching Doctors—or Selling to Them?" *Business Week* 4,095 (August 11, 2008): 26–28. Pharmaceutical companies often make contributions to medical communication companies that offer continuing education courses for doctors. This practice creates controversy because companies may use the courses to influence what doctors prescribe to their patients. This article discusses criticisms by physicians and ethicists of the practice and the plans of some companies to move away from them.

Weiss, Andrew M. "The Wholesale Sedation of America's Youth." *Skeptical Inquirer* 32, no. 6 (November/December, 2008): 31–36. The author expresses ethical and medical concerns over the high rates of prescription drug use by children, many under age five. He describes the upward trend in usage, the potential side effects that result, and a change in attitudes that makes use of drugs an accepted part of childhood. Further, as part of a magazine devoted to challenging commonly held beliefs, he argues that the evidence for the need and effectiveness of these drugs is weak.

Woodlock, Delanie. "Virtual Pushers: Antidepressant Internet Marketing and Women." *Women's Studies International Forum* 28, no. 4 (July/August 2005): 304–314. Few countries outside the United States allow DTC advertising for prescription drugs. According to this study, companies get around the restriction by creating internationally accessible Web sites.

The Web sites on antidepressants appear to market the products directly to women, often without clear medical justification.

WEB DOCUMENTS

Bass, Alison. "A Dose of Honesty in Prescription Drug Ads." Boston.com. Available online. URL: http://www.boston.com/bostonglobe/editorial_opinion/oped/articles/2008/06/02/a_dose_of_honesty_in_prescription_drug_ads. Posted June 2, 2008. The experience of the author's 83-year-old father illustrates the impact of misleading drug ads. He was put on the anemia drug Procrit in part because ads said it reduced fatigue and weakness. In fact, the drug is designed for cancer patients undergoing chemotherapy, and it increases the risks of heart failure—points easily missed in the ads. The author's father had a mild heart attack soon after starting the drug.

Carpenter, Siri. "The Epidemic of Overmedication: Use of Multiple Drugs, Especially in Older Adults, Can Exacerbate Ailments." MSNBC. Available online. URL: http://www.msnbc.msn.com/id/27645077. Updated November 17, 2008. The author describes the experiences of her own mother, who began to have memory problems that seemed related to the many drugs she took. The story makes the more general point that "The use of multiple, often unnecessary medications—especially among older people—is an entrenched, escalating, frightening, and mostly unexamined problem in modern health care."

Children and Adults against Drugging America. "Overmedicating of America." Available online. URL: http://www.chaada.org/Overmedicatingof America.html. Downloaded June 23, 2009. The name of this group makes clear the perspective they offer on overuse of prescription drugs. Although one-sided, this webpage summarizes key criticisms many make about high prescription rates and the role of drug companies in fostering overuse.

Cox, Lauren. "Top 7 Celebrity Drug Endorsements: Commercial or a Cause?" ABC News. Available online. URL: http://abcnews.go.com/Health/CelebrityCafe/story?id=7209401&page=1. Posted April 1, 2009. Celebrities commonly appear in prescription drug ads, and the FDA regulates these ads to some extent. However, critics point out that regulations do not cover another trend, publicizing drugs indirectly. Celebrities have used ads to raise awareness about public health problems, but companies that sell products for the problems benefit from the awareness and pay the celebrities a fee. Examples cited in the article include Marcia Cross of *Desperate Housewives* on migraine headaches, Kelsey Grammer of *Frasier* on irritable bowel syndrome, and former senator and presidential candidate Bob Dole on erectile dysfunction.

Donmoyer, Ryan J. "House Considering $37 Billion Drug Tax, Rangel Says." Bloomberg.com. Available online. URL: http://www.bloomberg. com/apps/news?pid=20601103&sid=aeEJZicjYE60. Updated June 16, 2009. The chair of the House of Representatives Ways and Means Committee, Democrat from New York Charles Rangel, offers two reasons for taxing drug advertising. One is to raise public funds for health care reform and another is to end what he views as a subsidy to drugmakers. The proposal is preliminary but reflects negative sentiment among some in Congress about drug companies and their advertising.

Kaiser Family Foundation. "Impact of Direct-to-Consumer Advertising on Prescription Drug Spending." Available online. URL: http://www.kff. org/rxdrugs/6084-index.cfm. Posted June 10, 2003. The impact is large according to the summary of results posted on this webpage. The study found with data for 2000 that "every $1 the pharmaceutical industry spent on DTC advertising in that year yielded an additional $4.20 in drug sales." Although a bit dated, the figures supply some facts to support claims about the influence of advertising on prescription drug use.

Ralston, Richard E. "Prescription Drug Advertising Is Good for All of Us." *Capitalism Magazine*. Available online. URL: http://www.capmag.com/article.asp?ID=4275. Posted June 25, 2005. While most decry the influence of ubiquitous drug ads, a minority view presented on this webpage makes the opposite case. The author believes that informing people about new drugs benefits those who might need them.

ScienceDaily. "Most TV Prescription Drug Ads Minimize Risk Information, Study Finds." Available online. URL: http://www.sciencedaily.com/releases/2008/01/080103161527.htm. Posted January 4, 2008. This article summarizes a study coming from the University of Georgia, Athens. The study finds that ads fail to provide balanced information, particularly concerning the risks of side effects. With a few exceptions, the ads did not violate the minimum requirements of the law but still failed to give consumers the information they need to make fully informed decisions about the use of a prescription drug.

U.S. Food and Drug Administration. "Prescription Drug Advertising: Questions and Answers." Available online. URL: http://www.fda.gov/Drugs/ResourcesForYou/Consumers/PrescriptionDrugAdvertising/UCM 076768.htm. Updated June 18, 2009. This helpful webpage answers questions such as: Does the FDA review and approve all advertisements for drugs before their release? Does the FDA approve ads for prescription drugs before they are seen by the public? And what must product-claim ads tell you?

Warner, Judith. "Overselling Overmedication." *New York Times*. Available online. URL: http://warner.blogs.nytimes.com/2008/02/14/overselling-overmedication. Posted February 14, 2008. This blog reviews several books decrying the excess use of prescription drugs but concludes that critics overstate their case. Warner suggests that people have always looked for drugs to help them cope, and that drugs today do a much better job of meeting medical and personal needs than in the past. In her view, the accusation that the search of drug companies for profits leads to excess drug use greatly oversimplifies the issue.

RISKS, SIDE EFFECTS, AND ABUSE

BOOKS

American Psychiatric Association. *Benzodiazepine Dependence Toxicity and Abuse*. Arlington, Va.: American Psychiatric Publishing, 1990. Although dated, this book sponsored by experts and focused on the facts addresses questions about the potential for excess prescription of benzodiazepines and high risks for dependence. Benzodiazepine tranquilizers such as Valium and Xanax commonly treat anxiety, insomnia, and seizures but are prone to misuse and addiction. The expert authors describe the potential hazards of this class of drugs and offer guidelines for appropriate prescription. They recognize the benefits of drugs for patients but also recognize the need for physicians to prescribe them carefully.

Bass, Alison. *Side Effects: A Prosecutor, a Whistleblower, and a Bestselling Antidepressant on Trial*. Chapel Hill, N.C.: Algonquin Books, 2008. A legal thriller as well as an indictment of drug company tactics in selling drugs, this book examines the efforts of the maker of Paxil, SmithKline Beecham at the time and later GlaxoSmithKline, to hide the risks of the antidepressant's side effects. In this case, the prescription of the drug to adolescents increased risks of suicide. The case eventually led to a suit in New York State and changes in FDA warnings about the drug.

Bremner, J. Douglas. *Before You Take That Pill: Why the Drug Industry May Be Bad for Your Health*. New York: Avery, 2008. According to this researcher and physician at Emory University, the risks of many prescription drugs outweigh the benefits. Rather than focusing on potential risks and protecting users, however, drug companies push doctors to prescribe their drugs and push for approval of new drugs without full attention to safety. More than other critiques of the drug industry, this book gives information on specific medications. It does not oppose use of pharmaceuticals but aims to make consumers fully informed about risks when making decisions.

Colvin, Rod. *Prescription Drug Addiction: The Hidden Epidemic*. Omaha, Neb.: Addicus Books, 1995. This book warned early of the trend toward addiction to prescription drugs. To help readers understand the problem, it contains the personal stories of people from diverse backgrounds who became addicted. Chapters cover topics such as treatment, support for families, obtaining fraudulent prescriptions, and law enforcement. The authors aim to give abusers of prescription drugs hope that they can overcome their addiction and find the help they need to reach this goal.

Drug Enforcement Administration, Last Acts Partnership, Pain & Policy Studies Group, University of Wisconsin. *Prescription Pain Medications: Frequently Asked Questions and Answers for Health Care Professionals, and Law Enforcement Personnel.* Washington, D.C.: U.S. Department of Justice Drug Enforcement Administration Diversion Control Program, 2004. Also available online. URL: http://www.painfoundation.org/eNews2004/0904/PainMedLegalFAQ.pdf. Downloaded May 29, 2009. An expert committee provides information in this document on balancing the need for pain control with the goal of preventing abuse of prescription drugs. The short work of 18 pages contains answers to 30 questions and a key to addiction-related terms. Among the questions asked are: What kinds of problems might patients encounter when obtaining opioid prescriptions, in having them filled, or in taking the prescriptions properly? What is the extent of opioid prescription abuse? And what requirements must physicians and pharmacists meet to comply with federal and state laws regulating opioids?

Hobson-Dupont, Jack. *The Benzo Book.* Nantucket, Mass.: Essex Press, 2006. The author unwittingly became addicted to a benzodiazepine his doctor prescribed, Xanax, and wants to help others taking similar tranquilizers and sleeping pills and dealing with the risk of becoming addicted. For many people, stopping "benzos" is like stopping cocaine or heroine, but most physicians do not realize the seriousness of the problem. While the book contains background information, a key part is the personal story of the author about becoming addicted to and getting off the drugs.

Institute of Medicine. *Standardizing Medication Labels: Confusing Patients Less. Workshop Summary.* Washington, D.C.: National Academies Press, 2008. The workshop findings summarized in this 100-page book begin with the fact that about half of patients taking prescription drugs misunderstand instructions on the correct dose or the warnings accompanying the mediation. The papers summarized here describe the problem and, more importantly, offer some recommendations on how to standardize drug labeling so that fewer mistakes result. Although they focus on specialized topics, the summaries of technical research and papers are clearly written.

Karch, Steven B. *Karch's Pathology of Drug Abuse.* 4th edition. Boca Raton: CRC Press, 2009. This comprehensive volume contains much technical information for toxicologists, forensic scientists, and pathologists. However, it also contains some sections on the history and epidemiology of drug abuse that nonspecialists may appreciate. The book covers illicit drugs like cocaine as well as prescription drugs, and it devotes several chapters to stimulants (including those for ADHD), opiates, and opioids.

Leavitt, Fred. *The Real Drug Abusers.* Lanham, Md.: Rowman & Littlefield, 2003. The author, a psychopharmacologist at California State University in Hayward, says that the public is woefully misinformed about the nature of drug abuse. Junkies, drug pushers, and addicted prostitutes get attention of the media, but the drug problem in the United States goes far beyond these images. Rather, it includes overmedication with psychiatric drugs, the emphasis on profits over progress by the drug companies, and mistakes in giving prescriptions. The book also covers topics that relate only tangentially to prescription drugs (for example, mistreatment of human subjects in medical studies, the effectiveness of the drug wars, and the marketing of caffeine, alcohol, and tobacco).

Meier, Barry. *Pain Killer: A "Wonder" Drug's Trail of Addiction and Death.* Emmaus, Pa.: Rodale, 2003. The author follows the rise of OxyContin as a miracle drug for those suffering from pain to its current reputation as a highly abused, addictive, and deadly drug. He calls release of the drug a public health disaster that led to an epidemic of addiction and crime. Much of the book traces the early history of the drug and its emergence as a major source of abuse. The maker of the drug, Purdue, received much criticism for claims that OxyContin is less addictive than other painkillers and for excessive promotions. As the drug became popular on the street, the company responded slowly in restricting its sales and usage.

Mogil, Cindy. *Swallowing a Bitter Pill: How Prescription and Over-the-Counter Drug Addictions Are Ruining Lives—My Story.* Far Hills, N.J.: New Horizon Press, 2001. This personal story goes beyond the statistics on prescription drug abuse to show how the problem can devastate the lives of the addicts. Mogil describes how she became addicted and how she managed to get pills to feed her addiction. More important, she describes steps to recovery. To help others, she founded Prescription (Rx) Anonymous, a recovery organization for prescription drug abusers and their families.

National Center on Addiction and Substance Abuse at Columbia University. *Women under the Influence.* Baltimore, Md.: Johns Hopkins University Press, 2006. Focused on substance abuse among girls and women, this book includes a chapter on illicit use of prescription drugs. The research reported in the volume compares the addiction and abuse of women to that of men. Although women abuse drugs less than men, the problem remains a significant one. Women tend to become addicted more quickly than men and benefit from different types of treatments.

Pinsky, Drew. *When Painkillers Become Dangerous: What Everyone Needs to Know about OxyContin and Other Prescription Drugs.* Center City, Minn.:

Hazelden, 2004. Although highly effective in giving relief from pain, Oxy-Contin is dangerously addictive. This book describes the trend toward abuse of painkillers like OxyContin and how addiction to the drugs can be treated. It also gives advice to family and friends of those with an addiction. At 150 pages, the book is short, clear, and focused on key issues.

United States Congress, Senate Committee on Governmental Affairs. *Legal Drugs, Illegal Purposes: The Escalating Abuse of Prescription Medications: Hearing before the Committee on Governmental Affairs, United States Senate, One Hundred Eighth Congress, First Session, August 6, 2003, Field Hearing in Bangor, Maine.* Washington, D.C.: U.S. Government Printing Office, 2004. Also available online. URL: http://frwebgate.access.gpo.gov/cgi-bin/getdoc.cgi?dbname=108_senate_hearings&docid=f:89040.pdf. Downloaded May 28, 2009. Witnesses from Maine at this hearing describe the local damage created by prescription drug abuse. Police, public health officials, and substance abuse recovery experts say something needs to be done about the problem. Senator Susan M. Collins of Maine says that no state has been hit harder by the epidemic of prescription drug abuse, and she highlights the alarming increase in abuse of OxyContin in rural regions and of methadone (a drug to treat addiction often used to feed an addiction).

United States Congress, Senate Committee on the Judiciary, Subcommittee on the Constitution. *Generation Rx: The Abuse of Prescription and Over-the-Counter Drugs: Hearing before the Subcommittee on the Constitution of the Committee on the Judiciary, United States Senate, One Hundred Tenth Congress, Second Session, March 12, 2008.* Washington, D.C.: U.S. Government Printing Office, 2009. Also available online. URL: http://frwebgate. access.gpo.gov/cgi-bin/getdoc.cgi?dbname=110_senate_hearings& docid=f:47336.pdf. Downloaded May 27, 2009. This hearing aims to publicize the growing national trend in abuse of prescription drugs. It includes the statements of witnesses from a variety of positions: Nora Volkow, Director of the National Institute on Drug Abuse; Derek Clark, Director of the Substance Abuse Council, Clinton, Iowa; Alexander De-Luca, Senior Consultant of the Pain Relief Network; and Steve Pasierb, President and CEO of the Partnership for a Drug-Free America. From the business side, speakers representing health care product makers and chain drugstores also offer statements. While most statements describe the seriousness of prescription drug abuse, representatives of patients using pain relievers say that the war on drugs has made it difficult for those with severe pain to get the drugs they need. Drugstore chains also are concerned that shutting down Internet sales of prescription drugs can harm legitimate businesses. The hearing thus emphasizes that enforcement needs to prevent the abuse of prescription drugs while protecting the ability of doctors to prescribe potentially addictive drugs for legitimate purposes.

United States General Accounting Office. *Prescription Drugs: OxyContin Abuse and Diversion and Efforts to Address the Problem: Report to Congressional Requesters.* Washington, D.C.: U.S. General Accounting Office, 2003. Also available online. URL: http://frwebgate.access.gpo.gov/cgi-bin/getdoc. cgi?dbname=gao&docid=f:d04110.pdf. Downloaded May 27, 2009. This report reviews the growing abuse of OxyContin, an opioid pain reliever introduced in 1995, and its diversion for illicit purposes. It notes that the prescription drug's potency makes it prone to abuse but also that manufacturers' heavy promotion of the drug and its high sales have increased opportunities to use it illicitly. The report also offers some recommendations on further steps that the government can take to monitor the manufacturing and sales of OxyContin and to limit the potential for products to be diverted. Many changes in enforcement have followed this report, but it still provides useful background and history on the problem.

Volkow, Nora D. *Prescription Drugs: Abuse and Addiction.* Bethesda, Md.: National Institute on Drug Abuse, 2005. Also available online. URL: http://www.nida.nih.gov/ResearchReports/Prescription/prescription. html. Downloaded April 20, 2009. This short, 12-page publication from the major government research institute on drug abuse presents information on the problem through a series of questions and answers. Sections on opioids, depressants, and stimulants describe the prescription drugs most often abused, their effects on the body, and their health risks. Other sections cover trends, responsibility, and treatment. This clearly written and relatively brief treatment is an excellent introductory source on the problem of prescription drug abuse.

Wartell, Julie, and Nancy G. La Vigne. *Prescription Fraud.* Washington, D.C.: U.S. Department of Justice, Office of Community Oriented Policing Services, 2004. Part of a series designed to help police fight crime more effectively, this 68-page book considers ways to prevent pharmaceutical diversion, or the illegal acquisition of prescription drugs for personal use or profit. It describes the seriousness of the problem and the kinds of drugs most often acquired for personal use or profit. Most of the book suggests ways to identify and respond to local prescription fraud by increasing the risk of detection, making it hard to commit the crime, and reducing rewards to offenders. The book also helps readers to understand the problem of prescription drug abuse by considering the point of view of the police.

ARTICLES

Arria, Amelia M., Kevin E. O'Grady, Kimberly M. Caldeira, Kathryn B. Vincent, Eric D. Wish. "Nonmedical Use of Prescription Stimulants and Analgesics: Associations with Social and Academic Behaviors among

College Students." *Journal of Drug Issues* 38, no. 4 (Fall 2008): 1,045–1,060. College students who use stimulants and pain relievers for nonmedical uses tend to have lower grades, skip more classes, and spend less time studying. The authors conclude that nonmedical users of prescription drugs compose a high-risk group for academic problems in college.

Baldauf, Sarah. "Former Pharma Pitchman: Beware of New Drugs. Interview with T. Nesi." *U.S. News & World Report* 145, no. 10 (November 3–10, 2008): 64. Tom Nesi, formerly the director of public affairs at Bristol-Myers Squibb, has an insider's view of the sales and marketing tactics used by pharmaceutical companies. Based on his experiences, he warns consumers to avoid taking free sample pills, exercise caution when offered a new medication, and learn about potential side effects. He also talks about the history of Vioxx, a drug removed form the market after research showed it caused heart attacks and strokes.

Bate, Roger. "The Deadly World of Fake Drugs." *Foreign Policy* 168 (September/October 2008): 56–62, 64–65. This article describes the growing industry in trafficking counterfeit pharmaceutical drugs. According to figures from the World Health Organization, 30 percent of drugs sold in Africa, Asia, and Latin America are phony. If the trend continues and the counterfeiters reach into high-income nations like the United States, the fake drugs would cause even greater harm by preventing people from getting the treatments they need.

Bernstein, Elizabeth. "New Addiction on Campus: Raiding the Medicine Cabinet." *Wall Street Journal* (March 25, 2008): D1. Also available online. URL: http://online.wsj.com/article/SB120639877117160751.html. Downloaded May 19, 2009. College students use prescription drugs such as Ritalin and Adderall to study and lose weight, but a recent trend suggests more dangerous abuse of addictive painkillers such as OxyContin, Vicodin, and Percocet. The author says that pharm parties are replacing keg parties for some students, who bring whatever pharmaceuticals they can find, mix them in a big bowl, and eat them like candy. Such abuse has clear dangers for health and well-being.

Byrne, Marilyn H., Laura Lander, and Martha Ferris. "The Changing Face of Opioid Addiction: Prescription Pain Pill Dependence and Treatment." *Health & Social Work* 34, no. 1 (February 2009): 53–56. This article describes the trend toward abuse of opioids and gives some interesting statistics on the groups most likely to abuse. It says that most new users of prescription drugs for nonmedical uses are white, female, and on average about 25 years old. The authors call for targeting abusers of prescription drugs for treatment and determining the most effective treatment strategies.

Carpenter, Siri. "Is Your Parent Over-Medicated?" *Prevention* 60, no. 12 (December 2008): 142–151. Prescription drug use has grown most among older persons, and this polypharmacy can have worrying side effects. According to this article, one fifth of persons age 65 and over take 10 or more drugs a week. With such high usage, adult children need to pay attention to the risk of overmedication of parents, particularly when the conditions seem to get worse rather than better with more drugs.

Cave, Damien. "Legal Drugs Kill Far More Than Illegal, Florida Says." *New York Times* (June 14, 2008): A10. Also available online. URL: http://www. nytimes.com/2008/06/14/us/14florida.html?scp=12&sq=prescription %20 drugs&st=cse. Downloaded May 18, 2009. Despite all the attention given to the illicit sale and use of cocaine in Florida, figures from the state show that prescription drugs kill more people. This news story summarizes a report from the Florida Medical Examiners Commission that found deaths from prescription drugs to be three times higher than deaths from all illicit drugs combined. The trends appear to be similar in other states, but the specific figures reported in the article on deaths from heroin, methamphetamine, and cocaine compared with deaths from Vicodin, OxyContin, Valium, and Xanax reveal the extent of abuse of prescription drugs.

Conte, Annemarie. "Rx for Disaster." *Good Housekeeping* 247, no. 4 (October 2008): 156–159, 220–225. This article in a women's magazine warns about rising teen use of prescription drugs not prescribed to them. Along with highlighting the seriousness of the problem, the article gives parents advice on dealing with the problems in their own families.

De Koff, Derek. "This Is My Brain on Chantix." *New York* 41, no. 6 (February 18, 2008): 30–33, 94. Chantix is a drug that helps smokers quit by preventing nicotine from attaching to brain cells and by moderating the withdrawal symptoms. Through personal experience, the author finds that Chantix also causes suicidal thoughts. The FDA has issued warnings about this side effect, citing 34 suicide deaths of Chantix patients.

DiConsiglio, John. "Generation Rx." *Scholastic Choices* 22, no. 1 (September 2006): 16–19. This article for teens emphasizes the risks of taking prescription drugs without guidance from a medical professional. To illustrate the risks, it tells the stories of several teens who became addicted to prescription drugs.

Field, Terry S., Kathleen M. Mazor, and Becky Briesacher. "Adverse Drug Events Resulting from Patient Errors in Older Adults." *Journal of the American Geriatrics Society* 55, no. 2 (February 2007): 271–276. This study finds that the complexity of seniors' medication regimes and the need on occasion to change those regimes lead to errors in taking prescription drugs. Patients have trouble following clinical instructions, particularly when they suffer from dementia and confusion. These errors often lead to adverse events and harm to patients.

"Finding Out about the Side Effects of Your Prescription Drugs." *Harvard Health Letter* 30 no. 6 (April 2005): 1–3. Rather than give advice on specific medications, this article describes ways to find and use information from package inserts, online documents, and other sources on drug side effects and hazards. It notes limitations of some types of information and encourages consumers to strive for better understanding of the consequences of taking medications.

Ford, Jason A. "Nonmedical Prescription Drug Use among Adolescents: The Influence of Bonds to Family and School." *Youth & Society* 40, no. 3 (March 2009): 336–352. What kinds of teens are most likely to abuse prescription drugs? It turns out from this study that they are the same kind of teens that abuse nonprescription drugs. Based on a 2005 national survey, the findings document that teens with weak ties to family and school most often misuse prescription drugs.

Harmon, Amy. "Young, Assured and Playing Pharmacist to Friends." *New York Times* (November 16, 2005): A1. Also available online. URL: http://www.nytimes.com/2005/11/16/health/16patient.html?_r=2&hp. Downloaded April 17, 2009. The stories of young adults who self-medicate (that is, without physician supervision) through trading and experimenting with drugs reveals the extent of changing attitudes toward prescription drugs. In using prescription drugs to deal with problems such as fatigue, depression, and anxiety, the subjects of this piece rely on their own research and the experiences of their friends rather than physicians.

Harris, Gardiner. "The Safety Gap: Chinese Drug Manufacturers." *New York Times Magazine* (November 2, 2008): 44–49. This article gives the background on contamination of ingredients from China that manufacturers used for some medications sold in the United States. Ingredients are often counterfeit or contaminated, but neither the FDA nor other U.S. agencies have the ability to inspect all Chinese factories. Another dilemma exacerbates the problem: Stricter controls on imported ingredients would increase prices, which in turn would make some drugs less accessible to users. The author nicely describes the difficulty in correcting drug safety problems in China.

Hellman, Deborah. "Pushing Drugs or Pushing the Envelope: The Prosecution of Doctors in Connection with Over-prescribing of Opium-based Drugs." *Philosophy & Public Policy Quarterly* 28, no. 1/2 (Winter/Spring 2008): 7–12. One recently adopted way to control the abuse of prescription drugs involves prosecuting doctors who prescribe them. Such prosecutions use the Controlled Substances Act to target the distribution by physicians of opium-based drugs not needed for medical purposes. The approach raises sticky problems in deciding when doctors have responsibility for how patients use the drugs they prescribe. The author argues that doctors may make mistakes in prescribing drugs, but these mistakes are not the same as pushing drugs.

Lenzer, Jeanne. "Medicine's Magic Bullets?" *Discover* 29, no. 7 (July 2008): 46–52. Rather than produce miracle cures, prescription drugs are more likely, according to this article, to cause adverse reactions. The author describes problems ranging from biased clinical trials to excessive claims of benefits in advertising that lead to the widespread use of unsafe drugs and make clear the need for FDA reforms.

Lord, Morgan. "8 Drugs Doctors Would Never Take." *Men's Health* 23, no. 5 (June 2008): 124–126. The author lists several drugs with potentially dangerous side effects and warns patients taking these drugs to consult with their doctors about the risks. The eight drugs are Advair, Avandia, Celebrex, Ketek, Prilosec, Nexium, Visine Original, and Pseudoephedrine.

Mackenzie, Peter. "Clinical: How to Avoid Costly Prescribing Errors." *GP: General Practitioner* (May 13, 2005): 86–88. This advice for physicians suggests giving more attention to avoiding prescription errors: Doctors should take more care in writing, dispensing, and monitoring the taking of drugs. The most important need is to warn patients of potential side effects or adverse reactions.

Mandavilli, Apoorva. "FDA Tackles Tainted Drugs from China." *Discover* 30, no. 1 (January 2009): 24. After several drugs were found to be contaminated by tainted ingredients imported from China, many called for stronger regulations on drugs manufactured outside the country. This article reviews the FDA response. For example, the FDA plans to set up offices in China, India, Latin America, Europe, and the Middle East.

Markel, Howard. "When Teenagers Abuse Prescription Drugs, the Fault May Be the Doctor's." *New York Times* (December 27, 2005): F5. Also available online. URL: http://www.nytimes.com/2005/12/27/health/27essa.html?scp=6&sq=prescription%20drugs&st=cse. Downloaded May 18, 2009. The ability of teens to abuse prescription drugs comes in part from Internet sales, trading with other teens, and extra pills kept around home by parents. However, the physician author of this essay also blames doctors for writing too many prescriptions. He believes that doctors should do more to check for a history of prescription drug abuse among patients and to keep prescriptions of controlled substances to minimal amounts.

"Mix-ups over Medicine." *Ebony* 64, no. 7 (May 2009): 38. This article lists a number of problems that can lead to mistakes in prescribing and taking medications. These include taking the wrong drug (particularly when the names of different drugs sound alike), taking the wrong dosage, and taking drugs that cause harm when combined with other drugs. The article provides a summary of the problems and what consumers can do to avoid them.

Neal, Jordan, and Carol Kaufmann. "A Fatal Combination: Brother's Misuse of Prescription Drugs." *Reader's Digest* 173 (October 2008): 19. Along with facts and arguments, evidence of the seriousness of prescription drug abuse comes from real-life stories. In this article, Jordan Neal tells of the death of her brother from a combination of a cold medication, OxyContin, and alcohol.

Phillips, David P., Gwendolyn E. C. Barker, and Megan M. Eguchi. "A Steep Increase in Domestic Fatal Medication Errors with Use of Alcohol and/or Street Drugs." *Archives of Internal Medicine* 168, no. 14 (July 28, 2008): 1,561–1,566. Also available online. URL: http://archinte.ama-assn.org/cgi/content/short/168/14/1561. Downloaded April 17, 2009. The authors of this study examined death certificates, particularly those listing the cause of fatal medication error, over a 22-year period. Their findings show that deaths from fatal medication errors have increased, in large part because abusers more often combine prescription drugs with street drugs and alcohol.

Rinaldo, Denise. "The Internet Drug Trade." *Scholastic Choices* 23, no. 2 (October 2007): 12–15. Relating stories about how two teenage girls became addicted to prescription drugs, this article focuses on access through the Internet. It criticizes sales of prescription drugs via the Internet because such sales foster problems of abuse.

Taylor, Phil. "High-wire Act: NFL's Clandestine Drug Culture." *Sports Illustrated* 108, no. 24 (June 16, 2008): 18–19. The clandestine drug culture of the title refers to the illegal use of prescription painkillers and anabolic steroids. Football players use the drugs to enhance performance rather than for recreation. The author suggests drug use could lead soon to an embarrassing scandal for the National Football League.

Van Zee, Art. "The Promotion and Marketing of OxyContin: Commercial Triumph, Public Health Tragedy." *American Journal of Public Health* 99, no. 2 (February 2009): 221–227. The title nicely summarizes the theme of this article. Drug companies have generated high sales of OxyContin with their promotion and marketing campaigns, even though studies failed to demonstrate that it worked much better than other pain relievers. However, the campaigns minimized the risk of addiction and fostered the public health tragedy of OxyContin abuse.

Viani, Lisa Owens. "Don't Flush the Ambien! Environmentally-Friendly Prescription Drug Disposal, San Mateo County, Calif." *Utne Reader* 146 (March/April, 2008): 82. To help protect water supplies and landfills from leakage of disposed prescription drugs, San Mateo has devised some environmentally friendly methods of disposal. According to the article, the country has set up a drop-off system for unused drugs and hopes other counties will adopt similar programs.

Prescription Drugs

Wu, Li-Tzy, Christopher L. Ringwalt, Paolo Mannelli, and Ashwin A. Pat-kar. "Prescription Pain Reliever Abuse and Dependence among Adoles-cents: A Nationally Representative Study." *Journal of the American Academy of Child and Adolescent Psychiatry* 47, no. 9 (September 2008): 1,020–1,029. According to the results of this study, 7 percent of youth ages 12 to 17 reported nonprescription use of prescription pain relievers and 1 percent met criteria for abuse or dependence on the prescription pain relievers. Although the results depend on potentially biased self-reports from youth, the reliance on a representative national sample al-lows the results to be generalized widely.

WEB DOCUMENTS

Associated Press. "FDA Panel Votes to Eliminate Vicodin, Percocet: Over-doses of Acetaminophen Also Lead Experts to Urge Lower Tylenol Doses." MSNBC. Available online. URL: http://www.msnbc.msn.com/id/31664450/ns/health-more_health_news. Updated July 1, 2009. Vico-din and Percocet are drugs that combine acetaminophen, the ingredient in Tylenol, with opiate-based products to manage pain. An expert panel convened by the FDA about the risks of high doses of acetaminophen says these prescription drugs are dangerous, sometimes deadly. The FDA need not follow the recommendations and has given no timetable for responding to them.

Blackstone, John. "Prescription for Drug Danger Online." Available online. URL: http://www.cbsnews.com/stories/2008/07/09/eveningnews/main4246544.shtml. Posted July 9, 2008. This news story reports that 85 percent of webpages selling drugs do not require a prescription. That obvi-ously makes it easy for children to get illegal access to prescription drugs.

Business Wire. "Ten Things You and Your Family Should Know about the Dangers of Prescription Painkillers, According to the Waismann Foun-dation." Available online. URL: http://www.opiates.com/media/prescription-painkiller-dangers.html. Posted September 7, 2004. This document aims to help parents become aware of the risks of this major source of prescription drug abuse. It encourages parents to talk with chil-dren about the risks and to look for signs of abuse.

Donn, Jeff. "Zicam Not Alone in Side Effect Reports." ABCNews.com. Available online. URL: http://abcnewscom/Health/wireStory?id=7863624. Posted June 17, 2009. Problems experienced by users of Zicam, an over-the-counter treatment for colds, reveal a gap in review and approval of drugs by the FDA, according to this Associated Press article. Since a 1938 law passed Congress, homeopathic remedies have not had to go through the approval process of prescription drugs. This article describes some examples of safety problems that have resulted. In the case of Zicam, the

FDA has warned consumers to stop using the product because it can permanently damage the sense of smell.

Donn, Jeff, Martha Mendoza, and Justin Pritchard. "Tons of Released Drugs Taint U.S. Water." ABCNews. Available online. URL: http://abcnews.com/US/wireStory?id-7376041. Posted April 20, 2009. This report from the Associated Press summarizes a detailed investigation of pollution by prescription drugmakers. The main point is sobering: "U.S. manufacturers, including major drugmakers, have legally released at least 271 million pounds of pharmaceuticals into waterways that often provide drinking water—contamination the federal government has consistently overlooked."

Landers, Susan J. "Dangerous Diversions: Specter of Prescription Drug Abuse Creates Tough Balancing Act for Doctors." AmedNews. Available online. URL: http://www.ama-assn.org/amednews/2008/03/17/hlsa0317.htm. Posted March 17, 2008. Physicians face problems in providing needed relief to patients in pain but may unwittingly contribute to prescription drug abuse. This article describes the problems and quotes experts on how to deal with them. It also notes that electronic monitoring of prescription drugs can help deal with patients who go to multiple doctors to get access to excess pain relievers.

National Academies of Science. "Medication Errors Injure 1.5 Million People and Cost Billions of Dollars Annually; Report Offers Comprehensive Strategies for Reducing Drug-Related Mistakes." News from the National Academies. Available online. URL: http://www8.national academies.org/onpinews/newsitem.aspx?RecordID=11623. Posted July 20, 2006. This press release summarizes a longer report from experts working with the National Academies of Science. The title summarizes the theme, and the report recommends a series of actions for patients, health care organizations, government agencies, and pharmaceutical companies to take in response to the high levels of medication errors.

National Institute on Drug Abuse. "Selected Prescription Drugs with Potential for Abuse." Available online. URL: http://www.drugabuse.gov/PDF/PrescriptionDrugs.pdf. Revised April 2005. This list includes drugs in categories of depressants such as barbiturates and benzodiazepines, opioids and morphine derivatives such as codeine and oxycodone, stimulants such as methamphetamines and methylphenidate, and other compounds such as anabolic steroids. Along with commercial and street names for the drugs, the document lists the effects and potential health consequences of the drugs.

Office of National Drug Control Policy. "Prescription for Danger." The Anti-Drug.com. Available online. URL: http://www.theantidrug.com/pdfs/prescription_report.pdf. Posted January 2008. The report gives particular attention to increasing abuse of prescription drugs by teens. It disputes the myth that prescription drugs are safer than street drugs and offers advice to parents on identifying abuse by their kids and getting treatment help. The document contains several useful charts on the extent of abuse.

———. "Proper Disposal of Prescription Drugs." Available online. URL: http://www.whitehousedrugpolicy.gov/publications/pdf/prescrip_disposal.pdf. Posted 2009. Flushing unused prescription drugs down the toilet contaminates the environment and perhaps even drinking water. This document describes several other ways, involving varying degrees of inconvenience, to dispose of the unused drugs properly.

———. "Teens and Prescription Drugs: An Analysis of Recent Trends on the Emerging Drug Threat." Available online. URL: http://eric.ed.gov/ERICDocs/data/ericdocs2sql/content_storage_01/0000019b/80/28/04/7d.pdf. Posted February 2007. This analysis warns of the trend among teens away from street drugs and toward prescription drugs. It presents several charts and graphs demonstrating the high level of illicit use of prescription drugs by teens, the ease of getting such drugs, and the potential for dependence. It also shows that most teens wrongly believe that using prescription drugs is safe.

CHAPTER 8

ORGANIZATIONS AND AGENCIES

The organizations and agencies listed in this chapter fall into four categories:

- federal government organizations,
- international organizations,
- pharmaceutical companies, and
- advocacy and professional organizations.

For each organization, the listings include the webpage and e-mail address. Rather than list their e-mail address, many organizations include a web-based form for submitting questions and comments via the Internet. In these cases, the text notes that e-mail is available via a web form. The listings then include phone numbers, postal addresses, and brief descriptions of the organizations.

FEDERAL GOVERNMENT ORGANIZATIONS

Center for Drug Evaluation and Research (CDER)
URL: http://www.fda.gov/
AboutFDA/CentersOffices/
CDER
E-mail: druginfo@fda.hhs.gov
Phone: (888) 463-6332
White Oak Building 51
10903 New Hampshire Avenue
Silver Spring, MD 20993
The unit within the FDA that regulates prescription drugs by testing the safety and effectiveness of new drugs, monitoring the risks of approved drugs, checking drug ads for truthfulness and balance, and providing information to professionals and consumers.

Centers for Medicare and Medicaid Services (CMS)
URL: http://www.cms.hhs.gov
E-mail: web form
Phone: (877) 267-2323

**7500 Security Boulevard
Baltimore, MD 21244**
Its mission is to ensure effective, up-to-date health care coverage and quality care for beneficiaries of Medicare and Medicaid, two programs that provide prescription drug benefits.

**Drug Enforcement
 Administration (DEA)**
URL: http://www.usdoj.gov/dea
E-mail: web form
Phone: (202) 307-1000
**8701 Morrissette Drive
Springfield, VA 22152**
Enforces controlled substances laws and regulations, including the illegitimate diversion and use of legally produced prescription drugs.

**Environmental Protection
 Agency (EPA)**
URL: http://www.epa.gov
Phone: (202) 272-0167
**Ariel Rios Building
1200 Pennsylvania Avenue NW
Washington, DC 20460**
Uses science, research, education, and assessment to protect human health and the environment and has recently examined environmental contamination by prescription drug residue.

**Federal Communications
 Commission (FCC)**
URL: http://www.fcc.gov
E-mail: fccinfo@fcc.gov
Phone: (888) 225-5322
**445 12th Street SW
Washington, DC 20554**

Regulates interstate and international communications by radio, television, wire, satellite, and cable, and once had responsibility for prescription drug advertisements but now has responsibility for over-the-counter drugs.

**Federal Trade Commission
 (FTC)**
URL: http://www.ftc.gov/bcp/
 consumer.shtm
E-mail: web form
Phone: (202) 326-2222
**600 Pennsylvania Avenue NW
Washington, DC 20580**
Enforces laws concerned with protection of consumer interests and has dealt with issues relating to Internet sales of drugs, direct-to-consumer drug ads, and competition in health services.

**Food and Drug Administration
 (FDA)**
URL: http://www.fda.gov
E-mail: webmail@oc.fda.gov
Phone: (888) 463-6332
**10903 New Hampshire Avenue
Silver Spring, MD 20993-0002**
The federal agency responsible for ensuring that human drugs are safe and effective and are accurately and honestly represented to the public.

**Government Accountability
 Office (GAO)**
URL: http://www.gao.gov
E-mail: contact@gao.gov
Phone: (202) 512-3000
**441 G Street NW
Washington, DC 20548**
An independent government agency that investigates how the federal

government spends taxpayer dollars and does research for Congress on, among many other topics, prescription drug safety and prices.

Health Care Financing Administration (HCFA)
URL: http://www.os.dhhs.gov/about/opdivs/hcfa.html
Phone: (410) 966-3000
200 Independence Avenue SW
Washington, DC 20201
An agency within the Department of Health and Human Services that oversees Medicare, the federal portion of Medicaid, and quality assurance for federal health care programs.

National Center for Health Statistics (NCHS)
URL: http://www.cdc.gov/nchs
E-mail: cdcinfo@cdc.gov
Phone: (800) 232-4636
3311 Toledo Road
Hyattsville, MD 20782
An agency within the Centers for Disease Control and Prevention that provides a wide variety of data and statistical information on health-related topics, including use of prescription drugs.

National Institute on Drug Abuse (NIDA)
URL: http://www.nida.nih.gov
E-mail: information@nida.nih.gov
Phone: (301) 443-1124
6001 Executive Boulevard, Room 5213
Bethesda, MD 20892-9561
Conducts, supports, and disseminates scientific research on drug abuse and addiction, including prescription drug abuse and addiction.

National Institutes of Health (NIH)
URL: http://www.nih.gov
E-mail: NIHinfo@od.nih.gov
Phone: (301) 496-4000
9000 Rockville Pike
Bethesda, MD 20892
The primary federal agency for conducting and supporting medical research, including research on the development and testing of medications and drugs.

Office of National Drug Control Policy (ONDCP)
URL: http://www.whitehouse drugpolicy.gov
E-mail: web form
Phone: (800) 666-3332
P.O. Box 6000
Rockville, MD 20849-6000
Establishes policy priorities and objectives for the nation's drug control program and coordinates drug-control activities of executive branch agencies.

U.S. Department of Commerce (DOC)
URL: http://www.commerce.gov
E-mail: TheSec@doc.gov
Phone: (202) 482-2000
1401 Constitution Avenue NW
Washington, DC 20230
Focuses on fostering and promoting commerce, economic development, and technological advancement and deals with issues involving international trade of prescription drugs.

U.S. Department of Health and Human Services (HHS)
URL: http://www.hhs.gov
E-mail: web form
Phone: (877) 696-6775
200 Independence Avenue SW
Washington, DC 20201
The cabinet department most concerned with issues of prescription drugs and the location of key agencies such as the Food and Drug Administration and the National Institutes of Health.

U.S. Department of Justice (DOJ)
URL: http://www.usdoj.gov
E-mail: AskDOJ@usdoj.gov
Phone: (202) 514-2000
950 Pennsylvania Avenue NW
Washington, DC 20530-0001
Enforces the laws of the United States, protects public safety, and has responsibility for prosecuting violations of federal prescription drug laws.

U.S. House Energy and Commerce Committee
URL: http://energycommerce. house.gov
Phone: (202) 225-2927
2125 Rayburn House Office Building
Washington, DC 20515
Lead committee for much legislation on prescription drug costs and safety.

U.S. Senate Special Committee on Aging
URL: http://aging.senate.gov
Phone: (202) 224-5364
G31 Dirksen Senate Office Building
Washington, DC 20510
Serves as a focal point in the Senate for discussion and debate on matters relating to older Americans and has presented findings and recommendations concerning prescription drug needs of the elderly.

INTERNATIONAL ORGANIZATIONS

Health Action International (HAI)
URL: http://www.haiweb.org
E-mail: info@haiweb.org
Phone: + 31 20 683 3684
Overtoom 60/III
1054 HK Amsterdam
The Netherlands
A network of groups in more than 70 countries that supports, among many other health-related goals, the equitable access to prescription drugs.

International Federation of Associations of Pharmaceutical Physicians (IFAPP)
URL: http://www.ifapp.org
E-mail: secretariat@ifapp.org
Phone: + 31 (0) 348 489 305
Kuipersweg 2T
3449 JA Woerden
The Netherlands
Fosters the development and international recognition of Pharmaceutical Medicine as a medical specialty and the development of training

and continuing education programs in the specialty.

International Society for Pharmacoepidemiology (ISPE)
URL: http://www.pharmacoepi. org
E-mail: ispe@paimgmt.com.
Phone: (301) 718-6500
5272 River Road, Suite 630
Bethesda, MD 20816
Promotes pharmacoepidemiology, a science that applies epidemiologic approaches to studying the use, effectiveness, value, and safety of pharmaceuticals.

International Society of Pharmacovigilance (ISoP)
URL: http://www.isoponline.org
E-mail: administration@ isoponline.org
Phone: + 44 (0) 203 256 0027
140 Emmanuel Road
London SW12 0HS
United Kingdom
Fosters the safe and proper use of medicines through the detection, evaluation, understanding, and prevention of adverse drug reactions or any other drug-related problems.

International Union of Basic and Clinical Pharmacology (IUPHAR)
URL: http://www.iuphar.org
E-mail: IUPHAR@kumc.edu
University of Kansas Medical Center
3901 Rainbow Boulevard, Mail Stop 4016
Kansas City, KS 66160
Represents the interests of pharmacologists (scientists who study

how drugs affect living organisms) throughout the world.

World Health Organization (WHO)
URL: http://www.who.int/en
E-mail: info@who.org
Phone: + 41 22 791 21 11
Avenue Appia 20
1211 Geneva 27
Switzerland
An agency of the United Nations that deals with health issues, including improvements in world access to prescription drugs.

World Intellectual Property Organization (WIPO)
URL: http://www.wipo.int
E-mail: web form
Phone: + 41 22 338 9111
34, chemin des Colombettes
CH-1211 Geneva 20
Switzerland
An agency of the United Nations with the goal of developing a system of intellectual property that protects the rights of patent developers and promotes the public interest.

World Trade Organization (WTO)
URL: http://www.wto.org
E-mail: enquiries@wto.org
Phone: (41-22) 739 51
Centre William Rappard
Rue de Lausanne 154
CH-1211 Geneva 21
Switzerland
An international organization with 153 member nations that deals with the rules of trade across nations and with disputes over patents and trade of prescription drugs.

PHARMACEUTICAL COMPANIES

Amgen
URL: http://www.amgen.com
E-mail: web form
Phone: (805) 447-1000
One Amgen Center Drive
Thousand Oaks, CA 91320-1799
A biotechnology company that uses recombinant DNA technology and molecular biology science to make medicines such as Epogen and Arenesp for anemia.

AstraZeneca
URL: http://www.astrazeneca.com
E-mail: web form
Phone: + 44 20 7304 5000
15 Stanhope Gate
London W1K 1LN
United Kingdom
A company resulting from the merger of Swedish AB and the British Zeneca Group in 1999, it is the maker of Arimidex for treatment of certain types of breast cancer, Crestor for high cholesterol, and Nexium (the purple pill) for heartburn relief.

Bristol-Myers Squibb
URL: http://www.bms.com
E-mail: web form
Phone: (800) 332-2056
345 Park Avenue
New York, NY 10154
The company's pharmaceuticals segment makes Plavix and Pravachol for cardiovascular problems, Taxol for cancer treatment, drugs such as Abilify for affective and other psychiatric disorders, Avapro for hypertension, and Reyataz for HIV.

Eli Lilly
URL: http://www.lilly.com
Phone: (317) 276-2000
Lilly Corporate Center
Indianapolis, IN 46285
Known for its breakthrough antidepressant drug Prozac and other drugs for psychiatric and mental health conditions, the company also makes Cialis for erectile dysfunction, Cymbalta for depression and anxiety, and Seconal for epilepsy and insomnia.

Genentech Roche
URL: http://www.gene.com
E-mail: web form
Phone: (650) 225-1000
1 DNA Way
South San Francisco, CA 94080-4990
A biotechnology company, recently having agreed to merge with Roche, that uses human genetic information to discover, develop, manufacture, and commercialize medicines such as Avastin for carcinoma of the rectum or colon and Herceptin for breast cancer.

Generic Pharmaceutical Association (GPhA)
URL: http://www.gphaonline.org
E-mail: web form
Phone: (703) 647-2480
2300 Clarendon Boulevard
Suite 400
Arlington, VA 22201
Represents the interests of manufacturers and distributors of generic drugs in scientific, government, and public affairs forums.

GlaxoSmithKline
URL: http://www.gsk.com
Phone: + 44 (0) 20 8047
980 Great West Road
Brentford, Middlesex, TW8 9GS
United Kingdom
With offices in North Carolina as well as Britain, the company makes Paxil to treat depression, Advair for asthma and chronic obstructive pulmonary disease, Avandia for diabetes, Levitra for erectile dysfunction, Tagamet for stomach acid, and AZT for treatment of HIV/AIDS.

IMS Health
URL: http://www.imshealth.
   com/portal/site/imshealth
E-mail: web form
Phone: (203) 845-5200
901 Main Avenue
Suite 612
Norwalk, CT 06851-1187
A private company that supplies data to clients on health care and prescription drugs.

Johnson & Johnson
URL: http://www.jnj.com
E-mail: web form
P.O. Box 726
Langhorne, PA 19047-0726
Along with over-the-counter health products such as Band-Aids, Listerine, Motrin, Nicoderm, Pepcid AC, Rogaine, Rolaids, Sudafed, Tylenol, and Visine, the company sells prescription drugs such as Haldol for schizophrenia, Topamax for epilepsy, Remicade for a variety of immune system diseases, and Zyrtec for allergies.

Merck
URL: http://www.merck.com
Phone: (908) 423-1000
One Merck Drive
P.O. Box 100
Whitehouse Station, NJ 08889-
   0100
It makes Cozaar and Hyzaar for hypertension; Vytorin, Zetia, and Zocor to lower cholesterol; Propecia for male-pattern baldness; Singulair for asthma; Fosamax for osteoporosis; and Gardasil, a vaccine for cervical cancer; but it is also well known for making Vioxx, a pain relief drug taken off the market for causing heart problems.

Novartis International AG
URL: http://www.novartis.com
Phone: + 41 61 324 11 11
CH-4002 Basel
Switzerland
Created by the merger of Ciba and Sandoz, it makes Diovan for hypertension, Gleevec for chronic myeloid leukemia, Zometa for cancer complications, Sandostatin for excess production of growth hormone, Femara for breast cancer, and Enablex for an overactive bladder.

Pfizer
URL: http://www.pfizer.com/
   home
E-mail: web form
Phone: (212) 733-2323
235 East 42nd Street
New York, NY 10017
The world's largest pharmaceutical company makes the anticholesterol statin drug Lipitor, the antidepressant Zoloft, and the erectile

dysfunction drug Viagra; the company acquired Wyeth on October 15, 2009.

Roche Group
URL: http://www.roche.com
E-mail: basel.webmaster@roche.com
Phone: + 41-61-688 1111
Konzern-Hauptsitz
Grenzacherstrasse 124
CH-4070 Basel
Switzerland
With its U.S. unit, Hoffman-La Roche, headquartered in Nutley, New Jersey, the company makes the tranquilizer Valium, the antibiotic Rocephin, Invirase for HIV/AIDS, Xenical for treatment of obesity, Tamiflu for influenza, and Boniva for treatment of osteoporosis.

Sanofi-Aventis U.S.
URL: http://www.sanofi-aventis.us
E-mail: web form
Phone: (800) 981-2491
55 Corporate Drive
Bridgewater, NJ 08807
It makes Allegra for allergies, Ambien for sleep problems, Plavix to prevent formation of clots that lead to heart attacks and strokes, Taxotere

for treatment of breast cancer, Actonel for osteoporosis, and Arava for rheumatoid arthritis symptoms such as joint swelling and tenderness.

Schering-Plough
URL: http://www.schering-plough.com
Phone: (908) 298-4000
2000 Galloping Hill Road
Kenilworth, NJ 07033-0530
Acquired by Merck on November 3, 2009, the company jointly manages Vytorin and Zetia for high cholesterol and makes Remicade for inflammatory disorders, Nasonex for allergies, and Temodar for brain tumors.

Wyeth
URL: http://www.wyeth.com
Phone: (973) 660-5500
5 Giralda Farms
Madison, NJ 07940
The company, acquired by Pfizer in October 2009 produced fenfluramine, the diet drug that was removed from the market for causing health problems, and makes Premarin and Prempro for estrogen replacement, Effexor for depression and anxiety disorders, Ativan for anxiety and insomnia, and Enbrel for arthritis.

ADVOCACY AND PROFESSIONAL ORGANIZATIONS

AARP
URL: http://www.aarp.org
E-mail: web form
Phone: (888) 687-2277
601 E Street NW

Washington, DC 20049
A leading organization for people age 50 and over that provides services and products for members, including information on prescrip-

tion drug prices, safety, and effectiveness.

American Medical Association (AMA)
URL: http://www.ama-assn.org
Phone: (800) 621-8335
515 North State Street
Chicago, IL 60654
An organization of physicians that works to promote medicine and public health, it makes recommendations for reducing drug costs, improving drug access, and regulating drug advertising.

American Pharmacists Association (APhA)
URL: http://www.pharmacist.com
E-mail: web form
Phone: (800) 237-2742
2215 Constitution Avenue NW
Washington, DC 20037
The largest association of pharmacists in the United States, it uses information, education, and advocacy to help members deliver optimal health care to patients.

BlueCross BlueShield Association (BCBSA)
URL: http://www.blueadvocacy.org/site/page/prescription_drugs
E-mail: blueadvocacy@blueadvocacy.org
Phone: (202) 626-4780
1310 G Street NW
Washington, DC 20005
This association of independent providers of health insurance has an Office of Policy and Representation (called Blue Advocacy) that makes

recommendations for prescription drug policy.

Center for Public Integrity
URL: http://www.publicintegrity.org
E-mail: web form
Phone: (202) 466-1300
910 17th Street NW
Suite 700
Washington, DC 20006
Produces original investigative journalism about significant public issues; its investigation of lobbying by pharmaceutical companies was highly critical of the power of the industry.

Kaiser Family Foundation (KFF)
URL: http://www.kff.org
E-mail: web form
Phone: (650) 854-9400
2400 Sand Hill Road
Menlo Park, CA 94025
A charitable organization that focuses on major health care issues facing the United States, including access to prescription drugs, by doing research and communicating facts, information, and analysis.

National Conference of State Legislatures (NCSL)
URL: http://www.ncsl.org
E-mail: ncslnet-admin@ncsl.org
Phone: (202) 624-5400
444 North Capitol Street NW
Suite 515
Washington, DC 20001
A resource to help state legislatures develop programs for their own states that reports on trends in prescription drug laws (and many other topics) among the 50 states.

National Organization for Rare Disorders (NORD)
URL: http://www.rarediseases.org
E-mail: orphan@rarediseases.org
Phone: (203) 744-0100
55 Kenosia Avenue
P.O. Box 1968
Danbury, CT 06813-1968
Helps people with rare diseases (affecting fewer than 200,000 Americans) and has advocated for government policies that encourage drug companies to develop orphan drugs for these rare diseases.

National Pharmaceutical Association (NPhA)
URL: http://www.npha.net
E-mail: npha@npha.net
Phone: (800) 944-6742
107 Kilmayne Drive
Suite C
Cary, NC 27511
A nationwide professional organization of pharmacists that represents the views of minority pharmacists.

Needy Meds
URL: http://www.needymeds.org
E-mail: web form
Phone: (978) 281-6666
P.O. Box 219
Gloucester, MA 01931
Helps prescription drug users get financial assistance to purchase medicines.

Patients not Patents
URL: http://www.patientsnotpatents.org
E-mail: jeff@patientsnotpatents.org
Phone: (202) 277.6213
1712 Eye Street NW

Suite 915
Washington, DC 20006
Seeks to educate the public about the effects of intellectual property laws on the availability of health care and prescriptions drugs.

Pharmaceutical Research and Manufacturers of America (PhRMA)
URL: http://www.phrma.org
E-mail: web form
Phone: (202) 835-3400
950 F Street NW
Washington, DC 20004
Represents leading pharmaceutical and biotechnology companies in the United States and advocates for public policies that support the efforts of companies to discover and market new medicines.

Prescription Access Litigation (PAL)
URL: http://www.prescriptionaccess.org
E-mail: pal@communitycatalyst.org
Phone: (617) 275-2931
30 Winter Street
10th Floor
Boston, MA 02108
Uses class action litigation and public education to challenge what it calls illegal pricing tactics and deceptive marketing by drug companies and others in the pharmaceutical industry.

Prescription Policy Choices (PPC)
URL: http://www.policychoices.org
Phone: (207) 622-3302

P.O. Box 204
Hallowell, ME 04347
A research and advocacy organization that evaluates alternative policies and programs, particularly those at the state level, in order to reduce prescription drug prices and increase access to medications.

Prescription Project
URL: http://www.prescription
  project.org
Phone: (617) 275-2853
30 Winter Street
Boston, MA 02108
This initiative of The Pew Charitable Trusts promotes consumer safety through reforms in the approval, manufacture, and marketing of prescription drugs and through projects to encourage evidence-based prescribing.

Public Citizen Health Research
  Group
URL: http://www.citizen.org/hrg
E-mail: web form
Phone: (202) 588-1000
1600 20th Street NW
Washington, DC 20009
Promotes changes in health care policy, oversight of drug safety, and bans or relabeling of unsafe or ineffective drugs.

PART III

APPENDICES

APPENDIX A

GUIDANCE FOR INDUSTRY: CONSUMER-DIRECTED BROADCAST ADVERTISEMENTS[1]

In this 1999 document, the FDA summarizes the rules for the advertisements presented on television and radio. The guidance sets limits on what drug companies can do in their ads but can also help viewers understand the FDA regulations.

I. INTRODUCTION

This guidance is intended to assist sponsors who are interested in advertising their prescription human and animal drugs, including biological products for humans, directly to consumers through broadcast media, such as television, radio, or telephone communications systems.[2]

II. BACKGROUND

The Federal Food, Drug, and Cosmetic Act (the Act) requires that manufacturers, packers, and distributors (sponsors) who advertise prescription human and animal drugs, including biological products for humans, disclose in advertisements certain information about the advertised product's uses and risks. For prescription drugs and biologics, the Act requires advertisements to contain "information in brief summary relating to side effects, contraindications, and effectiveness" (21 U.S.C. 352(n)). The resulting information disclosure is commonly called the *brief summary*.

The prescription drug advertising regulations (21 CFR 202.1) distinguish between print and broadcast advertisements. Print advertisements must include the brief summary, which generally contains each of the risk concepts from the product's approved package labeling. Advertisements broadcast through media such as television, radio, or telephone communications systems must disclose the product's major risks in either the audio or audio and visual parts of the presentation; this is sometimes called the *major statement*. This guidance does not address the major statement requirement.

Sponsors of broadcast advertisements are also required to present a brief summary or, alternatively, may make "adequate provision . . . for dissemination of the approved or permitted package labeling in connection with the broadcast presentation" (21 CFR 202.1(e)(1)). This is referred to as the *adequate provision* requirement. The regulations thus specify that the major statement, together with adequate provision for dissemination of the product's approved labeling, can provide the information disclosure required for broadcast advertisements.

The purpose of this guidance is to describe an approach that FDA believes can fulfill the requirement for *adequate provision* in connection with consumer-directed broadcast advertisements for prescription drug and biological products. The approach presumes that such advertisements:

- Are not false or misleading in any respect. For a prescription drug, this would include communicating that the advertised product is available only by prescription and that only a prescribing healthcare professional can decide whether the product is appropriate for a patient.
- Present a fair balance between information about effectiveness and information about risk.
- Include a thorough *major statement* conveying all of the product's most important risk information in consumer-friendly language.
- Communicate all information relevant to the product's indication (including limitations to use) in consumer-friendly language.

III. FULFILLING THE *ADEQUATE PROVISION* REQUIREMENT

A sponsor wishing to use consumer-directed broadcast advertisements may meet the adequate provision requirement through an approach that will allow most of a potentially diverse audience to have reasonably convenient access to the advertised product's approved labeling. This audience will include many persons with limited access to technologically sophisticated outlets (e.g., the Internet) and persons who are uncomfortable actively requesting additional product information or are concerned about being personally identified in their search for product information. One acceptable approach to disseminating the product's approved labeling is described below. This approach includes the following components.

Appendix A

A. Disclosure in the advertisement of an operating toll-free telephone number for consumers to call for the approved package labeling. Upon calling, consumers should be given the choice of:

- Having the labeling mailed to them in a timely manner (e.g., within 2 business days for receipt generally within 4–6 days); or
- Having the labeling read to them over the phone (e.g., by offering consumers a selection of prerecorded labeling topics).

B. Reference in the advertisement to a mechanism to provide package labeling to consumers with restricted access to sophisticated technology, such as the Internet, and those who are uncomfortable actively requesting additional product information or are concerned about being personally identified in their search for product information. One acceptable mechanism would be to provide the additional product information in the form of print advertisements appearing concurrently in publications that reach the exposed audience. The location of at least one of these advertisements would be referenced in the broadcast advertisement. If a print advertisement is part of an adequate provision procedure, it should supply a toll-free telephone number and an address for further consumer access to full package labeling. This mechanism of providing access to product labeling has the advantage of also providing considerable information in the form of the required brief summary and in the advertising text itself.

- When a broadcast advertisement is broadly disseminated, FDA believes that ensuring that passive and privacy-sensitive information seekers have adequate access to detailed product information is critical to complying with the *adequate provision* regulatory requirement. Thus, print advertisements associated with broadly disseminated broadcast advertisements should be comparably broadly disseminated in terms of the targeted audiences.

- An alternative mechanism for providing private access to product information would be to ensure the availability of sufficient numbers of brochures containing package labeling in a variety of publicly accessible sites (e.g., pharmacies, doctors' offices, grocery stores, public libraries). Brochures should be available at enough sites so that most consumers exposed to the broadcast advertisement can obtain the labeling without traveling beyond their normal range of activities. This alternative mechanism is likely to be logistically feasible only when the associated broadcast advertising campaign is relatively limited in audience reach.

C. Disclosure in the advertisement of an Internet webpage (URL) address that provides access to the package labeling.
D. Disclosure in the advertisement that pharmacists, physicians (or other health care providers), or veterinarians (in the case of animal drugs) may provide additional product information to consumers. This statement should communicate clearly that the referenced professional is a source of additional product information.

Telephone advertisements that make a product claim (not reminder advertisements) occur when there is a telephone communication between an individual and a product's sponsor where both a product name and a representation or suggestion relating to a product (e.g., its indication) are disclosed by the sponsor. Under these circumstances, such advertisements are subject to the disclosure requirements of the Act and the regulations. However, telephone advertisements are different from advertisements broadcast through television and radio. By participating in the telephone communication, the consumer has already indicated his or her willingness to discuss the topic or receive additional information. Consequently, adequate provision for disseminating product labeling in connection with telephone advertisements may be achieved with fewer of the components listed above. For such advertisements, adequate provision could consist of the availability of the option of having product labeling mailed to the caller in a timely manner (e.g., within 2 business days for receipt generally within 4–6 days), or having the labeling read to them over the phone (e.g., by allowing consumers to select from prerecorded labeling topics), as well as disclosing that health care providers are a source of additional product information.

When a broadcast advertisement is presented in a foreign language, the information sources that are part of the advertisement's "adequate provision" mechanism (i.e., print advertisements or brochures, web sites, toll-free telephone number recorded messages or operators) should be in the language of the broadcast ad. Regardless of the language used for the advertisement, current broadcast advertising regulations require the dissemination of approved product labeling, which, in most cases, must be in English, and is generally written in language directed to health care professionals. The Agency strongly encourages sponsors to consider the benefits of *also* providing consumers with nonpromotional, consumer-friendly product information in the language of the broadcast ad (e.g., FDA-approved patient labeling or accurate, consumer-friendly translations of product labeling information).

The FDA encourages sponsors who use this *adequate provision* mechanism to collect relevant data on consumer use and make their findings publicly known. FDA also encourages sponsors and other interested parties to make known their research relating to the overall effects of DTC promotion on the public health.

Appendix A

---

[1] This guidance has been prepared by the Intra-Agency Group on Advertising and Promotion at the Food and Drug Administration. This guidance represents the Agency's current thinking on procedures to fulfill the requirements for disclosure of product information in connection with consumer-directed broadcast advertisements for prescription human and animal drugs, and human biological products. It does not create or confer any rights for or on any person and does not operate to bind FDA or the public. An alternative approach may be used if such approach satisfies the requirements of the applicable statute, regulations, or both.

[2] This guidance is not intended to cover the advertising of restricted medical devices, which are subject to the requirements of section 502(r) of the Federal Food, Drug, and Cosmetic Act.

Source: U.S. Food and Drug Administration. Available online. URL: http://www.fda.gov/downloads/Drugs/GuidanceComplianceRegulatory Information/Guidances/ucm070065.pdf. Last updated August 1999.

APPENDIX B

GUIDANCE[1]: DRUG SAFETY INFORMATION—FDA'S COMMUNICATION TO THE PUBLIC

Meeting the FDA's key goal, to ensure the safety of prescription drugs, requires not only evaluation of risks before approval but also communicating safety information to the public. The first half of the 2007 document presented below explains how the agency works toward this goal.

This guidance represents the Food and Drug Administration's (FDA's) current thinking on this topic. It does not create or confer any rights for or on any person and does not operate to bind FDA or the public.

I. WHAT IS THIS GUIDANCE ABOUT?

This document provides guidance on how FDA is developing and disseminating information to the public regarding important drug safety issues, including emerging drug safety information.[2] As discussed in more detail below, an *important drug safety issue* is one that has the potential to alter the benefit/risk analysis for a drug in such a way as to affect decisions about prescribing or taking the drug. The term *emerging drug safety information* refers to information about an important drug safety issue that has not yet been fully analyzed or confirmed.

For many years, FDA has provided information on drug risks and benefits to healthcare professionals and patients when that information has generated a specific concern or prompted a regulatory action, such as a revision to the drug product's labeling. More recently, FDA has begun taking a more comprehensive approach to making information on potential drug risks available to the public earlier, in some cases while the Agency still is evaluating whether any regulatory action is warranted. FDA believes that timely communication of important drug safety information will give healthcare professionals, patients, consumers, and other interested persons access to the most current information concerning the potential risks and benefits of a marketed drug, helping them to make more informed individual treatment choices.

This Guidance[3] describes FDA's current approach to communicating important drug safety information, including emerging drug safety information, to the public and the factors that influence when such information is communicated. FDA may disseminate important drug safety information by other methods and at other times than those described in this guidance.

II. WHY IS FDA ISSUING THIS GUIDANCE?

FDA has been reexamining its risk communication program, including how and when we communicate emerging drug safety information to the public. We are issuing this guidance to reaffirm our commitment to communicating important information about drug safety in a timely manner, in some cases while the Agency still is evaluating whether any regulatory action is warranted.

FDA's risk communication efforts are part of a larger drug safety initiative that began in November 2004, when FDA announced an initiative to strengthen the safety program for marketed drugs. This initiative included: (1) sponsoring an independent study by the Institute of Medicine of the National Academies of the effectiveness of the drug safety system, with emphasis on postmarketing risk assessment and surveillance; (2) conducting workshops and Advisory Committee meetings regarding complex drug safety and risk management issues, including emerging concerns; and (3) publishing three risk management guidances.[4]

FDA augmented its drug safety initiative in February 2005 by creating an independent Drug Safety Oversight Board to enhance oversight of drug safety decision making within CDER. FDA also announced its commitment to "increase the transparency of the Agency's decision-making process by establishing new and expanding existing communication channels to provide targeted drug safety information to the public. These channels will be used to help ensure that established and emerging drug safety data are quickly available in an easily accessible form. The increased openness will enable patients and their healthcare professionals to make better-informed decisions about individual treatment options."[5]

To fulfill this commitment, FDA issued for comment a draft guidance titled *FDA's 'Drug Watch' for Emerging Drug Safety Information* in May

2005. In December 2005, FDA held a public hearing regarding "FDA's Communication of Drug Safety Information" that examined the various risk communication tools employed by FDA. Comments from participants emphasized that, increasingly, patients are taking a more active role in their health care. Patients want information about the drugs they are taking, and actively seek this information from various sources, including the Internet. Patients and their healthcare providers rely on information from these sources to make important prescribing and treatment decisions (including about consumer self-care). Because of its expertise and access to important information concerning the benefits and safety of medications, FDA is an important source of drug information.

FDA has carefully reviewed the comments it received on the draft guidance (30 comments were submitted to the public docket)[6] and during the public hearing. This final version of the guidance reflects our consideration of these comments, as well as our experience with posting emerging drug safety information.

Due to potential confusion between the proposed *Drug Watch* and FDA's existing *MedWatch* program, FDA no longer plans to use the name *Drug Watch* to describe the Web page that contains drug safety information. As discussed in more detail in section VII of this guidance, we have identified drugs that have been the subject of a Public Health Advisory or an Alert (see section VI.E of this guidance) on a single Web page linked from FDA's Web site. This is part of our ongoing effort to use and enhance existing FDA communications mechanisms to better convey important drug safety information to the public. In addition, we have revised this guidance to describe the various methods FDA currently uses to communicate established and emerging drug safety information to the public. It should be noted that we will continue to evaluate and enhance the effectiveness of the various methods we use to communicate about important drug safety issues, including the mechanisms described in this guidance and the presentation of drug safety information on the Agency's Web sites (http://www.fda.gov and http://www.fda.gov/cder). We intend to update this guidance, as appropriate, to reflect any substantial modifications to our communication of drug safety information to the public.

III. WHAT DRUG SAFETY INFORMATION DOES FDA COMMUNICATE?

FDA communicates information about *important drug safety issues,* and under the drug safety initiative, FDA has enhanced its efforts to communicate such information earlier in our decision making process (see section V of this guidance). An *important drug safety issue* is one that has the potential to alter the benefit/risk analysis for a drug in such a way as to affect decisions about prescribing or taking the drug. Examples of important drug safety issues include, but are not limited to:

- Serious adverse drug experiences[7] identified after approval or in the setting of a new use
- Additional serious or more frequent adverse drug experiences in a subpopulation of patients
- Medication errors

IV. HOW DOES FDA EVALUATE DRUG SAFETY INFORMATION?

All drugs have risks, and healthcare professionals and patients must balance the risks and benefits of a drug when making decisions about medical therapy. FDA monitors and reviews available safety information related to marketed drugs throughout each drug product's lifecycle. When a drug is approved, the product labeling includes, among other things, available information about the benefits and risks of the drug. After drug approval, the Agency may learn of new, or more frequent, serious adverse drug experiences from postapproval clinical studies or from clinical use. For example, additional adverse drug experiences, some of them serious, may be identified as a drug is used more widely and under more diverse conditions (e.g., concurrently with other drugs), or as the drug is prescribed for off-label uses.

As new information related to a marketed drug becomes available, the Agency reviews the data and evaluates whether there is a potential drug safety concern. When a potential drug safety concern arises, relevant scientific experts within the Agency engage in a prompt review and analysis of available data. Often, there is a period of uncertainty while FDA evaluates the new safety information to determine whether there is an important drug safety issue related to a specific drug or drug class and whether regulatory action is appropriate. During this period, FDA also is actively engaged in scientific efforts to gather additional safety information. The Drug Safety Oversight Board may be consulted and provide recommendations to the Director of the Center for Drug Evaluation and Research regarding the management and communication of an emerging drug safety issue. FDA also may consult an Advisory Committee regarding an emerging drug safety issue. Sponsors are also evaluating the new safety information and providing the results of their analyses to FDA during this time. As additional data relevant to an emerging drug safety issue become available (e.g., data from an ongoing study or data from available clinical databases), such data are considered in the analysis and decision-making process. Upon evaluation of additional data, further regulatory action, such as a revision to product labeling or a Risk Minimization Action Plan (RiskMAP), may be appropriate.

Interpretation of postmarketing safety data is complex, involving analysis of postapproval clinical data, detailed review of adverse drug experience reports in the context of relevant clinical studies, estimates of drug usage and adverse drug experience reporting rates, estimates of background rates of the adverse event, and other relevant information. Decisions about how to address a safety concern often are a matter of judgment, about which reasonable persons with relevant expertise may disagree. We engage in vigorous and comprehensive discussions within the Agency regarding potential drug safety issues to ensure that all points of view are considered prior to making a decision on how to proceed.

As the Agency evaluates a drug safety issue to determine whether regulatory action is warranted, we may communicate further information to the public at appropriate points in the decision-making process. Consistent with our public health mandate, we may advise the public of an emerging drug safety concern as well as the next steps the Agency may take regarding an important drug safety issue.

V. WHEN DOES FDA COMMUNICATE EMERGING DRUG SAFETY INFORMATION?

We use the term *emerging drug safety information* to describe information FDA is monitoring or analyzing that may have the potential to alter the benefit/risk analysis for a drug in such a way as to affect decisions about prescribing or taking the drug (i.e., an important drug safety issue), but that has not yet been fully analyzed or confirmed. Emerging drug safety information may be derived from data from postmarketing surveillance (for example, reported serious adverse drug experiences), clinical studies, clinical pharmacology studies, epidemiological studies, or the scientific literature. Such information may relate to new risks or new information on known risks.

For years, FDA and sponsors have disseminated emerging drug safety information. The Agency currently disseminates emerging drug safety information after having completed an analysis of available data and, in some cases, before having reached a decision about the need for a regulatory action. Agency communications about emerging drug safety information may help achieve certain longstanding public health goals, including enhanced vigilance on the part of healthcare professionals who may be prompted by the information to increase their reporting of safety observations to FDA. We are mindful of the potential public health implications of providing emerging drug safety information and are particularly concerned about possible consequences, such as inappropriate modification or discontinuation of useful treatment. We attempt to anticipate and address these possible consequences through our risk communications by describing the nature of a safety concern and what is known about its relationship to a particular drug and making recommendations for healthcare professionals and patients about how to monitor for and manage the concern. There will always be some tension between the goal of having people informed about potentially important information as early as possible and the goal of having that information thoroughly substantiated. Our goal is to make emerging drug safety information available to the public in a balanced, impartial manner so that health care professionals and patients can consider the information when making decisions about medical treatment despite uncertainties in the data. The Agency is committed to providing accurate, clear, reliable, and useful drug safety information.

FDA considers many factors in the course of evaluating an emerging drug safety concern and deciding whether emerging drug safety information should be made available to the public. These factors include, but are not limited to, the following:

- Reliability of the data
- Magnitude of the risk
- Seriousness of the event (e.g., severity and reversibility) relative to the disease being treated
- Plausibility of a causal relationship between the use of a drug and the adverse event[8]
- Extent of patient exposure (e.g., how broadly is the drug used)
- Potential to prevent or mitigate the risk in the patient population (e.g., monitoring)
- Effect on clinical practice
- Disproportionate impact on particular populations (e.g., children or the elderly)

Providing information about an emerging drug safety issue does not necessarily mean that FDA has concluded there is a causal relationship between the drug and the adverse events described. Communicating emerging drug safety information also does not necessarily mean that FDA is advising healthcare professionals to limit their prescribing of the drug at issue, rather it is intended to further inform such prescribing.

VI. HOW DOES FDA COMMUNICATE IMPORTANT DRUG SAFETY INFORMATION?

FDA uses a broad range of methods to communicate drug safety information to the public. Certain forms of communication are targeted to specific audiences (e.g., healthcare professionals or patients). Others are directed at more than one group to ensure widespread dissemination of information about important drug safety issues, including emerging drug safety issues. FDA is continuing to evaluate its communication efforts and will modify them to enhance their accessibility and effectiveness. We welcome public comment at any time suggesting ways to improve our safety communications. The table, below, summarizes the methods discussed in this section for FDA communication of drug safety information.

TABLE: SUMMARY OF SELECTED METHODS FOR FDA COMMUNICATION OF DRUG SAFETY INFORMATION

Type of Communication	Content	Target Audience
Professional labeling for prescription drugs	Summary of essential information needed for safe and effective use of the drug	Healthcare providers
Patient-directed labeling for prescription drugs (patient package inserts and Medication Guides)	Summary of essential information needed for safe and effective use of the drug	Patients
OTC "drug facts" labeling	Summary of essential information needed for safe and effective use of the drug	Consumers
Public health advisory	Information and advice regarding an emerging drug safety issue or other important public health information	General public
Patient information sheet	Concise summary in plain language of the most important information about a particular drug. Includes an Alert when appropriate to communicate an important, and often emerging, drug safety issue	Patients and/or consumers, lay caregivers, and interested members of the general public

Appendix B

Type of Communication	Content	Target Audience
Healthcare professional sheet	Concise summary of an important, and often emerging, drug safety issue, with background information about the detection of the issue and points to consider for clinical decision making	Healthcare professionals
Alerts on patient information and healthcare professional sheets	Summary of an important, and often emerging, drug safety issue; alerts are tailored to the needs of the primary target audience for each type of information sheet	Healthcare professionals, patients and/or consumers, lay caregivers, and interested members of the general public

[1] This guidance has been prepared by the Office of Regulatory Policy in the Center for Drug Evaluation and Research (CDER) at the Food and Drug Administration (FDA).

[2] The term *drug* as used in this guidance includes all drug and biological products regulated by CDER. Information about marketed drugs available on the Index to Drug-Specific Information Web page may include approved drugs used for labeled or unlabeled indications, or unapproved drugs.

[3] The draft version of this guidance was called *FDA's 'Drug Watch' for Emerging Drug Safety Information*.

[4] See the following guidance documents published in March 2005: *Premarketing Risk Assessment; Development and Use of Risk Minimization Action Plans;* and *Good Pharmacovigilance Practices and Pharmacoepidemiologic Assessment,* available at http://www.fda.gov/cder/guidance/index.htm.

[5] FDA Fact Sheet (February 15, 2005).

[6] See Docket No. 2005D-0062 (available at http://www.fda.gov/ohrms/dockets/dockets/05d0062/05d0062.htm).

[7] A *serious adverse drug experience* is defined as:

Any adverse drug experience occurring at any dose that results in any of the following outcomes: Death, a life-threatening adverse drug experience, inpatient hospitalization or prolongation of existing hospitalization, a persistent or significant disability/incapacity, or a congenital anomaly/birth defect. Important medical events that may not result in death, be life-threatening, or require hospitalization may be considered a serious adverse drug experience when, based upon appropriate medical judgment, they may jeopardize the patient or subject and may require medical or surgical intervention to prevent one of the outcomes listed in this definition. Examples of such medical events include allergic bronchospasm requiring intensive treatment in an emergency room or at home, blood dyscrasias or convulsions that do not result in inpatient hospitalization, or the development of drug dependency or drug abuse (21 CFR 314.80(a)).

8 See, e.g., guidance for industry on *Good Pharmacovigilance Practices and Pharmaco-epidemiologic Assessment* at pages 6 to 7 and 17 to 18.

Source: U.S. Food and Drug Administration. Available online. URL: http://www.fda.gov/downloads/Drugs/GuidanceComplianceRegulatoryInformation/Guidances/ucm072281.pdf. Last updated March 2007.

APPENDIX C

NIDA INFOFACTS: PRESCRIPTION AND OVER-THE-COUNTER MEDICATIONS

NIDA, or the National Institute on Drug Abuse, is the major federal research agency on drug abuse. As part of its mandate, it publicizes the dangers of drug abuse, including abuse of prescription drugs, to the public. This document lays out the basic facts on abuse of prescription and over-the-counter medications.

Prescription medications such as pain relievers, central nervous system (CNS) depressants (tranquilizers and sedatives), and stimulants are highly beneficial treatments for a variety of health conditions. Pain relievers enable individuals with chronic pain to lead productive lives; tranquilizers can reduce anxiety and help patients with sleep disorders; and stimulants help people with attention-deficit hyperactivity disorder (ADHD) focus their attention. Most people who take prescription medications use them responsibly. But when abused—that is, taken by someone other than the patient for whom the medication was prescribed or taken in a manner or dosage other than what was prescribed—prescription medications can produce serious adverse health effects, including addiction.

Patients, health care professionals, and pharmacists all have roles in preventing the abuse[1] of and addiction to prescription medications. For example, patients should follow the directions for use carefully; learn what effects and side effects the medication could have; and inform their doctor/pharmacist whether they are taking other medications [including over-the-counter (OTC) medications or health supplements], since these could potentially interact with the prescribed medication. The patient should read all information provided by the pharmacist. Physicians and other health care providers should screen for past or current substance abuse in the patient during routine examination, including asking questions about what other medications the patient is taking and why. Providers should note any rapid increases in the amount of a medication needed or frequent requests for refills before the quantity prescribed should have been finished, as these may be indicators of abuse.[1]

Similarly, some OTC medications, such as cough and cold medicines containing dextromethorphan, have beneficial effects when taken as recommended; but they can also be abused and lead to serious adverse health consequences. Parents should be aware of the potential for abuse of these medications, especially when consumed in large quantities, which should signal concern and the possible need for intervention.

COMMONLY ABUSED PRESCRIPTION MEDICATIONS

Although many prescription medications can be abused, the following three classes are most commonly abused:

- **Opioids**—usually prescribed to treat pain
- **CNS depressants**—used to treat anxiety and sleep disorders
- **Stimulants**—prescribed to treat ADHD and narcolepsy

OPIOIDS

What Are Opioids?

Opioids are analgesic, or pain-relieving, medications. Studies have shown that properly managed medical use (taken exactly as prescribed) of opioid analgesics is safe, can manage pain effectively, and rarely causes addiction.

Among the compounds that fall within this class are hydrocodone (e.g., Vicodin), oxycodone (e.g., OxyContin—an oral, controlled-release form of the drug), morphine, fentanyl, codeine, and related medications. Morphine and fentanyl are often used to alleviate severe pain, while codeine is used for milder pain. Other examples of opioids prescribed to relieve pain include propoxyphene (Darvon); hydromorphone (Dilaudid); and meperidine (Demerol), which is used less often because of its side effects. In addition to their effective pain-relieving properties, some of these medications can be used to relieve severe diarrhea (for example, Lomotil, also known as diphenoxylate) or severe coughs (codeine).

Appendix C

How Are Opioids Abused?

Opioids can be taken orally, or the pills may be crushed and the powder snorted or injected. A number of overdose deaths have resulted from the latter routes of administration, particularly with the drug OxyContin, which was designed to be a slow-release formulation. Snorting or injecting opioids results in the rapid release of the drug into the bloodstream, exposing the person to high doses and causing many of the reported overdose reactions.

How Do Opioids Affect the Brain?

Opioids act by attaching to specific proteins called opioid receptors, which are found in the brain, spinal cord, and gastrointestinal tract. When these compounds attach to certain opioid receptors in the brain and spinal cord, they can effectively change the way a person experiences pain.

In addition, opioid medications can affect regions of the brain that mediate what one perceives as pleasure, resulting in the initial euphoria or sense of well-being that many opioids produce. Repeated abuse of opioids can lead to addiction—a chronic, relapsing disease characterized by compulsive drug seeking and abuse despite its known harmful consequences.

What Adverse Effects Can Be Associated With Opioids?

Opioids can produce drowsiness, cause constipation, and, depending upon the amount taken, depress breathing. Taking a large single dose could cause severe respiratory depression or death.

These medications are only safe to use with other substances under a physician's supervision. Typically, they should not be used with alcohol, antihistamines, barbiturates, or benzodiazepines. Because these other substances slow breathing, their effects in combination with opioids could lead to life-threatening respiratory depression.

What Happens When You Stop Taking Opioids?

Patients who are prescribed opioids for a period of time may develop a physical dependence on them, which is not the same as addiction. Repeated exposure to opioids causes the body to adapt, sometimes resulting in tolerance (that is, more of the drug is needed to achieve the desired effect compared with when it was first prescribed) and in withdrawal symptoms upon abrupt cessation of drug use. Thus, individuals taking prescribed opioid medications should not only be given these medications under appropriate medical supervision, but they should also be medically supervised when stopping use in order to reduce or avoid withdrawal symptoms. Symptoms of withdrawal can include restlessness, muscle and bone pain, insomnia, diarrhea, vomiting, cold flashes with goose bumps ("cold turkey"), and involuntary leg movements.

Are There Treatments for Opioid Addiction?

Individuals who abuse or are addicted to prescription opioid medications can be treated. Initially, they may need to undergo medically supervised detoxification to help reduce withdrawal symptoms; however, that is just the first step. Options for effectively treating addiction to prescription opioids are drawn from research on treating heroin addiction. Behavioral treatments, usually combined with medications, have also been proven effective. Currently used medications are

- *Methadone*, a synthetic opioid that eliminates withdrawal symptoms and relieves craving, has been used successfully for more than 30 years to treat people addicted to heroin as well as opiates.
- *Buprenorphine*, another synthetic opioid, is a more recently approved medication for treating addiction to heroin and other opiates. It can be prescribed in a physician's office.
- *Naltrexone* is a long-acting opioid receptor blocker that can be employed to help prevent relapse. It is not widely used, however, because of poor compliance, except by highly motivated individuals (e.g., physicians at risk of losing their medical license). It should be noted that this medication can only be used for someone who has already been detoxified, since it can produce severe withdrawal symptoms in a person continuing to abuse opioids.
- *Naloxone* is a short-acting opioid receptor blocker that counteracts the effects of opioids and can be used to treat overdoses.

CNS DEPRESSANTS

What Are CNS Depressants?

CNS depressants (e.g., tranquilizers, sedatives) are medications that slow normal brain function. In higher doses, some CNS depressants can be used as general anesthetics or preanesthetics.

CNS depressants can be divided into three groups, based on their chemistry and pharmacology:

- *Barbiturates*, such as mephobarbital (Mebaral) and sodium pentobarbital (Nembutal), are used as preanesthetics, promoting sleep.
- *Benzodiazepines*, such as diazepam (Valium), alprazolam (Xanax), and estazolam (ProSom), can be prescribed to treat anxiety, acute stress

reactions, panic attacks, convulsions, and sleep disorders. For the latter, benzodiazepines are usually prescribed only for short-term relief of sleep problems because of the development of tolerance and risk of addiction.

- *Newer sleep medications,* such as zolpidem (Ambien), zaleplon (Sonata), and eszopiclone (Lunesta), are now more commonly prescribed to treat sleep disorders. These medications are nonbenzodiazepines that act at a subset of the benzodiazepine receptors and appear to have a lower risk for abuse and addiction.

How Are CNS Depressants Abused?

CNS depressants are usually taken orally, sometimes in combination with other drugs or to counteract the effects of other licit or illicit drugs (e.g., stimulants).

How Do CNS Depressants Affect the Brain?

Most of the CNS depressants have similar actions in the brain: they enhance the actions of the neurotransmitter gamma-aminobutyric acid (GABA)—neurotransmitters are brain chemicals that facilitate communication between brain cells. GABA works by decreasing brain activity. Although different classes of CNS depressants work in unique ways, it is ultimately their common ability to increase GABA activity that produces a drowsy or calming effect.

What Adverse Effects Can Be Associated With CNS Depressants?

Despite their beneficial effects for people suffering from anxiety or sleep disorders, barbiturates and benzodiazepines can be addictive and should be used only as prescribed.

CNS depressants should not be combined with any medication or substance that causes drowsiness, including prescription pain medicines, certain OTC cold and allergy medications, and alcohol. If combined, they can slow both heart rate and respiration, which can be fatal.

What Happens When You Stop Taking CNS Depressants?

Discontinuing prolonged use or abuse of high doses of CNS depressants can lead to serious withdrawal symptoms. Because the drug works by slowing the brain's activity, when one stops taking a CNS depressant, this activity can rebound to the point that seizures can occur. Someone who is either thinking about ending use of a CNS depressant, or who has stopped and is suffering withdrawal should seek medical treatment.

Are There Treatments for Addiction to CNS Depressants?

In addition to medical supervision during withdrawal, counseling in an in-patient or outpatient setting can help people who are overcoming addiction to CNS depressants. For example, cognitive-behavioral therapy has been used successfully to help individuals in treatment for abuse of benzodiaze-pines. This type of therapy focuses on modifying a patient's thinking, expectations, and behaviors while simultaneously increasing his or her skills for coping with various life stressors.

STIMULANTS

What Are Stimulants?

Stimulants (amphetamines [Adderall, Dexedrine] and methylphenidate [Concerta, Ritalin]) increase alertness, attention, and energy. They also increase blood pressure and heart rate, constrict blood vessels, increase blood glucose, and open up the pathways of the respiratory system. Historically, stimulants were prescribed to treat asthma and other respiratory problems, obesity, neurological disorders, and a variety of other ailments. As their potential for abuse and addiction became apparent, the prescribing of stimulants by physicians began to wane. Now, stimulants are prescribed for treating only a few health conditions, most notably ADHD, narcolepsy, and, in some instances, depression that has not responded to other treatments.

How Are Stimulants Abused?

Stimulants may be taken orally, but some abusers crush the tablets, dissolve them in water, and then inject the mixture; complications can arise from this because insoluble fillers in the tablets can block small blood vessels. Stimulants have been abused for both "performance enhancement" and recreational purposes (i.e., to get high).

How Do Prescription Stimulants Affect the Brain?

Stimulants have chemical structures that are similar to key brain neurotransmitters called monoamines, including dopamine and norepinephrine. Their therapeutic effect is achieved by slow and steady increases of dopamine that are similar to the natural production of this chemical by the brain. The doses prescribed by physicians start low and increase gradually until a therapeutic effect is reached. However, when taken in doses and routes other than those prescribed, stimulants can increase the brain's dopamine levels in a rapid and highly amplified manner—as do most other drugs of abuse—disrupting normal communication between brain cells, producing euphoria, and increasing the risk of addiction.

What Adverse Effects Are Associated With Stimulant Abuse?

Taking high doses of a stimulant can result in an irregular heartbeat, dangerously high body temperatures, and/or the potential for cardiovascular failure or seizures. Taking some stimulants in high doses or repeatedly can lead to hostility or feelings of paranoia in some individuals.

Stimulants should not be mixed with antidepressants, which may enhance the effects of a stimulant; or with OTC cold medicines containing decongestants, which may cause blood pressure to become dangerously high or may lead to irregular heart rhythms.

Are There Treatments for Stimulant Addiction?

Treatment of addiction to prescription stimulants is based on behavioral therapies proven effective for treating cocaine or methamphetamine addiction. At this time, there are no proven medications for the treatment of stimulant addiction.

Depending on the patient's situation, the first step in treating prescription stimulant addiction may be to decrease the drug's dose slowly and attempt to treat withdrawal symptoms (mood changes, sleep and appetite disturbances). This process of detoxification could then be followed with one of many behavioral therapies: contingency management, for example, improves treatment outcomes by enabling patients to earn vouchers for drug-free urine tests; the vouchers can be exchanged for items that promote healthy living. Cognitive-behavioral therapies—which teach patients skills to recognize risky situations, avoid drug use, and cope more effectively with problems—are proving beneficial. Recovery support groups may also be effective in conjunction with a behavioral therapy.

DEXTROMETHORPHAN (DXM)

What Is DXM?

DXM is the active ingredient found in OTC cough and cold medications. When taken in recommended doses, these medications are safe and effective.

How Is DXM Abused?

DXM is taken orally. In order to experience the mind-altering effects of DXM, excessive amounts of liquid or gelcaps must be consumed. The availability and accessibility of these products make them a serious concern, particularly for youth, who tend to be their primary abusers.

Prescription Drugs

What Are the Consequences Associated With the Abuse of DXM?

In very large quantities, DXM can cause effects similar to those of ketamine and PCP because these drugs affect similar sites in the brain. These effects can include impaired motor function, numbness, nausea/vomiting, and increased heart rate and blood pressure. On rare occasions, hypoxic brain damage—caused by severe respiratory depression and a lack of oxygen to the brain—has occurred due to the combination of DXM with decongestants often found in the medication.

WHAT ARE THE TRENDS IN THE ABUSE OF PRESCRIPTION DRUGS AND OTC MEDICATIONS?

Monitoring the Future (MTF) Survey[2]

Each year, the Monitoring the Future (MTF) survey assesses the extent of drug use among 8th-, 10th-, and 12th-graders nationwide. Nonmedical use of any prescription drug is reported only for 12th-graders, and in 2008, 15.4 percent reported past-year use. Prescription and OTC medications were the most commonly abused drugs by high school students after marijuana. In addition, they represent 6 of the top 10 illicit drugs reported by 12th-graders.

Prescription Painkillers. In 2002, MTF added questions to the survey about past-year nonmedical use of Vicodin and OxyContin. For Vicodin, past-year nonmedical use has remained stable at high levels for each grade since its inclusion in the survey.

RATE OF PAST-YEAR USE IN 2008

Drug Name	8th-Grade	10th-Grade	12th-Grade
Vicodin	2.9%	6.7%	9.7%
OxyContin	2.1%	3.6%	4.7%

CNS Depressants. Nonmedical use of tranquilizers (benzodiazepines and others) by 10th-grade students decreased between 2001 and 2008 for all prevalence periods (lifetime,[3] past-year, and past-month use). Use of sedatives (barbiturates), for which data are collected only from 12th-graders, has remained steady.

RATE OF PAST-YEAR USE IN 2008

Drug Name	8th-Grade	10th-Grade	12th-Grade
Tranquilizers	2.4%	4.6%	6.2%
Sedatives	—	—	5.8%

Appendix C

Stimulants. Nonmedical use of stimulants is broken up by the type of stimulant used: amphetamines, methamphetamine, or Ritalin. For all three stimulants surveyed, rates have decreased significantly among 8th-, 10th-, and 12th-graders in 2001–2008.

RATE OF PAST-YEAR USE IN 2008

Drug Name	8th-Grade	10th-Grade	12th-Grade
Amphetamines	4.5%	6.4%	6.8%
Methamphetamine	1.2%	1.5%	1.2%
Ritalin	1.6%	2.9%	3.4%

Cough Medicine. In 2006, a question about the use of cough and cold medicines to get high was asked for the first time.

RATE OF PAST-YEAR USE IN 2008

Drug Name	8th-Grade	10th-Grade	12th-Grade
Cough Medicine	3.6%	5.3%	5.5%

National Survey on Drug Use and Health (NSDUH)[4]

According to the 2007 NSDUH, an estimated 6.9 million persons, or 2.8 percent of the population, aged 12 or older had used prescription psycho-therapeutic medications nonmedically in the month prior to being surveyed. This includes 5.2 million using pain relievers (an increase from 4.7 million in 2005), 1.8 million using tranquilizers, 1.1 million using stimulants, and 350,000 using sedatives.

Past-month nonmedical use of prescription-type drugs among young adults aged 18 to 25 increased from 5.5 percent in 2002 to 6 percent in 2007. This was primarily due to an increase in pain reliever use, which was 4.1 percent in 2002 and 4.6 percent in 2007. However, nonmedical use of tranquilizers remained the same over the 6-year period.

Among persons aged 12 or older who used pain relievers nonmedically in the past 12 months, 56.5 percent reported that they got the drug most recently used from someone they knew and that they did not pay for it. Another 18.1 percent reported that they obtained the drug from one doctor. Only 4.1 percent purchased the pain reliever from a drug dealer or other stranger, and just 0.5 percent reported buying the drug on the Internet. Among those who reported getting the pain reliever from a friend or relative for free, 81 percent reported in a followup question that the friend or relative had obtained the drug from one doctor only.

Prescription Drugs

[1] A common vocabulary has not been established in the field of prescription drug abuse. Because much of the survey data collected in this area refer to nonmedical use of prescription drugs, this definition of "abuse," rather than that of the Diagnostic and Statistical Manual of Mental Disorders (DSM), is used. Also, because physical dependence to prescription medications can develop during medically supervised appropriate use, the term "addiction" is used to reflect dependence as defined by the DSM.

[2] These data are from the 2008 Monitoring the Future survey, funded by the National Institute on Drug Abuse, National Institutes of Health, Department of Health and Human Services, and conducted annually by the University of Michigan's Institute for Social Research. The survey has tracked 12th-graders' illicit drug use and related attitudes since 1975; in 1991, 8th- and 10th-graders were added to the study. The latest data are online at www.drugabuse.gov.

[3] "Lifetime" refers to use at least once during a respondent's lifetime. "Past year" refers to use at least once during the year preceding an individual's response to the survey. "Past month" refers to use at least once during the 30 days preceding an individual's response to the survey.

[4] NSDUH (formerly known as the National Household Survey on Drug Abuse) is an annual survey of Americans age 12 and older conducted by the Substance Abuse and Mental Health Services Administration. Copies of the latest survey are available at www.samhsa.gov and from NIDA at 877-643-2644.

Source: National Institute on Drug Abuse. Available online. URL: http://www.nida.nih.gov/infofacts/PainMed.html. Last updated July 2009.

APPENDIX D

THE FDA'S DRUG REVIEW PROCESS: ENSURING DRUGS ARE SAFE AND EFFECTIVE

Prescription drug users assume that products approved by the FDA are safe but know little about what goes into the review process. This document, updated July 10, 2009, describes the process and defines some commonly used terms.

The path a drug travels from a lab to your medicine cabinet is usually long, and every drug takes a unique route. Often, a drug is developed to treat a specific disease. An important use of a drug may also be discovered by accident

For example, Retrovir (zidovudine, also known as AZT) was first studied as an anti-cancer drug in the 1960s with disappointing results. It wasn't until the 1980s that researchers discovered the drug could treat AIDS, and the Food and Drug Administration approved the drug, manufactured by Glaxo-SmithKline, for that purpose in 1987.

Most drugs that undergo preclinical (animal) testing never even make it to human testing and review by the FDA. The drugs that do must undergo the agency's rigorous evaluation process, which scrutinizes everything about the drug—from the design of clinical trials to the severity of side effects to the conditions under which the drug is manufactured.

STAGES OF DRUG DEVELOPMENT AND REVIEW

Investigational New Drug Application (IND)—The pharmaceutical industry sometimes provides advice to the FDA prior to submission of an IND. Sponsors—companies, research institutions, and other organizations that take responsibility for developing a drug—must show the FDA results of preclinical testing they've done in laboratory animals and what they propose to do for human testing. At this stage, the FDA decides whether it is reasonably safe for the company to move forward with testing the drug in humans.

Clinical Trials—Drug studies in humans can begin only after an IND is reviewed by the FDA and a local institutional review board (IRB). The board is a panel of scientists and non-scientists in hospitals and research institutions that oversees clinical research.

IRBs approve the clinical trial protocols, which describe the type of people who may participate in the clinical trial, the schedule of tests and procedures, the medications and dosages to be studied, the length of the study, the study's objectives, and other details. IRBs make sure the study is acceptable, that participants have given consent and are fully informed of their risks, and that researchers take appropriate steps to protect patients from harm.

Phase 1 studies are usually conducted in healthy volunteers. The goal here is to determine what the drug's most frequent side effects are and, often, how the drug is metabolized and excreted. The number of subjects typically ranges from 20 to 80.

Phase 2 studies begin if Phase 1 studies don't reveal unacceptable toxicity. While the emphasis in Phase 1 is on safety, the emphasis in Phase 2 is on effectiveness. This phase aims to obtain preliminary data on whether the drug works in people who have a certain disease or condition. For controlled trials, patients receiving the drug are compared with similar patients receiving a different treatment—usually an inactive substance (placebo), or a different drug. Safety continues to be evaluated, and short-term side effects are studied. Typically, the number of subjects in Phase 2 studies ranges from a few dozen to about 300.

At the end of Phase 2, the FDA and sponsors try to come to an agreement on how the large-scale studies in Phase 3 should be done. How often the FDA meets with a sponsor varies, but this is one of two most common meeting points prior to submission of a new drug application. The other most common time is pre-NDA—right before a new drug application is submitted.

Phase 3 studies begin if evidence of effectiveness is shown in Phase 2. These studies gather more information about safety and effectiveness, studying different populations and different dosages and using the drug in combination with other drugs. The number of subjects usually ranges from several hundred to about 3,000 people.

Postmarketing study commitments, also called Phase 4 commitments, are studies required of or agreed to by a sponsor that are conducted after the FDA has approved a product for marketing. The FDA uses postmarketing study commitments to gather additional information about a product's safety, efficacy, or optimal use.

New Drug Application (NDA)—This is the formal step a drug sponsor takes to ask that the FDA consider approving a new drug for marketing in the United States. An NDA includes all animal and human data and analyses of the data, as well as information about how the drug behaves in the body and how it is manufactured.

When an NDA comes in, the FDA has 60 days to decide whether to file it so that it can be reviewed. The FDA can refuse to file an application that is incomplete. For example, some required studies may be missing. In accordance with the Prescription Drug User Fee Act (PDUFA), the FDA's Center for Drug Evaluation and Research (CDER) expects to review and act on at least 90 percent of NDAs for standard drugs no later than 10 months after the applications are received. The review goal is six months for priority drugs. (See "The Role of User Fees.")

There is also continuous interaction throughout the review process. For example, over roughly six years, the sponsor, Merck Research Laboratories of West Point, Pa., and the FDA had several face-to-face meetings and about 28 teleconferences regarding the asthma drug Singulair (montelukast sodium).

"It's the clinical trials that take so long—usually several years," says Sandra Kweder, M.D., deputy director of the Office of New Drugs in the CDER. "The emphasis on speed for FDA mostly relates to review time and timelines of being able to meet with sponsors during a drug's development," she says.

REVIEWING APPLICATIONS

Though FDA reviewers are involved with a drug's development throughout the IND stage, the official review time is the length of time it takes to review a new drug application and issue an action letter, an official statement informing a drug sponsor of the agency's decision.

Once a new drug application is filed, an FDA review team—medical doctors, chemists, statisticians, microbiologists, pharmacologists, and other experts—evaluates whether the studies the sponsor submitted show that the drug is safe and effective for its proposed use. No drug is absolutely safe; all drugs have side effects. "Safe" in this sense means that the benefits of the drug appear to outweigh the risks.

The review team analyzes study results and looks for possible issues with the application, such as weaknesses of the study design or analyses. Reviewers determine whether they agree with the sponsor's results and conclusions, or whether they need any additional information to make a decision.

Each reviewer prepares a written evaluation containing conclusions and recommendations about the application. These evaluations are then considered by team leaders, division directors, and office directors, depending on the type of application.

Reviewers receive training that fosters consistency in drug reviews, and good review practices remain a high priority for the agency.

Sometimes, the FDA calls on advisory committees made up of outside experts, who help the agency decide on drug applications. Whether an advisory committee is needed depends on many things.

"Some considerations would be if it's a drug that has significant questions, if it's the first in its class, or the first for a given indication," says Mark Goldberger, M.D., director of one of CDER's drug review offices. "Generally, FDA takes the advice of advisory committees, but not always," he says. "Their role is just that—to advise."

ACCELERATED APPROVAL

Traditional approval requires that clinical benefit be shown before approval can be granted. Accelerated approval is given to some new drugs for serious and life-threatening illnesses that lack satisfactory treatments. This allows an NDA to be approved before measures of effectiveness that would usually be required for approval are available.

Instead, less traditional measures called surrogate endpoints are used to evaluate effectiveness. These are laboratory findings or signs that may not be a direct measurement of how a patient feels, functions, or survives, but are considered likely to predict benefit. For example, a surrogate endpoint could be the lowering of HIV blood levels for short periods of time with anti-retroviral drugs.

Gleevec (imatinib mesylate), an oral treatment for patients with a life-threatening form of cancer called chronic myeloid leukemia (CML), received accelerated approval. The drug was also approved under the FDA's orphan drug program, which gives financial incentives to sponsors for manufacturing drugs that treat rare diseases. Gleevec blocks enzymes that play a role in cancer growth. The approval was based on results of three large Phase 2 studies, which showed the drug could substantially reduce the level of cancerous cells in the bone marrow and blood.

The sponsor, Novartis Pharmaceuticals Corp. of East Hanover, N.J., submitted the IND in April 1998. The FDA received the NDA in February 2001, and the drug was approved two-and-a-half months later in May 2001. Novartis has made commitments to conduct studies that confirm Gleevec's clinical benefit, such as increased progression-free survival in the treatment of CML.

Most drugs to treat HIV have been approved under accelerated approval provisions, with the company required to continue its studies after the drug is on the market to confirm that its effects on virus levels are maintained and that it ultimately benefits the patient. Under accelerated approval rules, if studies don't confirm the initial results, the FDA can withdraw the approval.

Because premarket review can't catch all potential problems with a drug, the FDA continues to track approved drugs for adverse events through a postmarketing surveillance program.

BUMPS IN THE ROAD

If the FDA decides that the benefits of a drug outweigh the risks, the drug will receive approval and can be marketed in the United States. But if there are problems with an NDA or if more information is necessary to make that determination, the FDA may decide that a drug is "approvable" or "not approvable."

A designation of approvable means that the drug can probably be approved, provided that some issues are resolved first. This might involve the sponsor and the FDA coming to a final agreement on what should go on the drug's labeling, for example. It could also involve more difficult issues, such as the adequacy of information on how people respond to various dosages of the drug.

A designation of "not approvable" describes deficiencies significant enough that it is not clear that approval can be obtained in the future, at least not without substantial additional data.

Common problems include unexpected safety issues that crop up or failure to demonstrate a drug's effectiveness. A sponsor may need to conduct additional studies—perhaps studies of more people, different types of people, or for a longer period of time.

Manufacturing issues are also among the reasons that approval may be delayed or denied. Drugs must be manufactured in accordance with standards called good manufacturing practices, and the FDA inspects manufacturing facilities before a drug can be approved. If a facility isn't ready for inspection, approval can be delayed. Any manufacturing deficiencies found would need to be corrected before approval.

"Sometimes a company may make a certain amount of a drug for clinical trials. Then when they go to scale up, they may lose a supplier or end up with quality control issues that result in a product of different chemistry," says the FDA's Kweder. "Sponsors have to show us that the product that's going to be marketed is the same product that they tested."

John Jenkins, M.D., director of CDER's Office of New Drugs, says, "It's often a combination of problems that prevent approval." Close communication with the FDA early on in a drug's development reduces the chance that an application will have to go through more than one cycle of review, he says. "But it's no guarantee."

The FDA outlines the justification for its decision in an action letter to the drug sponsor. When the action is either approvable or not approvable, CDER gives the sponsor a chance to meet with agency officials to discuss the deficiencies. At that point, the sponsor can choose to ask for a hearing, or correct any deficiencies and submit new information, or they can withdraw the application.

DRUG REVIEW STEPS

1. Preclinical (animal) testing.
2. An investigational new drug application (IND) outlines what the sponsor of a new drug proposes for human testing in clinical trials.
3. Phase 1 studies (typically involve 20 to 80 people).
4. Phase 2 studies (typically involve a few dozen to about 300 people).
5. Phase 3 studies (typically involve several hundred to about 3,000 people).
6. The pre-NDA period, just before a new drug application (NDA) is submitted. A common time for the FDA and drug sponsors to meet.
7. Submission of an NDA is the formal step asking the FDA to consider a drug for marketing approval.
8. After an NDA is received, the FDA has 60 days to decide whether to file it so it can be reviewed.
9. If the FDA files the NDA, an FDA review team is assigned to evaluate the sponsor's research on the drug's safety and effectiveness.
10. The FDA reviews information that goes on a drug's professional labeling (information on how to use the drug).
11. The FDA inspects the facilities where the drug will be manufactured as part of the approval process.
12. FDA reviewers will approve the application or find it either "approvable" or "not approvable."

THE ROLE OF USER FEES

Since the Prescription Drug User Fee Act (PDUFA) was passed in 1992, more than 1,000 drugs and biologics have come to the market, including new medicines to treat cancer, AIDS, cardiovascular disease, and life-threatening infections. PDUFA has allowed the Food and Drug Administration to bring access to new drugs as fast or faster than anywhere in the world, all while maintaining the same thorough review process.

Under PDUFA, drug companies agree to pay fees that boost FDA resources, and the FDA agrees to time goals for its review of new drug applications. Along with supporting increased staff, drug user fees help the FDA upgrade resources in information technology. The agency has moved toward an electronic submission and review environment, now accepting more electronic applications and archiving review documents electronically.

The goals set by PDUFA apply to the review of original new human drug and biological applications, resubmissions of original applications, and supplements to approved applications. The second phase of PDUFA, known as PDUFA II, was reauthorized in 1997 and extended the user fee program through September 2002. PDUFA III, which extends to Sept. 30, 2007, was reauthorized in June 2002.

PDUFA III allows the FDA to spend some user fees to increase surveillance of the safety of medicines during their first two years on the market, or three years for potentially dangerous medications. It is during this initial period, when new medicines enter into wide use, that the agency is best able to identify and counter adverse side effects that did not appear during the clinical trials.

In addition to setting time frames for review of applications, PDUFA sets goals to improve communication and sets goals for specific kinds of meetings between the FDA and drug sponsors. It also outlines how fast the FDA must respond to requests from sponsors. Throughout a drug's development, the FDA advises sponsors on how to study certain classes of drugs, how to submit data, what kind of data are needed, and how clinical trials should be designed.

THE QUALITY OF CLINICAL DATA

The Food and Drug Administration relies on data that sponsors submit to decide whether a drug should be approved. To protect the rights and welfare of people in clinical trials, and to verify the quality and integrity of data submitted, the FDA's Division of Scientific Investigations (DSI) conducts inspections of clinical investigators' study sites. DSI also reviews the records of institutional review boards to be sure they are fulfilling their role in patient protection.

"FDA investigators compare information that clinical investigators provided to sponsors on case report forms with information in source documents such as medical records and lab results," says Carolyn Hommel, a consumer safety officer in DSI.

DSI seeks to determine such things as whether the study was conducted according to the investigational plan, whether all adverse events were recorded, and whether the subjects met the inclusion/exclusion criteria outlined in the study protocol.

At the conclusion of each inspection, FDA investigators prepare a report summarizing any deficiencies. In cases where they observe numerous or serious deviations, such as falsification of data, DSI classifies the inspection as "official action indicated" and sends a warning letter or Notice of Initiation of Disqualification Proceedings and Opportunity to Explain (NIDPOE) to the clinical investigator, specifying the deviations that were found.

The NIDPOE begins an administrative process to determine whether the clinical investigator should remain eligible to receive investigational products and conduct clinical studies.

CDER conducts about 300–400 clinical investigator inspections annually. About 3 percent are classified in this "official action indicated" category.

The FDA has established an independent Drug Safety Oversight Board (DSOB) to oversee the management of drug safety issues and communication to the public about the risks and benefits of medicines. The board's responsibilities include conducting timely and comprehensive evaluations of emerging drug safety issues, selecting drugs to be placed on a Drug Watch Web site for health professionals and patients, and ensuring that experts—both inside and outside of the FDA—give their perspectives to the agency. The first meeting of the DSOB was held in June 2005.

Source: U.S. Food and Drug Administration. Available online. URL: http://www.fda.gov/Drugs/ResourcesForYou/Consumers/ucm143534.htm. Last updated July 10, 2009.

APPENDIX E

INSIDE CLINICAL TRIALS: TESTING MEDICAL PRODUCTS IN PEOPLE

Clinical trials have become the primary means to evaluate the safety of prescription drugs. They are required not only before approval but also after approval, when trials continue to identify any unrecognized problems. To encourage people to participate in these trials, the FDA describes what is involved and the benefits they provide in this document, updated on July 11, 2009.

WHAT IS A CLINICAL TRIAL?

Clinical trials, also known as clinical studies, test potential treatments in human volunteers to see whether they should be approved for wider use in the general population. A treatment could be a drug, medical device, or biologic, such as a vaccine, blood product, or gene therapy. Potential treatments, however, must be studied in laboratory animals first to determine potential toxicity before they can be tried in people. Treatments having acceptable safety profiles and showing the most promise are then moved into clinical trials.

Although "new" may imply "better," it is not known whether the potential medical treatment offers benefit to patients until clinical research on that treatment is complete. Clinical trials are an integral part of new product discovery and development and are required by the Food and Drug Administration before a new product can be brought to the market.

The FDA is committed to protecting the participants of clinical trials, as well as providing reliable information to those interested in participating. Recently, unethical behavior on the part of some researchers has shaken the public trust and prompted the federal government to establish regulations and guidelines for clinical research to protect participants from unreasonable risks.

Although efforts are made to control risks to clinical trial participants, some risk may be unavoidable because of the uncertainty inherent in clinical research involving new medical products. It's important, therefore, that people make their decision to participate in a clinical trial only after they have a full understanding of the entire process and the risks that may be involved.

WHY PARTICIPATE IN A CLINICAL TRIAL?

People volunteer to participate in clinical trials for different reasons. Some volunteer because they want to help advance medical knowledge. Others have tried all available treatments for their condition without success.

In a 2000 Harris Poll of cancer clinical trial participants, 76 percent of the respondents said they participated because they believed that the trial offered the best quality of care for their disease. Helping other people and receiving more and better attention for their own specific disease were other reasons cited.

People should not, however, be tempted to enroll in a clinical trial simply because a potential treatment is being offered free during a study, or because of the promise of money, says David Banks, an FDA pharmacist.

"People lured by compensation may overlook the known risks," Banks says. "Or [they may fail] to adequately appreciate the potential for discovery of serious new side effects during clinical testing of a new treatment." Banks also says that clinical trials "are generally not a means for patients to receive long-term treatment for their chronic disease." Still, he adds, "clinical trials often represent an option to seriously consider."

WHO CAN PARTICIPATE?

It's important to test medical products in the people they are meant to help. In the past, most new drug testing had been done on white men. Groups such as women, blacks, and Hispanics often were not adequately represented. It's important to test medical products in a wide variety of people because drugs can work differently in people of various ages, races, ethnicity, and gender. The FDA seeks to ensure that people from many different groups are included in clinical trials.

Trial guidelines, or eligibility requirements, are developed by the researchers and usually include criteria for age, sex, type and stage of disease, previous treatment history, and other medical conditions. Some trials involve people with a particular illness or condition to be studied, while others seek healthy volunteers. Inclusion or exclusion criteria—medical or social standards used to determine whether a person may or may not be allowed to enter a clinical trial—help identify appropriate participants and help to exclude those who may be put at risk by participating in a trial.

Volunteering for a clinical trial is no guarantee of acceptance. Similarly, there's no guarantee that an individual in a clinical trial will receive the drug or medical product being studied.

WHAT HAPPENS IN A CLINICAL TRIAL?

Every clinical trial is carefully designed to answer certain research questions. A trial plan called a protocol maps out what study procedures will be done, by whom, and why. Products are often tested to see how they compare to standard treatments or to no treatment. The FDA often provides extensive technical assistance to researchers conducting clinical trials, helping them design better trials that can characterize effects of a new product more efficiently, while reducing risks to those participating in the trials.

The clinical trial team includes doctors and nurses, as well as other health care professionals. This team checks the health of the participant at the beginning of the trial and assesses whether that person is eligible to participate. Those found to be eligible—and who agree to participate—are given specific instructions, and then monitored and carefully assessed during the trial and after it is completed.

Done at hospitals and research centers around the country, clinical trials are conducted in phases. Phase 1 trials try to determine dosing, document how a drug is metabolized and excreted, and identify acute side effects. Usually, a small number of healthy volunteers (between 20 and 80) are used in Phase 1 trials.

Phase 2 trials include more participants (about 100–300) who have the disease or condition that the product potentially could treat. In Phase 2 trials, researchers seek to gather further safety data and preliminary evidence of the drug's beneficial effects (efficacy), and they develop and refine research methods for future trials with this drug. If the Phase 2 trials indicate that the drug may be effective—and the risks are considered acceptable, given the observed efficacy and the severity of the disease—the drug moves to Phase 3.

In Phase 3 trials, the drug is studied in a larger number of people with the disease (approximately 1,000–3,000). This phase further tests the product's effectiveness, monitors side effects and, in some cases, compares the product's effects to a standard treatment, if one is already available. As more and more participants are tested over longer periods of time, the less common side effects are more likely to be revealed.

Sometimes, Phase 4 trials are conducted after a product is already approved and on the market to find out more about the treatment's long-term risks, benefits, and optimal use, or to test the product in different populations of people, such as children.

Phase 2 and Phase 3 clinical trials generally involve a "control" standard. In many studies, one group of volunteers will be given an experimental or "test" drug or treatment, while the control group is given either a standard treatment for the illness or an inactive pill, liquid, or powder that has no treatment value (placebo). This control group provides a basis for comparison for assessing effects of the test treatment. In some studies, the control group will receive a placebo instead of an active drug or treatment. In other cases, it is considered unethical to use placebos, particularly if an effective treatment is available. Withholding treatment (even for a short time) would subject research participants to unreasonable risks.

The treatment each trial participant receives is often decided by a process called randomization. This process can be compared to a coin toss that is done by computer. During clinical trials, no one likely knows which therapy is better, and randomization assures that treatment selection will be free of any preference a physician may have. Randomization increases the likelihood that the groups of people receiving the test drug or control are comparable at the start of the trial, enabling comparisons in health status between groups of patients who participated in the trial.

In conjunction with randomization, a feature known as blinding helps ensure that bias doesn't distort the conduct of a trial or the interpretation of its results. Single-blinding means the participant does not know whether he or she is receiving the experimental drug, an established treatment for that disease, or a placebo. In a single-blinded trial, the research team does know what the participant is receiving.

A double-blinded trial means that neither the participant nor the research team knows during the trial which participants receive the experimental drug. The patient will usually find out what he or she received at a pre-specified time in the trial.

WHAT ARE THE RISKS?

Some treatments being studied can have unpleasant, or even serious, side effects. Often these are temporary and end when the treatment is stopped. Others, however, can be permanent. Some side effects appear during treatment, and others may not show up until after the study is over. The risks depend on the treatment being studied and the health of the people participating in the trial. All known risks must be fully explained by the researchers before the trial begins. If new risk information becomes available during the trial, participants must be informed.

HOW ARE PEOPLE PROTECTED?

Most clinical trials are federally regulated with built-in safeguards to protect participants. Today, the Office for Human Research Protections (OHRP) in the Department of Health and Human Services (HHS) leads the department's programs for the protection of human research participants and oversees human protection in HHS-funded research.

"It's important that we have the rapport with the public that allows them to trust us with this program," says Bernard A. Schwetz, D.V.M., Ph.D., director of the OHRP. He adds, "Without people willing to participate, there won't be any clinical trials."

The FDA has authority over clinical trials for drug, biologic, and medical device products regulated by the agency. This authority includes studies that are HHS-funded (with joint oversight by the FDA and the OHRP), as well as studies that are solely funded by industry or by private parties. Many clinical trials are not subject to FDA regulation but are monitored by the institution sponsoring the trial, such as a hospital. (See "Institutional Review Boards.")

To help protect the rights and welfare of volunteers and verify the quality and integrity of data submitted for review, the FDA performs inspections of clinical trial study sites and anyone involved in the research, says David A. Lepay, M.D., Ph.D., senior advisor for clinical science and director of the FDA's Good Clinical Practice Program. Lepay says that the quality of clinical trials has improved markedly since the agency started inspecting them back in 1977.

"Between FDA, the help of other government agencies, the review by institutional review boards, the required monitoring of studies by industry or private sponsors, and the required oversight and reporting by investigators and their staff," Lepay says, "a lot of people are looking out for the research subject's safety."

WHAT IS INFORMED CONSENT?

The FDA requires that potential participants be given complete information about the study. This process is known as "informed consent," and it must be in writing. (See "Information Required for Informed Consent.")

The informed consent process provides an opportunity for the researcher and patient to exchange information and ask questions. Patients invited to enter a trial are not obligated to join, but can consent to participate if they find the potential risks and benefits acceptable. A consent form must be signed by the participant prior to enrollment and before any study procedures can be performed.

Participants also have the right to leave a study at any time. At the same time, people need to know that circumstances may arise under which their participation may be terminated by the researcher, without their consent.

For example, Schwetz says that sometimes it becomes evident early on that a trial is not working and researchers know they are not going to get enough meaningful information to make continuation worthwhile. In addition, if an unexpected change occurs in the health status of a participant, such as toxic effects or sudden kidney problems that may have developed, it "would not be in the best interest of the patient to continue, and certainly not consistent with what the investigator is trying to study," he says. In any case, the circumstances must be described in the consent document.

WHERE TO GET INFORMATION ON CLINICAL TRIALS

It is often difficult for patients to learn about opportunities to participate in clinical trials. Doctors and patient advocacy groups can be valuable resources for patients in search of clinical trial information. Newspapers, particularly in large cities, often carry clinical trial recruitment advertisements. A call to the relevant department at nearby university medical centers can lead to information about clinical trials currently recruiting patients.

The Web site ClinicalTrials.gov also provides patients, family members, health care professionals, and members of the public easy access to information on clinical trials for a wide range of diseases and conditions. The National Institutes of Health (NIH), through its National Library of Medicine, has developed this site in collaboration with all NIH institutes and the FDA.

The site contains information on thousands of clinical studies sponsored by the NIH, other federal agencies, and the pharmaceutical industry in about 100,000 locations worldwide. Studies listed in the database are conducted primarily in the United States and Canada, but include locations in about 90 countries. ClinicalTrials.gov gives information about a trial's purpose, who may participate, locations, and phone numbers for more details. In addition, a glossary is available that will help people become familiar with the most common clinical trial terms.

Appendix E

THE BOTTOM LINE

While it's true that clinical trials offer no guarantees, when standard treatments fail, or none exist, clinical research trials sometimes can offer hope. People can reduce the confusion and uncertainty that often comes with deciding whether or not to participate in a clinical trial by obtaining all the information available on various Web sites, through phone calls, within FDA, HHS, and NIH offices, and from patient advocacy organizations.

The bottom line: Know and understand the different types of trials, which questions to ask, and your rights as a trial participant. Find out what risks there may be, and determine what level of risk you are willing to accept before you agree to enroll in a clinical trial for medical research.

INFORMATION REQUIRED FOR INFORMED CONSENT

The FDA requires that people be told

- that the study involves research of an unproven drug, biologic (such as a vaccine, blood product, or gene therapy), or medical device
- the purpose of the research
- how long the participant will be expected to participate in the study
- what will happen in the study and which parts of the study are experimental
- possible risks or discomforts to the participant
- possible benefits to the participant
- other procedures or treatments that might be advantageous to the participant instead of the treatment being studied
- that the FDA may look at study records, but the records will be kept confidential
- whether any compensation and medical treatments, if any, are available if the participant is injured, what those treatments are, where they can be found, and who will pay for the treatment
- the person to contact with questions about the study, participants' rights, or if the participant gets hurt
- that participation is voluntary and that participants can quit the study at any time without penalty or loss of benefits to which they are otherwise entitled.

INSTITUTIONAL REVIEW BOARDS

Clinical trial procedures are reviewed by institutional review boards (IRBs). These boards are composed of at least five members that include scientists, doctors, and lay people, and they must approve every clinical trial taking place within their jurisdiction—usually a hospital. The purpose of an IRB review is to ensure that appropriate steps are taken to protect the rights and welfare of participants as subjects of research. If the risks to participants are found to be too great, the IRB will not approve the research, or it will specify changes that must be made before the research can be done.

IRBs also review participant inclusion and exclusion requirements to be sure that appropriate people have been identified as eligible for the trial. They often look at how and where recruitment for clinical trials will occur. IRBs review the adequacy of the informed consent document to ensure that it includes all the elements required by law, and that it is at an appropriate reading level and understandable to study participants.

Source: U.S. Food and Drug Administration. Available online. URL: http://www.fda.gov/Drugs/ResourcesForYou/Consumers/ucm143531.htm. Last updated July 11, 2009.

APPENDIX F

STRATEGIES TO REDUCE MEDICATION ERRORS: WORKING TO IMPROVE MEDICATION SAFETY

Errors in giving and taking prescription drugs are a serious problem. In this document, updated July 11, 2009, the FDA describes its approach in dealing with the problem.

When Jacquelyn Ley shattered her elbow on the soccer field, her parents set out to find her the best care in Minneapolis. "We drove past five other hospitals to get to the one we wanted," says Carol Ley, M.D., an occupational health physician. Her husband, an orthopedic surgeon, made sure Jacquelyn got the right surgeon. After a successful three-hour surgery to repair the broken bones, Jacquelyn, who was 9 at the time, received the pain medicine morphine through a pump and was hooked up to a heart monitor, breathing monitor, and blood oxygen monitor. Her recovery was going so well that doctors decided to turn off the morphine pump and to forgo regular checks of her vital signs.

Carol Ley slept in her daughter's hospital room that night. When she woke up in the middle of the night and checked on her, Jacquelyn was barely breathing. "I called her name, but she wouldn't respond," she says. "I shook her and called for help." The morphine pump hadn't been shut down, but had accidentally been turned up high. The narcotic flooded Jacquelyn's body. She survived the overdose, but it was a close call. "If three more hours had gone by, I don't think Jacquelyn would have survived," Ley says. "Fortunately, I woke up."

Ley was pleased with the way the hospital handled the error. "They came right out and said the morphine pump was incorrectly programmed, they

259

told me the steps they were going to take to make sure Jacquelyn was OK, and they also told me what they were going to do to make sure this kind of mistake won't happen again. And that's very important to me." The hospital began using pumps that are easier to use and revamped nurses' training. Ley believes there were many contributors to the error, including the fact that it was Labor Day weekend and there were staff shortages. "It goes to show that this can happen to anyone, anywhere," says Ley, who now chairs the board of the National Patient Safety Foundation.

MULTIPLE FACTORS

Since 1992, the Food and Drug Administration has received nearly 30,000 reports of medication errors. These are voluntary reports, so the number of medication errors that actually occur is thought to be much higher. There is no "typical" medication error, and health professionals, patients, and their families are all involved. Some examples:

A physician ordered a 260-milligram preparation of Taxol for a patient, but the pharmacist prepared 260 milligrams of Taxotere instead. Both are chemotherapy drugs used for different types of cancer and with different recommended doses. The patient died several days later, though the death couldn't be linked to the error because the patient was already severely ill.

An older patient with rheumatoid arthritis died after receiving an overdose of methotrexate—a 10-milligram daily dose of the drug rather than the intended 10-milligram weekly dose. Some dosing mix-ups have occurred because daily dosing of methotrexate is typically used to treat people with cancer, while low weekly doses of the drug have been prescribed for other conditions, such as arthritis, asthma, and inflammatory bowel disease.

One patient died because 20 units of insulin was abbreviated as "20 U," but the "U" was mistaken for a "zero." As a result, a dose of 200 units of insulin was accidentally injected.

A man died after his wife mistakenly applied six transdermal patches to his skin at one time. The multiple patches delivered an overdose of the narcotic pain medicine fentanyl through his skin.

A patient developed a fatal hemorrhage when given another patient's prescription for the blood thinner warfarin.

These and other medication errors reported to the FDA may stem from poor communication; misinterpreted handwriting; drug name confusion; confusing drug labels, labeling, and packaging; lack of employee knowledge; and lack of patient understanding about a drug's directions. "But it's important to recognize that such errors are due to multiple factors in a complex medical system," says Paul Seligman, M.D., director of the FDA's Office of

Pharmacoepidemiology and Statistical Science. "In most cases, medication errors can't be blamed on a single person."

A medication error is "any preventable event that may cause or lead to inappropriate medication use or patient harm while the medication is in the control of the health care professional, patient, or consumer," according to the National Coordinating Council for Medication Error Reporting and Prevention. The council, a group of more than 25 national and international organizations, including the FDA, examines and evaluates medication errors and recommends strategies for error prevention.

A REGULATORY APPROACH

The public took notice in 1999 when the Institute of Medicine (IOM) released a report, "To Err Is Human: Building a Safer Health System." According to the report, between 44,000 and 98,000 deaths may result each year from medical errors in hospitals alone. And more than 7,000 deaths each year are related to medications. In response to the IOM's report, all parts of the U.S. health system put error reduction strategies into high gear by re-evaluating and strengthening checks and balances to prevent errors.

In addition, the U.S. Department of Health and Human Services (HHS) and other federal agencies formed the Quality Interagency Coordination Task Force in 2000 and issued an action plan for reducing medical errors. In 2001, former HHS Secretary Tommy G. Thompson announced a Patient Safety Task Force to coordinate a joint effort to improve data collection on patient safety. The lead agencies are the FDA, the Centers for Disease Control and Prevention, the Centers for Medicare and Medicaid Services, and the Agency for Healthcare Research and Quality.

The FDA enhanced its efforts to reduce medication errors by dedicating more resources to drug safety, which included forming a new division on medication errors at the agency in 2002. "FDA works to prevent medication errors before a drug reaches the market and monitors any errors that may occur after that," says Jerry Phillips, R.Ph., former director of the FDA's Division of Medication Errors and Technical Support.

Here's a look at key areas in which the FDA is working to reduce medication errors.

Bar code label rule: After a public meeting in July 2002, the FDA decided to propose a new rule requiring bar codes on certain drug and biological product labels. Health care professionals would use bar code scanning equipment, similar to that used in supermarkets, to make sure that the right drug in the right dose and route of administration is given to the right patient at the right time.

Prescription Drugs

"It's a promising way to automate aspects of medication administration," says Robert Krawisz, former executive director of the National Patient Safety Foundation. "The technology's impact at VA hospitals so far has been amazing." The Department of Veterans Affairs (VA) already uses bar codes nationwide in its hospitals, and the result has been a drastic reduction in medication errors. For example, the VA medical center in Topeka, Kan., has reported that bar coding reduced its medication error rate by 86 percent over a nine-year period.

Here's how it works: When patients enter the hospital, they get a bar-coded identification wristband that can transmit information to the hospital's computer, says Lottie Lockett, R.N., a nursing administrator at the Houston VA Medical Center. Nurses have laptop computers and scanners on top of medication carts that they bring to patients' rooms. Nurses use the scanners to scan the patient's wristband and the medications to be given. The bar codes provide unique, identifying information about drugs given at the patient's bedside. "Before giving medications, nurses use the scanner to pull up a patient's full name and social security number on the laptops, along with the medications," Lockett says. "If there is not a match between the patient and the medication or some other problem, a warning box pops up on the screen."

The FDA's final rule on bar code labeling was published on Feb. 26, 2004. The rule, which took effect on April 26, 2004, applies to prescription drugs, biological products (other than blood, blood components, and devices regulated by the Center for Biologics Evaluation and Research), and over-the-counter (OTC) drugs that are commonly used in hospitals. Manufacturers, repackers, relabelers, and private label distributors of prescription and OTC drugs would be subject to the bar code requirements. The agency continues to study whether it also should develop a rule requiring bar code labeling on medical devices.

Drug name confusion: To minimize confusion between drug names that look or sound alike, the FDA reviews about 300 drug names a year before they are marketed. "About one-third of the names that drug companies propose are rejected," says Phillips. The agency tests drug names with the help of about 120 FDA health professionals who volunteer to simulate real-life drug order situations. "FDA also created a computerized program that assists in detecting similar names and that will help take a more scientific approach to comparing names," Phillips says.

After drugs are approved, the FDA tracks reports of errors due to drug name confusion and spreads the word to health professionals, along with recommendations for avoiding future problems. For example, the FDA has reported errors involving the inadvertent administration of methadone, a drug used to treat opiate dependence, rather than the intended Metadate ER (methylphenidate) for the treatment of attention-deficit/hyperactivity disorder (ADHD). One report involved the death of an 8-year-old boy after a possible medication error at the dispensing pharmacy. The child, who was being treated for ADHD, was found dead at home. Methadone substitution was the suspected cause of death. Some FDA recommendations regarding drug name confusion have encouraged pharmacists to separate similar drug products on pharmacy shelves and have encouraged physicians to indicate both brand and generic drug names on prescription orders, as well as what the drug is intended to treat.

The last time the FDA changed a drug name after it was approved was in 2004 when the cholesterol-lowering medicine Altocor was being confused with the cholesterol-lowering medicine Advicor. Now Altocor is called Altoprev, and the agency hasn't received reports of errors since the name change. Other examples of drug name confusion reported to the FDA include:

- Serzone (nefazodone) for depression and Seroquel (quetiapine) for schizophrenia
- Lamictal (lamotrigine) for epilepsy, Lamisil (terbinafine) for nail infections, Ludiomil (maprotiline) for depression, and Lomotil (diphenoxylate) for diarrhea
- Taxotere (docetaxel) and Taxol (paclitaxel), both for chemotherapy
- Zantac (ranitidine) for heartburn, Zyrtec (cetirizine) for allergies, and Zyprexa (olanzapine) for mental conditions
- Celebrex (celecoxib) for arthritis and Celexa (citalopram) for depression.

Drug labeling: Consumers tend to overlook important label information on OTC drugs, according to a Harris Interactive Market Research Poll conducted for the National Council on Patient Information and Education and released in January 2002. In May 2002, an FDA regulation went into effect that aims to help consumers use OTC drugs more wisely.

The regulation requires a standardized "Drug Facts" label on more than 100,000 OTC drug products. Modeled after the Nutrition Facts label on foods, the label helps consumers compare and select OTC medicines and follow instructions. The label clearly lists active ingredients, uses, warnings, dosage, directions, other information, such as how to store the medicine, and inactive ingredients.

As for health professionals, the FDA proposed a new format in 2000 to improve prescription drug labeling for physicians, also known as the package insert. One FDA study showed that practitioners found the labeling to be lengthy, complex, and hard to use. The proposed redesign would feature a user-friendly format and would highlight critical information more clearly. The FDA is still reviewing public comments on this proposed rule. The agency also has been working on a project called DailyMed, a computer system that will be available without cost from the National Library of Medicine next year. DailyMed will have new information added daily, and will allow health professionals to pull up drug warnings and label changes electronically.

Error tracking and public education: The FDA reviews medication error reports that come from drug manufacturers and through MedWatch, the agency's safety information and adverse event reporting program. The agency also receives reports from the Institute for Safe Medication Practices (ISMP) and the U.S. Pharmacopeia, or USP (see "Who Tracks Medication Errors?").

A recent ISMP survey on medication error reporting practices showed that health professionals submit reports more often to internal reporting programs such as hospitals than to external programs such as the FDA. According to the ISMP, one reason may be health professionals' limited knowledge about external reporting programs.

The FDA receives and reviews about 300 medication error reports each month and classifies them to determine the cause and type of error. Depending on the findings, the FDA can change the way it labels, names, or packages a drug product. In addition, once a problem is discovered, the FDA educates the public on an ongoing basis to prevent repeat errors.

In 2001, the agency released a public health advisory to hospitals, nursing homes, and other health care facilities about the hazards of mix-ups between medical gases, which are prescription drugs. In one case, a nursing home in Ohio reported four deaths after an employee mistakenly connected nitrogen to the oxygen system.

The ISMP reports medication errors through various newsletters that target health professionals in acute care, nursing, and community/ambulatory care. The ISMP also has launched a newsletter for consumers called Safe Medicine.

In December 2003, the USP released an analysis of medication errors captured in 2002 by its anonymous national reporting database, Med-MARX. Of the errors reported to MedMARX, slightly more than one-third reached the patient and involved a geriatric patient. Many of these medication errors were found to be harmful.

WHAT CONSUMERS CAN DO

In one case reported to the ISMP, a doctor called in a prescription for the antibiotic Noroxin (norfloxacin) for a patient with a bladder infection. But the pharmacist thought the order was for Neurontin (gabapentin), a medication used to treat seizures. The good news is that the patient read the medication leaflet stapled to his medication bag, noticed the drug he received is used to treat seizures, and then asked about it. ISMP president Michael Cohen, R.Ph., Sc.D., says, "You should expect to count on the health system to keep you safe, but there are also steps you can take to look out for yourself and your family."

- Know what kind of errors occur. The FDA evaluated reports of fatal medication errors that it received from 1993 to 1998 and found that the most common types of errors involved administering an improper dose (41 percent), giving the wrong drug (16 percent), and using the wrong route of administration (16 percent). The most common causes of the medication errors were performance and knowledge deficits (44 percent) and communication errors (16 percent). Almost half of the fatal medication errors occurred in people over 60. Older people are especially at risk for errors because they often take multiple medications. Children are also a vulnerable population because drugs are often dosed based on their weight, and accurate calculations are critical.

- Find out what drug you're taking and what it's for. Rather than simply letting the doctor write you a prescription and send you on your way, be sure to ask the name of the drug. Cohen says, "I would also ask the doctor to put the purpose of the prescription on the order." This serves as a check in case there is some confusion about the drug name. If you're in the hospital, ask (or have a friend or family member ask) what drugs you are being given and why.

- Find out how to take the drug and make sure you understand the directions. If you are told to take a medicine three times a day, does that mean eight hours apart exactly or at mealtimes? Should the medicine be stored at room temperature or in the refrigerator? Are there any medications, beverages, or foods you should avoid? Also, ask about what medication side effects you might expect and what you should do about them. And read the bottle's label every time you take a drug to avoid mistakes. In the middle of the night, you could mistake ear drops for eye drops, or accidentally give your older child's medication to the baby if you're not careful. Use the measuring device that comes with the medicine, not spoons from the kitchen drawer. If you take multiple medications and have trouble keeping them straight, ask your doctor or pharmacist about compliance aids, such as containers with sections for daily doses. Family members can help by reminding you to take your medicine.

- Keep a list of all medications, including OTC drugs, as well as dietary supplements, medicinal herbs, and other substances you take for health reasons, and report it to your health care providers. The often-forgotten things that you should tell your doctor about include vitamins, laxatives, sleeping aids, and birth control pills. One National Institutes of Health study showed a significant drug interaction between the herbal product St. John's wort and indinavir, a protease inhibitor used to treat HIV infection. Some antibiotics can lower the effectiveness of birth control pills. If you see different doctors, it's important that they all know what you are taking. If possible, get all your prescriptions filled at the same pharmacy so that all of your records are in one place. Also, make sure your doctors and pharmacy know about your medication allergies or other unpleasant drug reactions you may have experienced.

• If in doubt, ask, ask, ask. Be on the lookout for clues of a problem, such as if your pills look different than normal or if you notice a different drug name or different directions than what you thought. Krawisz says it's best to be cautious and ask questions if you're unsure about anything. "If you forget, don't hesitate to call your doctor or pharmacist when you get home," he says. "It can't hurt to ask."

WHO TRACKS MEDICATION ERRORS?

THE FOOD AND DRUG ADMINISTRATION

Accepts reports from consumers and health professionals about products regulated by the FDA, including drugs and medical devices, through Med-Watch, the FDA's safety information and adverse event reporting program. (800) 332-1088
www.fda.gov/medwatch/how.htm

INSTITUTE FOR SAFE MEDICATION PRACTICES

Accepts reports from consumers and health professionals related to medication. Publishes Safe Medicine, a consumer newsletter on medication errors. 1800 Byberry Road, Suite 810 Huntingdon Valley, PA 19006-3520 (215) 947-7797
www.ismp.org/Pages/Consumer.html

U.S. PHARMACOPEIA

The Medication Errors Reporting (MER) Program, in cooperation with the Institute for Safe Medication Practices, is a voluntary national medication error reporting program.
12601 Twinbrook Parkway
Rockville, MD 20852 (800) 23-ERROR (233-7767)
www.usp.org

Appendix F

MedMARX

USP's anonymous medication error reporting program used by hospitals. These data are not submitted to the FDA.
www.medmarx.com

HOSPITAL STRATEGIES

Hospitals and other health care organizations work to reduce medication errors by using technology, improving processes, zeroing in on errors that cause harm, and building a culture of safety. Here are a couple of examples.

Pharmacy intervention: It was a challenge for health care providers, especially surgeons, at Fairview Southdale Hospital in Edina, Minnesota, to ensure that patients continued taking their regularly prescribed medicines when they entered the hospital, says Steven Meisel, Pharm.D., director of medication safety at Fairview Health Services. "Surgeons are not typically the original prescribers," he says. The solution was to have pharmacy technicians record complete medication histories on a form. In a pilot program, the technicians called most patients on the phone a couple of days before surgery. A pharmacist reviewed the information, and then the surgeon decided which medications should be continued. After three months, the number of order errors per patient dropped by 84 percent, and the pilot program became permanent.

Computerized Physician Order Entry (CPOE): Studies have shown that CPOE is effective in reducing medication errors. It involves entering medication orders directly into a computer system rather than on paper or verbally. The Institute for Safe Medication Practices conducted a survey of 1,500 hospitals in 2001 and found that about 3 percent of hospitals were using CPOE, and the number is rising. Eugene Wiener, M.D., medical director at the Children's Hospital of Pittsburgh, says, "There is no misinterpretation of handwriting, decimal points, or abbreviations. This puts everything in a digital world."

The Pittsburgh hospital unveiled its CPOE system in October 2002. Developed by the hospital and the Cerner Corp. in Kansas City, Missouri, Children'sNet has replaced most paper forms and prescription pads. Wiener says that, unlike with adults, most drug orders for children are generally based on weight. "The computer won't let you put an order in if the child's weight isn't in the system," he says, "and if the weight changes, the computer notices." The system also provides all kinds of information about potential drug complications that the doctor might not have thought about. "Doctors always have a choice in dealing with the alerts," Wiener says. "They can choose to move past an alert, but the alert makes them stop and think based on the specific patient indications."

PATIENT SAFETY PROPOSALS

In March 2003, the Department of Health and Human Services announced two new FDA strategies that will use state-of-the-art technology to improve patient safety.

- **Bar codes:** Just as the technology is used in retail and other industries, required bar codes would contain unique identifying information about drugs. When used with bar code scanners and computerized patient information systems, bar code technology can prevent many medication errors, including administering the wrong drug or dose, or administering a drug to a patient with a known allergy. The requirement took effect in April 2004.

- **Safety reporting:** A proposed revamping of safety reporting requirements aims to enhance the FDA's ability to monitor and improve the safe use of drugs and biologics. In 2003, the FDA published a proposed rule. The rule, if enacted, would improve the quality and consistency of safety reports, require the submission of all suspected serious reactions for blood and blood products, and require reports on important potential medication errors.

Source: U.S. Food and Drug Administration. Available online. URL: http://www.fda.gov/Drugs/ResourcesForYou/Consumers/ucm143553.htm. Last updated July 11, 2009.

INDEX

Locators in **boldface** indicate main topics. Locators followed by *c* indicate chronology entries. Locators followed by *b* indicate biographical entries. Locators followed by *g* indicate glossary entries. Locators followed by *t* indicate tables.

A

AARP 33, 212–214
Abbott Laboratories 27, 37
abuse of prescription drugs
  60–63
  bibliography **192–204**
  Comprehensive Drug
    Abuse Prevention and
    Control Act 76–78,
    109*c*
  Heath Ledger and 122
  Rush Limbaugh and
    122
  NIDA Infofacts **231–241**
  state legislation 87
accelerated approval. *See*
  fast-track drug approval
access. *See* cost of
  prescription drugs
Access to Benefits Coalition
  24
ACE (angiotensin-
  converting enzyme) 29
ACE-inhibitor medications
  19, 20, 52
acetaminophen 52, 116*c*
active ingredients 80, 125*g*
Actonel 37, 41
Adams, Samuel Hopkins 6,
  106*c*
Adderall 44, 45
addiction 7, 12, 62, 74, 122
addictive drugs 8, 125*g*
adequate provision
  requirement 220–222
ADHD (attention deficit/
  hyperactivity disorder)
  44–45, 115*c*

adulterated drugs 73, 80,
  106*c*, 125*g*
*Adulteration of Various
  Substances Used in Medicine
  and the Arts* (Beck) 5, 104*c*
Advair 36, 117*c*
Advair Diskus 21
Adverse Event Reporting
  System 52, 125*g*
adverse events. *See* side
  effects
advertising. *See also* direct-
  to-consumer ads
  in 1800s 5
  bibliography **143,
    179–192**
  blockbuster drugs 28
  FDA and 108*c*, 110*c*,
    114*c*
  House investigation of
    115*c*
  and increase in drug
    use 65
  industry spending on 28
  Kefauver-Harris Act 76
  David Kessler and 121
  online research
    resources **139**
  patent medicines 5–6
  prescription drug use
    and **40–43**
  Pure Food and Drug
    Act 73
  research accounting
    and 27
  state legislation 87
  *Virginia Board of
    Pharmacy v. Virginia*

*Citizens Consumer
  Council* 89–91, 109*c*
Advil 38
advocacy organizations
  212–215
agencies. *See* organizations
  and agencies
aging 25, 64–65
Agriculture, U.S.
  Department of 7, 73
AIDS activists 13
alcohol 6
Aleve 55, 112*c*
Allegra 37
alpha-adrenergic blockers 29
AMA. *See* American Medical
  Association
Amaryl 58
Ambien 37
American Home Products
  57. *See also* Wyeth
American Medical
  Association (AMA) 213
  drug approval program
    7, 106*c*
  and DTC ads 16, 18,
    111*c*, 114*c*
  Joshua Sharfstein and
    124
American Pharmacists
  Association (APhA) 213
American Recovery and
  Reinvestment Act of 2009
  29
Amgen 32, 38, 79, 210
amoxicillin 21
amphetamines 44, 45
analgesics 125*g*

Index

Index

Index

Index

Prescription Drugs

Index

Index